THE A TO Z OF

AUTISM SPECTRUM DISORDERS

Carol Turkington
Ruth Anan, Ph.D.

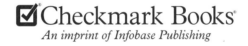
Checkmark Books®

An imprint of Infobase Publishing

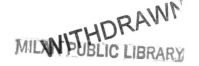

The A to Z of Autism Spectrum Disorders

Copyright © 2007 by Carol Turkington

Checkmark Books
An imprint of Infobase Publishing
132 West 31st Street
New York NY 10001

ISBN-10: 0-8160-7122-5
ISBN-13: 978-0-8160-7122-7

Library of Congress Cataloging-in-Publication Data
Turkington, Carol.
The encyclopedia of autism spectrum disorders / Carol Turkington, Ruth Anan.
p. ; cm.
Includes bibliographical references and index.
ISBN 0-8160-6002-9 (hc : alk. paper)—ISBN 0-8160-7122-5 (pb : alk. paper)
1. Autism—Encyclopedias.   I. Anan, Ruth. II. Title. III. Title: Autism spectrum disorders.
[DNLM: 1. Autistic Disorder—Encyclopedias—English.   WM 13 T939e 2007]
RC553.A88T87 2007
616.85′882003—dc22   2005027227

Checkmark Books are available at special discounts when purchased in bulk quantities for businesses, associations, institutions, or sales promotions. Please call our Special Sales Department in New York at (212) 967-8800 or (800) 322-8755.

You can find Facts On File on the World Wide Web at http://www.factsonfile.com

Text and cover design by Cathy Rincon

Printed in the United States of America

VB Hermitage 10 9 8 7 6 5 4 3 2 1

This book is printed on acid-free paper.

CONTENTS

FOREWORD

Autism spectrum disorders are pervasive developmental disabilities in which the core impairments have a profound influence on children's development. A relative or total absence of reciprocal social interactive skills is the primary symptom seen in young children with autism spectrum disorders. Unlike typically developing toddlers, who make almost nonstop bids for parental attention, these children make less frequent eye contact and direct fewer facial expressions toward their parents. They also fail to share their interest in things they see through pointing and holding up objects for their parents to see. Typically developing toddlers usually accompany these actions with sounds (and, later, actual words) to draw their parents' attention. In addition, they usually alternate their gaze between an object of interest and a parent's face. This stands in stark contrast with the way that an autistic child has trouble initiating a shared focus of attention. Likewise, children with autism have trouble responding to their parents' bids for shared attention.

A significant problem with communication is another core symptom in autistic spectrum disorders. Preschoolers diagnosed with autism may demonstrate delays in spoken language or may be completely nonverbal. They may simply echo what is said to them without meaning. Some children may be able to speak but demonstrate a lack of pragmatic communication skills. In other words, they may be able to respond to direct questions but cannot engage in back-and-forth conversations. They may recite pieces of dialogue from videos or books, using these phrases out of context. Children with more advanced language skills may demonstrate more subtle impairments. Their language may be stilted, or they may carry on monologues about topics of interest to them, without regard to whether or not anyone is following their discourse. Pretend play and nonvocal communication using gestures and facial expression are generally also delayed.

In contrast to these two "negative symptoms," or absences of specific skills, the third symptom of autistic spectrum disorders involves behavioral excess. Children diagnosed with autism may engage in repetitive mannerisms, such as flapping their hands, flicking their fingers in front of their eyes, pacing back and forth, running on tiptoe, and so on. Objects may be used in unusual ways, such as spinning or tapping them or repeatedly flicking a doll's eyes open and shut. Some children demonstrate an excessive interest in unusual topics, becoming fascinated with sprinkler systems or vacuums. Children diagnosed with autism also may be rigid, insisting on following specific rituals, demanding to perform activities in an exact order, or following the same route to a destination. When unable to engage in these ritualistic behaviors, they become highly anxious or upset.

Other behavioral excesses, although not part of the core diagnostic symptoms of autism, also may occur. Repetitive actions sometimes evolve into self-injurious behaviors, such as head-banging, hand-biting, or face-slapping. Children unable to effectively communicate their wants or needs may scream, scratch, or hit. Parents, in their haste to end these disruptive actions, may attempt to placate their children by offering desired objects or activities following aggression or self-injury, thereby inadvertently rewarding undesirable behaviors.

Effective treatment for autistic spectrum disorders must target these three core areas of impairment: communication, reciprocal social interactions, and atypical behaviors.

Although the specific causes of autistic spectrum disorders are still largely unknown, there is consensus that autism is a biologically based, neurodevelopmental disorder with a strong genetic component. In the last decade, symptoms of autism have been identified in younger and younger children, with diagnoses now being made as early as 18–24 months of age. Parents of newly diagnosed preschoolers often retrospectively report that their children showed negative symptoms, such as absent or impaired social and language skills much earlier.

As a result, routine screening for autism spectrum disorders is now recommended by many professional organizations, including the American Academy of Pediatrics, the American Academy of Neurology, and the National Research Council of the National Academy of Science. Increasingly sensitive screening instruments have been developed to identify children at risk, who are then referred to interdisciplinary diagnostic centers. According to current best-practice guidelines, comprehensive evaluation should include a combination of medical, developmental, and behavioral information.

A primary goal of early identification of autism spectrum disorders is to implement interventions as soon as possible—and the earlier treatment begins, the more progress can be made. To date, the most dramatic changes occur when children receive early and intensive behavioral intervention. The National Academy of Science recommends "a minimum of 25 hours per week, 12 months a year, in which the child is engaged in systematically planned and developmentally appropriate educational activity toward defined objectives" (National Research Council, 2002, p. 6). Clinical guidelines developed by the New York State Department of Health and Early Intervention advocate a minimum of about 20 hours per week of individualized behavioral intervention using applied behavioral analysis techniques.

Although experts widely agree that intervention should be both intensive and implemented at an early age, there is a lack of consensus regarding exactly what form it should take. Of all treatment options, intervention using principles of behavior analysis has the strongest support from research. A considerable number of studies have documented substantial treatment gains in children receiving intensive, behaviorally based intervention. Furthermore, there is evidence suggesting that treatment based on principles of behavior analysis is superior to equally time-intensive intervention using other methods.

Treatment programs using behaviorally based techniques vary considerably in their emphasis on formal discrete trial teaching versus more naturalistic teaching strategies. Discrete-trial training is highly directive, with the adult providing the instruction and delivering the appropriate consequence based on the child's response. Discrete trials are typically conducted at a table, but can be embedded within enjoyable play activities and daily routines. Sometimes criticized as an artificial manner of instruction, discrete trial teaching nevertheless has been shown to be an effective and efficient way to teach skills. However, it is also essential to use systematic methods of generalizing these skills into natural settings in order to ensure their effective use.

Other behavioral teaching methods, such as naturalistic environment training, emphasize a child-initiated interaction in a less structured environment. The common premise of naturalistic behavioral approaches to treatment is that targeted skills should be taught in the child's environment, in a conversational or play context. Reinforcers should be related to the child's current interest, and teaching trials should be interspersed with other enjoyable activities. For example, when used to teach communication skills, the adult provides the desired item only after the child uses a specific form of communication. Children with limited ability to imitate vocal sounds at first may learn functional communication skills using either signs or pictures.

Current trends in treatment emphasize the necessity of intervention based on valid research. Therefore, based on currently available research, effective intervention for children with autism should come from the field of applied behavior analysis. Furthermore, it should provide the specific blend of behavioral strategies best suited for each individual child at each particular stage of learning. Such intervention must be of suitable intensity to be effective. In addition, treatment must begin as soon as it is recognized that a child has an autism spectrum disorder, with the goal of improving each child's eventual level of functioning as much as possible.

For children with autism, this often translates into more than 20 hours of weekly one-on-one intervention. While expensive, cost-benefit analyses demonstrate that "front-loading" expenses (in other words, providing the highest intensity of intervention during the preschool years) actually saves money in the long run.

—Ruth Anan, Ph.D.
Director, Early Childhood Program
Center for Human Development

ACKNOWLEDGMENTS

The creation of this encyclopedia involved the help and guidance of a wide range of experts, without whom it could not have been possible. Thanks to the staffs of the National Institutes of Health; the American Academy of Pediatrics; American Academy of Allergy, Asthma & Immunology; American Academy of Child and Adolescent Psychiatry; American Association of People with Disabilities; American Occupational Therapy Association; American Psychiatric Association; American Psychological Association; American Speech-Language-Hearing Association; Autism Network International; Autism Research Institute; Autism Society of America; Childhood Apraxia of Speech Association of North America; and Children and Adults with Attention Deficit Disorder. Also the Children's Health Information Network, Council for Exceptional Children, Council for Learning Disabilities, Dana Alliance for Brain Initiatives, ERIC Clearinghouse on Disabilities and Gifted Education, Family Center for Technology and Disabilities, Family Education Network, Federation for Children with Special Needs, Federation of Families for Children's Mental Health, the Food and Drug Administration, Learning Disabilities Association, National ADD Association, National Adoption Center, National Alliance for Autism Research, National Aphasia Association, National Association for the Education of Young Children, National Association of the Deaf, National Center for Learning Disabilities, National Health Information Center, National Information Center for Children and Youth with Disabilities, National Institute of Child Health and Human Development, National Institute of Mental Health, National Vaccine Information Center, and the Obsessive-Compulsive Foundation.

Thanks to my agents, Gene Brissie and Ed Claflin; to my editor, James Chambers; to Sarah Fogarty, Grace Persico, and Vanessa Nittoli at Facts On File; and to Kara and Michael. And a very special thank you to the entire staff at Luciano's!

INTRODUCTION

Not until the middle of the 20th century was there a name for a disorder that now appears to affect at least one of every 500 children in America—a disorder that disrupts families and leads to unfulfilled lives for many children. In 1943, Dr. Leo Kanner of the Johns Hopkins Hospital studied a group of 11 children with baffling symptoms and came up with the label "early infantile autism." At the same time, German scientist Dr. Hans Asperger described a milder form of the same disorder that today bears his name: Asperger's syndrome.

Today, these disorders are listed in the *Diagnostic and Statistical Manual of Mental Disorders* (fourth edition, text revision; *DSM-IV-TR*) as two of the five pervasive developmental disorders, more often referred to today as autism spectrum disorders (ASDs). All five of these disorders on the autism continuum are characterized by varying degrees of impairment in communication skills, social interactions, and restricted, repetitive, and stereotyped patterns of behavior. The ASDs range from a severe form, called autistic disorder (more commonly known as the classic "autism"), to a milder form—Asperger's syndrome. If a child has symptoms of either of these disorders but does not meet the specific criteria for either, the diagnosis is called pervasive developmental disorder–not otherwise specified (PDD-NOS). Other rare, very severe disorders that are included in the autism spectrum disorders are Rett disorder and childhood disintegrative disorder.

Autism is a baffling brain disease usually appearing before a child's third birthday—sometimes as early as 18 months—profoundly affecting communication and social skills and impairing the child's ability to play, speak, and relate to the world. Parents are usually the first to notice unusual behaviors in their child. In some cases, the baby seems "different" from birth, unresponsive to people or focusing intently on one item for a long time. The first signs of an ASD can sometimes appear in children who seem to have been developing normally. When an engaging, babbling toddler suddenly becomes silent, withdrawn, self-abusive, or indifferent to social overtures, parents know immediately that something is wrong. Research has shown that parents are usually correct about noticing developmental problems, although they may not realize the specific nature or degree of the problem.

While autism was always one of the most common developmental disabilities, in the past several years an apparent increase in the number of children diagnosed with the disorder has schools straining to provide services and health officials urgently seeking the cause of the condition.

The U.S. Department of Education reports a 173 percent increase in autistic children served under the Individuals with Disabilities Education Act between the 1992–93 school year (when 15,580 children were counted) and 1997–98, when the figure jumped to 42,500. The situation appears to be particularly acute in California, where a 273 percent increase was recorded in the number of autistic children entering various state treatment centers between 1987 and 1998. Critics have argued that the increase is due to a change in the definition of autism (it is now much more broadly defined) or better or earlier diagnostic techniques. Opponents insist the increase is real and occurs for some as-yet-unknown reasons. The debate continues, and research is ongoing. In the meantime, thousands of very real families struggle every day with the challenges inherent in this heart-breaking condition that seems to isolate children in a remote, unreachable world.

Much about autism is debatable and often controversial, including the varied theories for its cause (vaccines, viruses, environmental toxins, faulty genes, diet) and potential treatments (drugs, hug therapy, aversive therapy, behavioral therapy, squeeze boxes, psychotherapy, vitamin therapy, or special diets). Even the terminology used in the area of autism spectrum disorders has undergone dramatic change. The ways that experts describe individuals and their symptoms have grown more diagnostically accurate, and ongoing refinement of legislation better protects the rights of those with autism and other severe disabilities. Clearly, there is an enormous amount of information desperately needed by people with autism and their families, teachers, and doctors.

In *The A to Z of Autism,* we have tried to present this information in a clear, balanced, concise format easily understood by the general reader, containing the latest findings, treatments, and methods of managing symptoms. Where there is controversy, we have tried to present both sides. Where there is ongoing research, we have pointed out the directions it may take.

This book has been designed as a guide and reference to a wide range of issues in the field of autism and contains entries discussing the various types and subtypes of autism, symptoms, suggested causes and treatments, leading scientists, lifestyle and estate planning issues, and the latest research. Appendixes include major autism-related organizations, a "Read More about It" section featuring special books with autism information written for patients and their families, a list of ongoing current clinical trials into autism spectrum disorders, and lists of state autism-related resources. A glossary of basic medical terms and an index are also included.

The book includes topics in three key areas:

Autism spectrum disorders

- autistic disorder (autism) (both low- and high-functioning)
- Asperger's syndrome
- Rett disorder
- pervasive developmental disorder–not otherwise specified (PDD-NOS)
- childhood disintegrative disorder

Legal discussions of relevant topics

- Disabilities Education Act
- Americans with Disabilities Act
- Rehabilitation Act of 1973
- special needs trusts
- estate planning

School-related entries

- independent education evaluations
- individualized education programs
- individualized transition plans
- assessments and screening tools

Readers should keep in mind, however, that changes occur rapidly in this field. A bibliography has been provided for readers who seek additional sources of information. Information in this book comes from the most up-to-date sources available and includes some of the most recent research in the field of learning disabilities, culled from leading textbooks and professional journals, in addition to the personal experience of the expert coauthor. It is not a substitute for prompt assessment and treatment by experts trained in the diagnosis of autism spectrum disorders.

—Carol Turkington
Cymru, Pennsylvania

ENTRIES A–Z

ability test Test of ability, such as an intelligence test, that measures an individual's aptitude to perform a task, manipulate information, or solve problems. Typically, tests of ability are used to assess specific performance abilities or potential for future learning rather than stored information. Among the most commonly used ability tests are the Wechsler Intelligence Scale for Children, either revised or third edition (WISC-R or WISC-III), the Scholastic Aptitude Test (SAT), which is widely used in college admissions processes, and the Woodcock-Johnson-III cognitive battery, which is commonly used in public school settings to define a baseline of aptitude against which achievement can be measured in determining whether a learning disability is present.

Ability tests can be physical or mental. They can test verbal or non-verbal areas, and are also frequently used to assess potential employees for specific tasks. Depending on the nature of the test, various professionals may be involved in its administration. Specific clinical training in psychology is required to administer the Wechsler or other intelligence tests, while the Woodcock-Johnson may be given by school guidance counselors with appropriate training. Standardized tests, such as the SAT, must be administered in specific contexts according to specific testing procedures, but overseeing such tests requires no formal professional training.

Ability tests have particular importance in relation to the Americans with Disabilities Act, which protects individuals with disabilities from discrimination, especially in the workplace. Ability tests designed to assess mechanical abilities, clerical abilities, and other job-related abilities can prevent equal access. Individuals can request alternative assessment of their abilities if they can provide documentation of a disability and they are otherwise qualified for a position.

Achenbach Childhood Behavior Checklist (CBCL) A standardized assessment designed to investigate social competence and behavior problems in children aged four to 18 as reported by parents. The CBCL can be filled out by parents or administered by an interviewer. It consists of 118 items related to the child's behavior problems that are scored on a three-point scale ranging from "not true" to "often true." There are also 20 social competency items used to obtain parents' reports of the amount and quality of their child's participation in sports, hobbies, games, activities, organizations, jobs and chores, friendships, how well the child gets along with others, how well the child plays and works alone, and school functioning. It was developed by psychologists Thomas M. Achenbach and Craig Edelbrock.

activities of daily living Personal-care activities necessary for everyday living, such as eating, bathing, grooming, dressing, and toileting. People with autism may not be able to perform these activities without help. Professionals often assess a person's activities of daily living as a way of determining what type of care is needed.

adaptive living skills Skills used in everyday living, such as gross and fine motor skills, eating and food preparation, toileting, dressing, personal self-care, domestic skills, time and punctuality, money and value, home and community orientation, and work skills. Techniques from the field of APPLIED

BEHAVIOR ANALYSIS often are used to teach adaptive living skills to individuals with autism.

ADD   See ATTENTION DEFICIT DISORDER.

Adderall   See DEXTROAMPHETAMINE/AMPHETAMINE.

adults with autism   Some adults with AUTISM SPECTRUM DISORDER (ASD), especially those with high-functioning autism or with ASPERGER'S SYNDROME, are able to work successfully in mainstream jobs. Nevertheless, communication and social problems often cause difficulties in many areas of life, and these adults will continue to need encouragement and support in their struggle for an independent life.

Many others with ASD can work in sheltered workshops under the supervision of managers trained in working with persons with disabilities. A nurturing environment at home, at school, and later in job training and at work, helps individuals with ASD continue to learn and to develop throughout their lives.

The public schools' responsibility for providing services ends when the student with ASD reaches the age of 22. The family is then faced with the challenge of finding living arrangements and employment to match the needs of this person, as well as the programs and facilities that can provide support services. Long before a child finishes school, parents should identify the best programs and facilities for the young adult.

Living Arrangements

Independent living   Some adults with ASD are able to live entirely on their own, while others can live semi-independently in their own home or apartment if they have help with personal finances, coping with government services, and so on. This assistance can be provided by family, a professional agency, or another type of provider.

Living at home   Government funds are available for families who choose to have their adult child with ASD live at home, including SUPPLEMENTAL SECURITY INCOME (SSI), Social Security Disability Insurance (SSDI), and Medicaid waivers. Informa-

tion about these programs is available from the U.S. Social Security Administration.

Foster and skill-development homes   Some families open their homes to provide long-term care to unrelated adults with autism. If the home teaches self-care and housekeeping skills and arranges leisure activities, it is called a "skill-development" home.

Supervised group living   People with disabilities often live in group homes or apartments staffed by professionals who help the individuals with basic needs, such as meal preparation, housekeeping, and personal care. Higher functioning people with autism may be able to live in a home or apartment with a few visits from staffers each week. These high-functioning individuals generally prepare their own meals, go to work, and conduct other daily activities on their own.

Institutions   Although the trend in recent decades has been to avoid placing people with disabilities into long-term-care institutions, this alternative is still available for people with autism who need intensive, constant supervision. Unlike many of the institutions years ago, today's facilities are far more humane and consider residents as individuals with human needs. Residents are typically offered opportunities for recreation and simple but meaningful work.

akathisia   A condition of inner restlessness and an inability to keep still, also known as "restless legs." Akathisia may be a side effect of some neuroleptic drugs.

allergy to cow's milk   Although the cause of autism is not known, some experts believe that an allergy to cow's milk may play a role in exacerbating the condition. However, not all researchers and experts agree about whether this theory is scientifically valid and whether there is a link between diet and autism symptoms.

Nevertheless, sometimes parents report behavioral improvements when their children stop drinking milk. Some researchers have found evidence of higher levels of certain peptides in the urine of children with autism, which may mean that some peptides from foods containing casein (such as dairy products) have not been broken down completely. Brain function may be disturbed if protein is not broken down or absorbed correctly. As yet, researchers are not sure why these proteins do not break down.

Experts caution that parents of an autistic child who want to try a milk-free diet to see if it improves symptoms should first consult a gastroenterologist and nutritionist who can give advice on proper nutrition.

aloofness   Social indifference is common in people with autism, making them appear uninterested in social interaction, although scientists are not completely sure why. One of the striking characteristics of autism is "face blindness," meaning that the patient is unable to "read" a person's face to detect emotional cues. This often results in impaired social behavior.

Many experts believe that the root cause of impaired social behavior typical of people with autism is probably related to a glitch in the brain. Some research suggests it could be a specific problem in the opioid signaling system. Brain opiates help a person understand positive outcomes and positive rewards, such as those that occur in pleasant social exchanges. Mice studies suggest that when opiate receptors are destroyed, the mice pups do not respond normally to their mothers.

American Sign Language (ASL)   A visual-gestural language initially developed as a primary means of communication among individuals with hearing problems in the United States. ASL has a unique grammar and syntax and is unrelated to English, although it reflects English influences. This visual language requires many nonmanual features, including facial expressions and body language. It also includes finger spelling (the manual alphabet) to spell out words, including proper names and technical phrases. Sign language is also used to teach people with autism and other DEVELOPMENTAL DIS-ABILITIES who have little or no communication skill.

Teaching autistic children how to use sign language is not as common as it once was due to the increase in computerized communication systems. Teaching sign language to people with autism does not interfere with learning to talk; in fact, research suggests that teaching sign language along with speech will speed up verbal communication.

People with different levels of autism can be taught to use sign language. Many aberrant behaviors associated with autism such as aggression, tantrums, self-injury, anxiety, and depression are often caused by frustration over the inability to communicate. Teaching people to use sign language decreases these problem behaviors and also may improve their attentiveness to social gestures.

Teaching sign language and speech at the same time is often referred to as signed speech, simultaneous communication, or total communication. Although there are several different forms of sign language, when using signed speech, experts say it is best to use the "Signing Exact English" or "Signed English" method, which uses the same syntax as spoken language. This method helps reinforce the syntactic rules of spoken language. For example, a statement using both Signed English and speech would be: "pet the cat." In contrast, the syntax of American Sign Language would be: "cat pet." Since most people do not understand sign language, some experts believe it is better to use a form of picture system or computerized communication device in addition to Signed Speech to enable communication with those who do not understand the signs. Signed English often uses the first letter of the word (also called initialization) with the basic movement of the sign to give hints to the intended word. This system also includes markers for prefixes, suffixes, plural endings and tenses, together with signs for articles, infinitives, and all forms of the verb "to be." This system is not used by deaf adults except for some initial signs that have found their way into popular usage.

Many linguists believe that it is only when sign language differs completely from English that it may properly be called American Sign Language, although some use ASL as a catchall term to describe an entire range of manual communication. At one end of the sign language continuum is finger spelling, in which hand shapes are used to spell out each word of the English language while speaking or moving the lips. This method (also called the Rochester method, or visible English) can be tiring to use and interpret. Further along the continuum are manually coded English systems, which use finger spelling but also include signs and markers. The most common forms of this system are Signed English and Signed Exact English.

In the middle of the sign language continuum is a system called Pidgin Sign English, the system used most often by hearing people learning to communicate with deaf people. This combines English with the vocabulary and nonmanual features of ASL, and is the preferred method of communication by many deaf people.

When used in the true sense of the word, ASL means the patterns used by deaf persons when they communicate in sign in a non-English style. Neither articles nor speech are used, although finger spelling is used for proper names.

One possible reason why teaching sign language and speech helps a child learn to speak more quickly is that both forms of communication stimulate the same area of the brain. Thus, when using Signed Speech, the area of the brain involved in speech production is stimulated from two sources (signing and speaking) rather than from one source (signing or speaking) alone.

Americans with Disabilities Act (ADA)   Legislation enacted in July 1990 that prohibits discrimination against individuals with disabilities, including autism. It guarantees equal opportunity for people with disabilities in terms of jobs, public accommodations, transportation, and telecommunications, as well as other state services.

The ADA represents a significant addition to the scope of protections defined by the Civil Rights Act of 1964, which was not designed to protect the rights of those with disabilities. It also augments other laws that address issues of disability and access to education and employment opportunities, such as the INDIVIDUALS WITH DISABILITIES EDUCATION ACT (IDEA) and the REHABILITATION ACT OF 1973 (RA).

While the ADA covers many areas of possible discrimination (including schools), it is used primarily to protect individuals with disabilities on the job. The IDEA and RA offer more specific protections and regulations in regard to schools.

On the job, employers are required to provide fair opportunities to those with disabilities if they are "otherwise qualified" for a position. For example, a person who is partly blind cannot perform the essential functions of airline pilots. A person in a wheelchair, however, may be able to perform the essential functions of a bookkeeper, and therefore should not be discriminated against based on physical limitations.

In addition, employers and schools may be required to provide accessibility to buildings for those who have physical disabilities. Employers with more than 15 employees also may be required to provide accommodations for employees with specific needs based on their disability, such as equipment or more frequent breaks. "Disability" is an important term from a legal perspective, as it distinguishes those with temporary or less severe limitations from those for whom a physical or mental impairment limits major life activities.

However, the ADA clearly protects educational institutions and employers from requirements to provide accommodations that cause unreasonable burdens or that represent significant lowering of educational standards.

Anafranil   See CLOMIPRAMINE.

Angelman syndrome (AS)   A childhood disorder characterized by HYPERACTIVITY, seizures, excessive laughter, and developmental delays. Initially presumed to be rare, Angelman syndrome is now believed to affect thousands of children who are undiagnosed or misdiagnosed as having autism or other childhood disorders.

In 1965, English physician Harry Angelman, M.D., first described three children with a set of characteristics now known as Angelman syndrome, including stiff, jerky gait; lack of speech; excessive laughter; and seizures. Other cases were eventually published, but the condition was considered to be extremely rare, and many physicians doubted its existence. The first reports from North America appeared in the early 1980s, and since then many new reports have appeared. In the United States and Canada, there are about 1,000 diagnosed individuals, but it has been reported throughout the world among divergent racial groups. In North America, most cases seem to be of Caucasian origin.

Symptoms and Diagnostic Path

Hyperactivity and a short attention span are probably the most typical behaviors, affecting boys and girls about equally. Infants and toddlers may be continually active, constantly keeping their hands or toys in their mouths or moving from object to object. In extreme cases, the constant movement can cause accidental bruises. In older children, there may be grabbing, pinching and biting. A child's attention span can be so short that it interferes with social interaction, since the child cannot pay attention to facial and other social cues. Excessive laughter is also quite common, which seems to be a reaction to physical or mental stimuli. Parents may first notice this laughter at the age of one to three months. Giggling, chortling and constant smiling soon develop and appear to represent normal reflexive laughter, but cooing and babbling are delayed.

Other symptoms include

- developmental delay
- severe speech impairment with almost no use of words
- movement or balance disorder
- easily excitable personality, often with HAND-FLAPPING movements
- abnormally small head
- seizures

Angelman syndrome is usually not recognized at birth or in infancy, since the developmental problems are hard to spot at that time. Parents may first suspect the diagnosis after reading about AS or meeting a child with the condition. The most common age of diagnosis is between age three and seven, when the characteristic behaviors and features become evident.

Treatment Options and Outlook

Persistent and consistent behavior modification helps decrease or eliminate unwanted behavior. In milder cases, the child's attention span may be sufficient to learn sign language and other communication techniques. For these children, educational and developmental training programs are much easier to structure and are generally more effective.

Most children do not receive drug therapy for hyperactivity although some may benefit from use of medications such as methylphenidate (Ritalin).

animal therapy A type of treatment sometimes used for people with autism, that may include horseback riding or swimming with dolphins.

Some experts believe that therapeutic horseback riding programs (sometimes referred to as hippotherapy) may provide both physical and emotional benefits, improve coordination and motor development, and create a sense of well-being and self-confidence. However, no studies using control groups have found animal therapy to be significantly effective for children with autism.

Dolphin therapy was first tried in the 1970s by David Nathanson, a psychologist who believed that interactions with dolphins would increase a child's attention span, enhancing cognitive processes. In anecdotal studies, he found that children with disabilities learned faster and retained information longer when they were with dolphins compared to children who learned in a classroom setting.

See also DOLPHIN-ASSISTED THERAPY.

antidepressants Medications used to treat depression that also may be used to treat patients with autism in order to reduce the frequency and intensity of repetitive behavior; decrease irritability, tantrums, and aggression; and improve eye contact and responsiveness. Antidepressants used to treat autism include amitriptyline (Elavil), bupropion (Wellbutrin), CLOMIPRAMINE (Anafranil), FLUVOXAMINE (Luvox), and FLUOXETINE (Prozac).

Side Effects

There can be a wide variety of possible side effects, depending on the type of antidepressant used. Side effects include insomnia, dizziness, drowsiness, sexual problems, excitability or nervousness, seizures, and weight loss or gain.

antiepileptic medication A class of medications normally prescribed to control seizures in patients with epilepsy. These medications also can be used to help control aggressive behaviors in patients with autism. They help to stabilize brain activity and therefore assist in the control of behavior.

The administration of antiepileptic medications often requires regular blood testing in order to ensure that liver or bone marrow damage does not occur. Since these medications are designed to treat seizure activity, they are often prescribed for children who suffer a seizure disorder as well as autism.

Depakote (valproate), which can lessen explosive behaviors and aggression, is a common antiepileptic used in autistic patients. Side effects include sedation and nausea. In rare cases, however, Depakote can cause liver damage, so close attention must be paid to the drug levels in the bloodstream.

Tegretol (carbamazapine) is equally as effective as Depakote, but it can cause a skin rash and bone marrow problems; for this reason, regular blood tests are required.

Neurontin (gabapentin) and Lamictal (lamotrigine) are other medications that show potential to help patients with autism but have not been studied sufficiently to be recommended for use with children. They appear to provide the same benefits as Depakote, as well as the same side effects, but insufficient data exist on their overall effect.

antihypertensives Medications, prescribed to treat high blood pressure, that have shown promise in treating aggressive behaviors in patients with autism. Although experts are not sure how these medications work, for some children they do stem aggressiveness and emotional outbursts.

Of the antihypertensives, Inderal (propranolol) and Visken (pindolol) both seem to lessen aggression and explosions. Their side effects include sedation, aggravation of asthmatic symptoms, and lightheadedness or fainting due to a drop in blood pressure. A physician should be consulted if signs of low blood pressure appear.

antipsychotics One of the main drug classes prescribed for the treatment of autism, which can help control aggression and HYPERACTIVITY along with behavioral problems and withdrawal. More typically these drugs treat psychotic behavior in psychiatric patients. The fact that this drug works both for autism and psychiatric illness does not mean that the two conditions are related, however.

Risperdal (RISPERIDONE) is the most common antipsychotic used for autistic patients, lessening aggression, agitation, and explosive behavior. Side effects include sedation, weight gain, dizziness, and muscular stiffness.

Zyprexa (olanzapine) relieves the same symptoms as Risperdal and causes the same side effects, except for muscular stiffness. It has not been as widely studied, however.

Seroquel (quetiapine) has many of the same effects as Risperdal with the same side effects, except that patients are less likely to gain weight on this drug. However, this medication has not been widely studied in individuals with autism.

Side Effects

In addition to the side effects mentioned above, other side effects of antipsychotics may include anxiety, fatigue, headache, and insomnia.

aphasia The loss or diminished ability to use or understand words, affecting speaking as well as reading or writing skills. Aphasia, ranging from mild to severe, can be common in individuals with severe autism.

applied behavior analysis (ABA) A form of therapy based on the theory that behavior rewarded is more likely to be repeated than behavior ignored. DISCRETE TRIAL TRAINING is part of this approach. ABA is a process of systematically applying interventions based on the principles of learning theory to improve reading, academics, social skills, communication, and ADAPTIVE LIVING SKILLS. This approach generally involves therapists who work intensely, one-on-one with a child for 20 to 40 hours a week. In a simple step-by-step manner, therapists teach skills such as identifying colors. The sessions usually begin with formal, structured drills, such as learning to point to a color when its name is given; and then, after some time, there is a shift toward generalizing skills to other situations and environments.

The one-on-one, individualized programs of applied behavior analysis break down learning tasks into the smallest, most basic parts, and build upon them incrementally. Differences between programs can be significant.

Educational/behavioral therapies are often effective in children with autism; ABA is usually the most effective. These methods can and should be used together with biomedical interventions, as together they offer the best chance for improvement.

ABA methods are used to support persons with autism to

- increase behaviors
- teach new skills
- teach self control and self-monitoring procedures
- generalize or to transfer behavior from one situation or response to another
- restrict or narrow conditions under which interfering behaviors occur
- reduce self injury or unnecessary repetition of movements

Parents, siblings, and friends may play an important role in helping strengthen the development of children with autism. Typical preschool children learn primarily by play, and the importance of play is critical in teaching language and social skills. Ideally, many of the techniques used in ABA, SENSORY INTEGRATION, and other therapies can be extended throughout the day by family and friends.

In one study of ABA published by autism expert Ivar Lovaas at UCLA in 1987, trained graduate students worked for two years of intensive, 40 hours per week behavioral intervention with 19 young autistic children ranging from 35 to 41 months of age. Almost half of the children improved so much after the ABA therapy that they were indistinguishable from typical children, and these children went on to lead fairly normal lives. Of the other half, most had significant improvements, but a few did not improve much.

ABA programs are most effective when started before age five, but they also can be helpful to older children. They are especially effective in teaching nonverbal children how to talk. Most experts agree that behavioral interventions involving one-on-one interactions are usually helpful, sometimes bringing very positive results. With older individuals, ABA is often used to teach ADAPTIVE LIVING SKILLS. Therapists should prompt as much as necessary to achieve a high level of success, with a gradual fading of prompts. There must be proper training of therapists, ongoing supervision, and regular team meetings to maintain consistency among therapists and check for problems. To ensure adequate training, experts recommend that clinicians overseeing ABA be board-certified behavior analysts. Most importantly, the sessions should be fun for the children in order to maintain their interest and motivation.

The effectiveness of ABA-based interventions with persons with autism is well documented, with more than 30 years of research studies. Parents are encouraged to be trained in ABA so they can provide the therapy themselves as well as hire other people to help.

apraxia   Loss of the ability to coordinate, sequence, and execute purposeful movements and gestures not caused by weakness or paralysis. Experts believe that apraxia is caused by damage to the cerebral cortex, including problems in development of the cortex in certain developmental disorders such as RETT DISORDER. Apraxia may affect any voluntary movements, such as those needed for eye gaze, walking, or speaking.

See also APRAXIA OF SPEECH.

apraxia of speech   A neurologically based speech disorder that may occur in people with autism. A person with this disorder has trouble planning and producing the precise, highly refined and specific series of movements of the tongue, lips, jaw, and palate that are necessary for intelligible speech. Apraxia of speech also may be called verbal apraxia, developmental apraxia of speech, or verbal dyspraxia.

Symptoms and Diagnostic Path

Research suggests that up to nine percent of children with autism will never develop speech; of those who do speak, 43 percent begin to talk by the end of their first year, 35 percent begin to talk sometime between their first and second year, and 22 percent begin to talk some time during their third year or after. Only 12 percent are totally nonverbal by age five. With appropriate interventions, there is reason to hope that children with autism can learn to talk, at least to some extent.

In typical speech/language development, the child's receptive and expressive skills develop at the same time. A child with apraxia of speech generally experiences a wide gap between receptive and expressive language abilities, so that the child's ability to understand language (receptive ability) may be normal, but expressive speech is seriously unclear, deficient, or completely absent.

Treatment Options and Outlook

Children with apraxia of speech can and do improve. The factors that appear to contribute to a prognosis include the individual characteristics of the child, such as receptive language, cognitive ability, desire to communicate, attention span, and the age at which appropriate treatment is begun (preschool age is best). Also important is the existence of other medical, speech and/or language issues, and how much the family is willing to participate in therapy and follow-through. With appropriate help, most children with apraxia of speech improve their expressive speech ability, although in some cases the child never really learns to speak intelligibly.

A child's treatment outcome is very difficult to predict, in part because no two children with apraxia are alike. Treatments that are most effective include those that include lots of practice and repetition with corrective feedback, a focus on targeted oral-motor patterns, sensory input for control of the movement sequences, sensory prompts such as visual, touch, and kinesthetic cues, use of rhythm and melody, and focus on speech sequences versus individual sounds.

Many experienced speech-language pathologists use an eclectic approach, incorporating several of the methods mentioned above and using them based on the individual child's needs. There is no one "program" that is right for every child with apraxia.

Children with apraxia of speech reportedly do not progress well in their actual speech production with therapy tailored for other articulation problems or with language stimulation approaches. Additionally, in young children the motor/sensory techniques and drills should be woven into play. Children with apraxia need frequent one-on-one therapy and lots of repetition of sounds, sound sequences, and movement patterns in order to incorporate them and make them automatic.

Many therapists recommend the use of sign language, picture books, and other means to augment speech in the child who is not clearly understood. This approach may be called "total communication." Having the child pair a vocal word attempt with a sign enhances the chance that the listener will be able to "catch" the communication (if the spoken word is not understood, perhaps the sign will be). Having others understand the communication can offer children motivation and the feeling of success in using their voice to communicate. Even very young children with apraxia of speech are aware of their problem. Providing successful communication experiences encourages the child.

Also, for children with apraxia of speech, signs can become important visual cues to help them know how to place their mouths in order to produce the desired word. When pairing of spoken word and sign is consistent, the child may come to associate the visual image of the sign with the placement of their articulators. For this reason, parents should not be afraid about using sign language with their child; children will drop the signs on their own as their speech becomes understood.

Another way parents can help autistic children learn to talk is by using the Picture Exchange Communication System (PECS), which involves pointing to a set of pictures or symbols on a board. In addition, parents can try encouraging the child to sing with a videotape or audiotape.

Asperger, Hans (1906–1980) Austrian pediatrician who published the first definition of ASPERGER'S SYNDROME (AS) in 1944. At an early age, young Hans showed special talents in language, and already in early school years he was known for his frequent poetic quotations. Considered to be aloof as a child, he earned his medical degree in 1931 and assumed directorship of the play-pedagogic station at the university children's clinic in Vienna in 1932. He married in 1935 and had five children.

Asperger had a special interest in "psychically abnormal" children. He identified a pattern of behavior and abilities that he saw mostly in boys, including a lack of empathy, little ability to form friendships, one-sided conversation, intense absorption in a special interest, and clumsy movements. Asperger called children with AS "little professors" because of their ability to talk about a subject with great detail. He described the syndrome in a paper submitted for publication in 1943, based on investigations of more than 400 children with "autistic psychopathy." However, since he did not travel widely and all his publishing was in German, Asperger's name was less known than that of Leo Kanner, who described infantile autism also in 1943. Although Asperger was not aware of Kanner's work on autism, he did use the word *autism* in his work.

In people with Asperger's syndrome, deficits in social interaction and unusual responses to the environment, similar to those in autism, are observed. Unlike in autism, however, cognitive and communicative development are within the normal or near-normal range in the first years of life, and verbal skills are usually an area of relative strength.

In 1946 he became director of the children's clinic. In 1977 Asperger became professor emeritus, delivering his last lecture six days before his death. His list of publications includes 359 items, most of which concern autistic psycopathy and death.

Asperger died before the syndrome that bears his name became widely recognized. The first person to use the term *Asperger's syndrome* in a paper was Lorna Wing, whose piece was published in 1981. Asperger's work was not internationally recognized until the 1990s.

See also KANNER, LEO.

Asperger's syndrome (AS) A condition characterized by sustained problems with social interactions and social relatedness, and the development of restricted, repetitive patterns of interests, acti-

vities, and behaviors. Asperger's syndrome is usually considered a subtype of high-functioning autism but without the delays in cognitive or language development. Although the correct modern term is Asperger's disorder, according to the *Diagnostic and Statistical Manual IV-TR* (the manual used to diagnose mental conditions), it is also sometimes called Asperger syndrome or Asperger's syndrome.

The disorder is named after Hans Asperger, a Viennese pediatrician who first documented this cluster of characteristics in the 1940s.

Asperger's disorder is one of five conditions grouped under the umbrella category of PERVASIVE DEVELOPMENTAL DISORDER (PDD) because those with any of the five conditions share a number of characteristics: restricted interests and activities that tend to be repetitive and impairments in social interaction, imaginative activity, verbal and nonverbal communication skills. The other four disorders in the PDD group include autism, RETT DISORDER, CHILDHOOD DISINTEGRATIVE DISORDER, and PERVASIVE DEVELOPMENTAL DISORDER–NOT OTHERWISE SPECIFIED (PDD-NOS). The umbrella term of pervasive developmental disorders was first used in the 1980s to describe this class of disorders with similar symptoms or characteristics; Asperger's was first classified as a PDD in 1994.

Asperger's was believed to be a milder variant of autism, but without the delays in cognitive or language development. In 1994 Asperger's was first classified as a pervasive developmental disorder (a designation that also includes AUTISTIC DISORDER).

Differentiating individuals with this condition from those with high-functioning autism remains difficult, and experts disagree as to whether they are actually different disorders. Inconsistencies in the way the term has been used and the lack, until quite recently, of recognized official definitions has made it difficult to interpret the research available on this condition. Even now, some clinicians will use the term to refer to people with autism who have IQs in the normal range, or to adults with autism, or to those with PDD-NOS, regardless of whether their early language development was normal, as the *DSM-IV-TR* requires for a diagnosis of Asperger's disorder. Although researchers emphasize differences from autism, such as in terms of better communication (particularly verbal) skills, the symptoms overlap considerably. The learning profile of individuals with Asperger's disorder is often consistent with a nonverbal learning disability (more difficulties with visual-perceptual problem-solving than language-based tasks and related social deficits).

Attention problems are often seen in children with Asperger's. Sometimes clinicians overlook social impairment, and mistakenly diagnose attention deficit hyperactivity disorder (ADHD) rather than Asperger's. Some children with pervasive developmental disorders, such as Asperger's disorder, may also meet the diagnostic criteria for ADHD. However, ADHD should only be diagnosed in Asperger's if the ADHD symptoms are more pronounced than those that could be attributed to Asperger's.

As all the pervasive developmental disorders (except for Rett disorder) Asperger's is believed to be more common in boys, although more research needs to be done to understand its genetic origins. According to the National Institutes of Health, Asperger's disorder occurs in one out of every 500 Americans—more often than multiple sclerosis, Down syndrome, or cystic fibrosis. It is estimated that more than 400,000 families are directly affected by this condition.

While biological factors are of crucial importance in the etiology of autism, so far brain imaging studies with Asperger's cases have found no consistent pattern or evidence of any type of lesion, and no single location of any lesion.

Associated medical conditions such as FRAGILE X SYNDROME, tuberous sclerosis, neurofibromatosis, and hypothyroidism (sluggish thyroid) are less common in Asperger's disorder than in classical autism. Therefore, scientists suspect there may be fewer major physical brain problems associated with Asperger's than with autism.

Symptoms and Diagnostic Path

Often there are no obvious delays in language or cognitive development, or in age-appropriate self-help skills. While these individuals may possess attention deficits, problems with organization, and an uneven profile of skills, they usually have average and sometimes gifted intelligence.

Individuals with Asperger's syndrome may have problems with social situations and in developing peer relationships. They may have noticeable difficulty with nonverbal communication, impaired use of social gestures, facial expressions, and EYE CONTACT. There may be certain repetitive behaviors or rituals. Though grammatical, speech is peculiar due to abnormal inflection and/or repetition. Clumsiness is common. Individuals with this disorder usually have a limited area of interest, such as single-minded obsessions about cars, trains, door knobs, hinges, astronomy, or history, that usually excludes more age-appropriate, common hobbies.

Asperger's vs. autism   When compared to autism, Asperger's disorder usually appears later in life, with less severe social and communication problems. Clumsiness and single-minded interests are more common and verbal IQ is usually higher than performance IQ (in autism, the reverse is usually true). The outcome is usually more positive than for autism. Children with Asperger's disorder have impaired social interactions similar to those of children with autism, as well as stereotyped or repetitive behaviors and mannerisms and nonfunctional rituals. However, language skills are normal and sometimes superior to those of an average child, although their speech is usually described as peculiar, such as being stilted and focusing on unusual topics. Children with Asperger's usually have normal IQ.

Most of the individuals with Asperger's syndrome are interested in having friends, but lack the social skills to begin or maintain a friendship. While high-functioning autistic individuals also may be social but awkward, they are typically less interested in having friends. In addition, high-functioning autistic individuals are often delayed in developing speech/language.

Treatment Options and Outlook

While there is no cure, early intervention has been proven to be effective. The need for academic and social supports increases through the school years, and by adolescence many children develop symptoms of depression and anxiety. It is important to continue supports into adulthood to ensure affected adults can lead productive lives.

Symptoms can be managed using individual psychotherapy to help the individual to process the feelings aroused by being socially handicapped. Other treatments may include parent education and training, BEHAVIORAL MODIFICATION, social skills training, educational interventions, and medication.

Medical treatments may include the following:

- for hyperactivity, inattention and impulsivity: stimulants such as methyphenidate, dextro-amphetamine, methamphetamine, pemoline, CLONIDINE, and tricyclic antidepressants (DESIP-RAMINE, nortriptyline)

- for irritability and aggression: mood stabilizers (valproate, carbamazepine, lithium), beta-blockers (nadolol, propranolol), neuroleptics (RISPERIDONE, HALOPERIDOL)

- for preoccupations, rituals and compulsions: antidepressants (FLUVOXAMINE, FLUOXETINE, CLO-MIPRAMINE)

- for anxiety: antidepressants (sertraline, fluox-etine, imipramine, clomipramine, nortriptyline)

assessment   A general term that covers a wide range of activities, instruments, and approaches involved in evaluating prior performance, describing present abilities and behaviors, and predicting future performance and behaviors. "Assessment" differs from "testing," which reflects performance on particular tasks at a specific time. Instead, assessment interprets overall patterns and relationships among testing results and other observations.

Several standardized tests and checklists have been developed to help assess the behavior of children with possible autism, and can be used in various ways. They can help determine if autism is likely, so that a decision can be made to seek a specific diagnosis. At other times, they may be used as part of the formal diagnostic process. Finally, in certain instances some of these instruments may be used to rate the severity of symptoms, which may help assess interventions, periodic monitoring of the child's progress, and outcomes.

A neuropsychological assessment might include a more comprehensive group of tests designed to identify functioning in specific areas, such as memory or visual processing. In most cases, such standardized testing is used together with case histories, interviews, and details on actual performance at school, among friends, and at home. Assessment may also incorporate testing in specific areas of brain function, or include testing designed to identify emotional, psychological, and personality factors that may be involved in learning difficulties. The field of assessment is in a state of continuous development in order to discover more accurate methods of evaluating performance and behavior.

Types of Autism Assessments

There are several individual autism assessment tests currently available for use in the United States that have been specifically designed to assess children with possible autism. All of these tests rely on either information about the child's behavior provided by a parent, direct observation of the child by a professional, or a combination of these methods. The specific autism tests include

- *AUTISM BEHAVIOR CHECKLIST (ABC):* a behavior checklist completed by a parent

- *AUTISM DIAGNOSTIC INTERVIEW–REVISED (ADI-R):* a structured interview

- *CHILDHOOD AUTISM RATING SCALE (CARS):* a test combining parent reports and direct observation by the professional

- *AUTISM DIAGNOSTIC OBSERVATION SCALE (ADOS):* a test using direct observation of the child's behavior as elicited by the examiner

Behavior checklists such as the ABC include lists of questions completed by parents and later scored by a professional. Structured interviews (such as the various versions of the ADI) include a set of questions and interviews that professionals use to question parents. Tests that rely on direct observation of the child by a professional (such as the PL-ADOS) often outline specific ways for the examiner to elicit responses from the child. These tests also have a standardized method for scoring the observed behaviors. CARS combines both historical information from a parent and direct observation of the child by the professional; CARS also provides a total score that can rate the severity of behavior.

assistive augmentative communication   Any symbol system of communication that relays a message and that can be used to add to more typical forms of communication when these methods are impaired. This might involve using unaided methods, such as gestures or American Sign Language, or aided techniques, such as alphabet or picture boards. A person communicates using these boards by "pointing" to each letter or picture, either with a finger or eye gaze (where the person looks at the word or picture he wants to communicate).

The more complex methods are electronic aids or recorded messages activated by buttons—some of which rely on complex electronic computer technology, also called speech generating devices (SGD), voice output communication aids (VOCA), or voice output devices.

Assistive Technology Act of 1998   This law, also known as P.L. 105-394, replaced the Technology-Related Assistance for Individuals with Disabilities Act of 1988. This act addresses the assistive-technology needs of individuals with disabilities.

attention   The focus of consciousness on something in the environment, or on a sensation or an idea. The length of time a child can pay attention to something (the attention span) increases with age, interest, and intelligence level. Attention includes a number of elements which are essential to all activities, including the following:

- *arousal:* being ready to receive stimuli
- *vigilance:* being able to select stimuli from those presented over a period of time
- *persistence or continuity:* being able to sustain a mental effort and select stimuli that are presented often
- *monitoring:* checking for and correcting errors

Breakdowns in these different elements can cause a variety of problems. A breakdown in vigilance, for example, might cause someone to select or focus on the wrong details. A breakdown in monitoring might lead to repeated careless errors. Persistence or continuity is necessary for a complex task to be completed.

attention deficit disorder (ADD)   A condition that is sometimes used to describe attention problems in the absence of hyperactivity. ADD is no longer a recognized medical term; the medical community now refers to ADD as *attention deficit hyperactivity disorder, primarily inattentive subtype,* as opposed to the more common *ADHD, combined subtype* or *ADHD, primarily impulsive/hyperactive subtype.*

atypical autism   A general term for conditions that are close to but do not quite fit the set of conditions of autism or other specific conditions.

See also PERVASIVE DEVELOPMENTAL DISORDER–NOT OTHERWISE SPECIFIED.

atypical learner   A general term for a child who is different from the typical student in physical, intellectual, social, or emotional development, and who differs in mental characteristics, sensory abilities, communication abilities, or social behavior to the extent that SPECIAL EDUCATION services are required.

auditory integration training (AIT)   A somewhat controversial treatment method used with people who have auditory processing problems, which reduces sensitivity to specific sound frequencies. The treatment is used to help people with autism, dyslexia, attention deficit hyperactivity disorder (ADHD), vestibular processing problems, and reading problems. About 40 percent of autistic children are reported to show very sensitive hearing. Auditory training is designed to overcome the hypersensitivity.

The training was developed by French otolaryngologist Guy Bérard, who believes that abnormal auditory processing occurs when there is a discrepancy between how well someone hears different sound frequencies. For example, a person with auditory processing problems may be hypersensitive to the frequencies 2,000 and 8,000 Hertz, but hear all the other frequencies normally. Auditory processing problems seem to be linked to a defect in the brainstem's reticular activating system, responsible for regulating information from the auditory and vestibular systems and focusing on certain types of sensory input.

Researchers who believe that AIT is effective suspect that many children diagnosed with autism and other problems have an AUDITORY PROCESSING DISORDER. This condition is particularly common if the child has SENSORY INTEGRATION DYSFUNCTION, such as touch sensitivity. AIT is thought to help improve attention span deficits, to correct poor auditory discrimination skills, and to improve the ability to follow directions, all of which are common problems in autistic children.

Other experts believe that dyslexia may also affect the auditory processing system. Brain scans of dyslexic people show fewer neurons on the left side of the medial geniculate nucleus, one of the most important parts of the auditory system and an area that processes fast-changing sounds. AIT focuses on training the child to improve discrimination of this type of sound.

The Training Process

The first step in AIT is to schedule an audiogram to determine whether the person has auditory sensitivity. After the first five hours of treatment, the child will get a second audiogram to determine if the sensitivities are still present and whether new sensitivities have developed. A final audiogram is given after the completion of the listening sessions. The goal of the training is that all frequencies should be perceived equally well and the sensitivities should be eliminated.

The training begins with twice-a-day, 30-minute sessions for 10 days. During the first five hours of training, each ear receives the same sound level input. For children with a speech or hearing impairment, the sound level is reduced in the left ear during the second five hours of training. The left hemisphere is responsible for processing speech and language; since the right ear is connected more directly to the left hemisphere, a higher sound level in the right ear will stimulate the left hemisphere. Using a cassette or CD player, the child listens to unpredictable, modulated music that has been specially processed. This is believed to stimulate the reticular activating system. If the child is sensitive to certain frequencies, these frequencies are filtered out. The special music is sup-posed to train the child to filter out unimportant sounds in order to focus on certain frequencies. It works by allowing a sound-sensitive child to adapt to sounds. Adaptation is a built-in mechanism, which after continued exposure to a stimulus reduces the perception of that stimulus. This may result in better sound discrimination. Because the vestibular system is also integrated in this part of the brain, the unique sounds used in AIT also may produce better posture, balance, and spatial orientation.

To be effective, the music used for AIT should cover a wide range of frequencies and have a good tempo or beat. Most music does not meet these criteria. AIT experts have reviewed more than 1,000 CDs and created a list of 70 CDs that can be used in AIT training—mostly jazz, pop, reggae, and contemporary rock. Very few classical pieces fit the requirements.

Effectiveness

Current research has not proven the benefits of this treatment. Studies into the effectiveness of the training have been inconclusive; some researchers using anecdotal studies have found benefit and others have not. There have been no controlled studies supporting AIT. Since the training is not invasive, however, some experts believe there is little to be lost by trying the approach. Although the treatment period is short (just two weeks), it is expensive (on average, about $2,000). Because of the lack of research supporting its efficacy, the ethical guidelines of the American Speech/Language/Hearing Association prohibit clinicians from charging money for this experimental treatment.

AIT is not without problems. Some patients report behavior changes, including agitation, hyperactivity, and rapid mood swings. Experts do not know why, but this type of reaction occurs with other forms of sensory integration training as well. Many children become less compliant, perhaps as a result of a tendency to become overfocused and hence, more reluctant to change tasks.

auditory processing disorder (APD)   Difficulty in processing information is a common problem for individuals with autism. An auditory processing disorder is a complex problem that occurs in the brain system responsible for recognizing and interpreting sounds, so that the person may not recognize slight differences between word sounds, even though the sounds themselves are loud and clear. One auditory processing problem occurs when a person hears speech sounds but does not perceive the meaning. For example, if someone says the word "horse," the person may hear the speech sound, but does not understand the meaning of the sound. APD is also called central auditory processing disorder, auditory perception problem, auditory comprehension deficit, central auditory dysfunction, central deafness, or word deafness. These kinds of problems are more likely if there is a lot of background noise, or if the person with APD is listening to complex information.

Although the lack of speech comprehension may be misinterpreted as an unwillingness to comply, in fact the person with autism may not be able to understand the meaning of words at that particular time.

Scientists still do not understand exactly how attention, memory, and sensory interpretation interact, or how they malfunction in cases of auditory processing disorders. In particular, experts do not understand the underlying cause of auditory processing problems in autism, but autopsy research has shown that an area in the limbic system called the hippocampus is not well developed in autistic individuals. The hippocampus is responsible for sensory processing as well as learning and memory. Information is transferred from the senses to the hippocampus, where it is processed and then transferred to areas of the cerebral cortex for long-term storage. Since auditory information is processed in the hippocampus, the information may not be properly transferred to long-term memory in autistic individuals.

Auditory processing problems also may be linked to several autistic characteristics. Autism is sometimes described as a social-communication problem. Processing auditory information is a critical component of social communication. Other characteristics that may be associated with auditory processing problems include anxiety or confusion in social situations, inattentiveness, and poor speech comprehension.

The better autistic children understand auditory information, the better they can comprehend their environment, both socially and academically.

Symptoms and Diagnostic Path

People with auditory processing difficulty typically have normal hearing and intelligence. However, they may have

- attention and memory problems related to oral information
- poor academic performance
- problems with multistep directions
- poor listening skills
- behavior problems
- need for more time to process information
- confusion over syllable sequences and problems developing vocabulary and understanding language
- problems with reading, comprehension, spelling, and vocabulary

A teacher or pediatrician may be the first person to notice symptoms of an auditory processing disorder in a child. A doctor can help rule out possible diseases that can cause some of these same symptoms. To determine whether the child has a functional hearing problem, an audiologist will administer tests to determine the softest sounds and words a person can hear and how well people can recognize sounds in words and sentences.

A speech-language pathologist can find out how well a child understands and uses language. The audiologist (who helps with functional problems of hearing and processing) and the speech-language pathologist (focused on language) may work as a team with a child.

Treatment Options and Outlook

Several strategies are available to help children with auditory processing difficulties, including:

- *auditory trainers:* electronic devices that allow a person to focus attention on a speaker and reduce the interference of background noise, often used in classrooms where the teacher wears a microphone to transmit sound and the child wears a headset to receive the sound. Children who wear hearing aids can use them in addition to the auditory trainer.

- *environmental modifications:* arranging classroom acoustics, placement, and seating
- *exercises:* methods that can boost language-building skills, increasing the ability to learn new words and improve a child's language base
- *auditory memory enhancement:* techniques that help children learn to condense complex information into a simpler form that is easier to remember

augmentative communication A method of communication used with people with autism, in which the spoken word is combined with the presentation of photographs, symbols, or gestures to help the person make his needs, feelings, and ideas known.

See also ASSISTIVE AUGMENTATIVE COMMUNICATION.

autism See AUTISTIC DISORDER.

autism, early onset Children whose symptoms of autism appear during the first year of life. (Children whose symptoms appear between ages one and two are referred to as having "late-onset" or "regressive" autism. Although some researchers argue that the regression is not real or that congenital autism was simply unnoticed by the child's parents, many parents do report that their children had completely normal speech, behavior, and social skills until some time between one and two years of age.)

One recent study compared 53 autistic children with 48 typical peers. The parents of the early-onset autism group reported a significant delay in reaching developmental milestones, including age of crawling (a two-month delay), sitting up (two-month delay), walking (four- to five-month delay), and talking (11-month delay or more). In contrast, the late-onset autism group reached developmental milestones at the same time as typical children up to the appearance of their autistic symptoms.

Prior to 1990, about two-thirds of children with autism had noticeable symptoms during the first year of life, and one-third regressed sometime after age one. Starting in the 1980s, the trend has reversed, so that today fewer than one-third are now early onset and two-thirds become autistic in their second year. Some experts believe these results suggest that something happens between ages one and two (such as increased exposure to an environmental toxin).

See also AUTISM, LATE ONSET.

autism, late onset The appearance of autistic symptoms at between 12 and 24 months of age, after an apparently normal developmental period. About two-thirds of children with autism do not exhibit any symptoms until about age two, reversing a trend through the 1980s in which most children with autism showed symptoms at an early age.

Today, many parents report that their child seemed to develop normally from birth to about age one or two, and then suddenly began to regress until eventually autism was diagnosed. Although some researchers argue that the regression is not real or that congenital autism was simply unnoticed by the child's parents, many parents do report that their children had demonstrated completely normal speech, behavior, and social skills until some time between one and two years of age.

One recent study compared 53 autistic children with 48 typical peers. The parents of the early-onset autism group reported a significant delay in reaching developmental milestones, including age of crawling (a two-month delay), sitting up (two-month delay), walking (four to five month delay), and talking (11-month delay or more). In contrast, the late-onset autism group reached developmental milestones at the same time as typical children up to the appearance of their autistic symptoms.

Prior to 1990, about two-thirds of children with autism experienced symptoms early, and one-third regressed sometime after age one year. Starting in the 1980s, the trend has reversed, so that today fewer than one-third show early onset and two-thirds become autistic in their second year. Some experts believe these results suggest that something happens between ages one and two (such as increased exposure to an environmental toxin).

See also AUTISM, EARLY ONSET.

Autism and Developmental Disabilities Monitoring Network (ADDM)   A group of 10 different projects that are developing or improving programs to track the number of children with autistic spectrum disorders (ASDs), funded by the Centers for Disease Control and Prevention (CDC). The goal of the ADDM network is to provide comparable, population-based estimates of the prevalence rates of autism and related disorders in different sites over time. The 11 states that are part of the ADDM network are Alabama, Arizona, Arkansas, Florida, Missouri/Illinois, New Jersey, South Carolina, Utah, West Virginia, and Wisconsin.

Alabama

The Alabama Autism Surveillance Program (AASP) takes place in different sites around the state in an attempt to monitor the number of children born in 1994 who lived in Alabama in 2002 and who had a diagnosis of AUTISM SPECTRUM DISORDER, MENTAL RETARDATION, and/or cerebral palsy. This surveillance system will provide the first steps in establishing an accurate count of the number of children in Alabama with these developmental disabilities. The investigators are members of the Department of Maternal and Child Health of the School of Public Health at the University of Alabama at Birmingham.

The study began with the northern 32 counties in Alabama, but could expand to cover the entire state. About 36,000 babies are born in this area each year. This study initially focused on children eight years of age, with plans to include children from ages three through 10 years.

In the 2001–02 school year, 1,233 Alabama students were classified as having autism and received special education services. That number was 0.17 percent of the 731,095 children enrolled in Alabama public schools on December 1, 2002.

Arizona

The Arizona Autism Spectrum Surveillance Program (AASSP) takes place in different sites around the state in an attempt to monitor the number of children with an ASD. This five-year epidemiologic study will help establish, for the first time, an accurate count of the number of Arizona children with autism. The study began in Maricopa County, where 55,000 babies are born each year, but it could expand to include Pima County.

In the 2000–01 school year, 1,213 Arizona students had autism and received special education services. That number was 0.14 percent of the 893,334 children enrolled in Arizona public schools on October 1, 2000.

The investigators of this study are members of the Department of Pediatrics and College of Public Health at the University of Arizona.

Arkansas

The Arkansas Autism Project is designed to identify and track the number of children in Arkansas with ASDs to help establish how many Arkansas children actually have autism. The entire state of Arkansas is included in this monitoring project, although at first, most attention will be directed to the larger school districts in the state and children seen at the autism clinic at the University of Arkansas for Medical Science (UAMS) Department of Pediatrics. This project will initially focus on children eight years of age, with plans to include children from three through ten years of age.

Although currently there is no accurate count of the number of Arkansas children with autism, the Arkansas Autism Society works with about 700 children and families within the state. The Arkansas Department of Education has seen an increase in the number of children receiving services who are classified as having autism. In the 2002–03 school year, 109 eight-year-olds (about three in 1,000) are being served in the public school system.

The Arkansas Autism Society provides information about autism and forms the basis for support groups for the families of children with autism. An autism clinic at the Dennis Development Center at UAMS provides diagnostic evaluations for children. The investigators for this study are members of the University of Arkansas for Medical Sciences, working in collaboration with the CDC and the Arkansas Department of Health.

Florida

The University of Miami Autism and Developmental Disabilities Monitoring project is a study coordinated with the Florida Department of Health to monitor the number of children with an ASD in south Florida, which will help establish for the first time an accurate count of the number of south Florida children with autism. The project will initially focus on Miami-Dade County, where about 32,000 babies are born each year. The study includes children four through eight years of age. During the 2000–01 school year, there were 4,971 students with autism receiving special education services, with 1,120 students receiving services in Miami-Dade County. During the 1999–2000 school year, the prevalence of autism in Miami-Dade County was 2.7 per 1,000 students.

Investigators are members of the University of Miami Department of Psychology, in association with the University of Miami, Center for Autism and Related Disabilities.

Missouri/Illinois

The Missouri/Illinois Autism and Developmental Disabilities Monitoring project takes place in different sites around the state in an attempt to monitor the number of children with ASD, mental retardation, or both, and to determine how many children with ASD or mental retardation have epilepsy. This research will establish an accurate count of children with these disabilities in the metropolitan St. Louis area. The project will include eight counties in the St. Louis metropolitan area: St. Louis, St. Louis City, St. Charles, Franklin, and Jefferson (in Missouri) and Madison, St. Clair, and Monroe (in Illinois), where 33,000 live births occur a year. In the 2001–02 school year, Missouri served 2,051 students and Illinois served 5,175 students with autism. In 2001–02, 1,102 students within the metropolitan St. Louis area were identified by their school system as having autism.

The investigators are members of the School of Medicine at Washington University, and the study is a joint program with the CDC, the Missouri Department of Health and Senior Services, Illinois Department of Public Health, and many other agencies and organizations that serve children with ASD and their families.

New Jersey

The New Jersey Autism Study is trying to monitor the number of eight-year-old children in New Jersey with an ASD with this multi-year epidemiologic study. The study includes Essex, Union, Hudson, and Ocean counties, but may expand to include other parts of the state. There are about 35,000 babies born in this four-county area each year. During the 2001–02 school year, 3,526 New Jersey students with autism were given special education services. In 1998, one CDC study found that 6.7 of every 1,000 children in Brick Township (in Ocean County) had an ASD.

The investigators are members of the Department of Pediatrics at the New Jersey Medical School who are working with the CDC, the New Jersey State Department of Education, and the New Jersey Governor's Council on Autism.

South Carolina

The South Carolina Developmental Disabilities Surveillance Program is a population-based study that will include information from a variety of sources to establish the rate of ASDs in the eastern half of the state, along the Coastal and Pee Dee regions, including 23 counties. About 25,000 babies are born in this area each year. The investigators are members of the Departments of Pediatrics and Epidemiology and College of Health Professions at the Medical University of South Carolina. During the 2000–01 school year, the State Department of Education reported serving 973 South Carolina students with autism. Although the exact number of people with autism is not known, the South Carolina Autism Division knows of 1,682 persons with autism living in the state.

Utah

The Utah Registry of Autism and Developmental Disabilities is a population-based project that will monitor the number of children in Utah with ASDs and mental retardation. The primary focus of the project is a CDC-sponsored public health registry of eight-year-old children with ASDs or mental retardation centering on Davis, Salt Lake, and Utah Counties, where about 70 percent of Utah's inhabitants live. At the same time, the Utah Department of Health will develop a self-reporting registry to include all ages in the entire state. About 33,000 babies are born in the three-county area each year (about 47,000 in the entire state), and during the 2001–02 school year, the Utah Office of Education reported serving 830 students with autism. The UCLA–University of Utah Epidemiologic Survey of

Autism Prevalence Study in 1983 estimated the incidence rate of autism in Utah to be four in 10,000.

The researchers are members of the Utah Department of Health's Children with Special Health Care Needs Bureau and the University of Utah School of Medicine's Department of Psychiatry. The study is working together with the CDC, the Utah Department of Health, and the University of Utah School of Medicine's Department of Psychiatry.

Other ASD programs in Utah include the Autism Society of Utah; the Utah Parent Center; the Carmen B. Pingree School for Children with Autism; the Utah Department of Health's Children with Special Health Care Needs Bureau; the Utah Division of Services for People with Disabilities; the University of Utah's Child, Adolescent, and Young Adult Specialty Clinic; and the University of Utah's Neurobehavior Clinic.

West Virginia

The West Virginia Autism Study is an investigation to determine and monitor the number of children born in 1992 with an ASD who lived in West Virginia in 2000, when they were eight years old. The entire state of West Virginia is included in the study, where about 30,500 babies are born each year. During the 2000–01 school year, there were 326 students with autism who were receiving special education services in West Virginia. A pilot study conducted in 1999–2000 in a six-county area found that nearly 21 of every 10,000 children aged three to 21 years had an ASD. The investigators are members of the West Virginia Autism Training Center in the College of Education and Human Services at Marshall University.

Wisconsin

The Wisconsin Surveillance of Autism and Other Developmental Disorders System takes place in different sites around the state in an attempt to monitor the number of eight-year-old children with an autism spectrum disorder, mental retardation, or both and to determine how many children with ASD or mental retardation have epilepsy. This surveillance system will help establish for the first time an accurate count of the number of Wisconsin children and families affected by these disorders. The study will initially include 10 counties of southeast-

ern Wisconsin (Kenosha, Racine, Milwaukee, Ozaukee, Waukesha, Jefferson, Rock, Dane, Green, and Walworth) but could expand to include the entire state. About 33,000 babies are born in these counties each year, and about half of the state's population live here.

In the 2002–03 school year, 3,083 of Wisconsin's 881,231 public school students had autism and received special education services, while 12,750 had some type of cognitive disability. The number of Wisconsin children receiving special education services for autism tripled from 1997 to 2002. It is clear more people are being identified with an ASD now than in the past, but public health professionals do not know how common these disorders are in Wisconsin, or whether the increase in the number of children identified with ASDs is due to better diagnosis or true increases.

The Waisman Center of the University of Wisconsin–Madison and the Medical College of Wisconsin offer programs dedicated to developmental disabilities research, diagnosis, and treatment.

This project is a collaboration between the Wisconsin Department of Health and Family Services and investigators from the Waisman Center and Department of Population Health Sciences of the University of Wisconsin–Madison. The study is a joint undertaking with the CDC, the Wisconsin State Department of Public Instruction, and many other agencies and organizations that serve children with developmental disabilities and their families.

autism behavior checklist (ABC)   Screening questionnaire for autism that is completed by a parent. This checklist is an individual autism assessment instrument specifically designed to screen children for possible autism; it is currently available for use by U.S. clinicians. This screening measure relies on historical information about the child's behavior (usually provided by a parent). Tests that rely on historical information may be in the form of behavior checklists. The ABC is a type of behavior checklist that includes lists of questions to be completed by parents and later scored by a professional.

The ABC was first published in 1980 and is part of a broader tool called the AUTISM SCREENING INSTRU-

MENT FOR EDUCATIONAL PLANNING–SECOND EDITION (ASIEP-2). The ABC is designed to be completed independently by a parent or a teacher familiar with the child, who then returns it to a trained professional for scoring and interpretation. Although it is primarily designed to identify children with autism within a population of school-age children with severe disabilities, the ABC has been used with children as young as three years of age.

The ABC has 57 questions divided into five categories:

- sensory
- relating
- body and object use
- language
- social and self-help

The ABC appears to have limited usefulness in identifying children with autism who are under the age of three. When used in conjunction with other diagnostic instruments and methods, the ABC may have some usefulness as a symptom inventory to be completed by parents or teachers.

Autism Diagnostic Interview–Revised (ADI-R) A diagnostic semi-structured interview for a clinician to use to help diagnose children suspected of having AUTISTIC DISORDER or a PERVASIVE DEVELOPMENTAL DISORDER. The original version of this test (Autism Diagnostic Interview) was published in 1989 and was intended primarily for research purposes, providing behavioral assessment for subjects with a chronological age of at least five years and a mental age of at least two years.

The ADI-R, published in 1994, is shorter and more appropriate for younger children than the ADI. It is appropriate for children with mental ages from about 18 months into adulthood, and is linked to the criteria found in the DIAGNOSTIC AND STATISTICAL MANUAL IV-TR. The ADI-R takes from one and a half to two hours to administer.

Both the ADI and the ADI-R focus on the three key areas defining autism: reciprocal social interaction, communication and language, and repetitive, stereotyped behaviors.

The ADI-R is useful for formal diagnosis as well as treatment and educational planning. It can help clinicians to differentiate autism from other developmental disorders and in assessing syndrome boundaries.

To administer ADI-R, an experienced clinical interviewer questions a parent who is familiar with the developmental history and current behavior of the child being evaluated. Composed of 93 items, the ADI-R focuses on three functional domains—language and communication, reciprocal social interactions, and restricted, repetitive, and stereotyped behaviors and interests.

Interview questions cover eight content areas, including the subject's background (including family, education, previous diagnoses, and medications), an overview of the subject's behavior, early development milestones, language acquisition and loss of language or other skills, current language function, social development and play, and interests and behaviors.

The ADI-R may be useful as part of a multidisciplinary intake assessment in diagnosing young children with possible autism. Because of the time needed to administer the ADI-R and the extensive training needed, this test may not be a practical assessment method in all clinical situations.

A structured parent interview such as the ADI-R can help get the most out of a parent's ability to remember, but it is not a substitute for direct observation of the child by a professional. Experts agree it is important to supplement structured parent interviews with direct observation of the child.

autism diagnostic observation scale (ADOS) A semi-structured assessment of communication, social interaction and play or imaginative use of materials for individuals suspected of having autism or other AUTISM SPECTRUM DISORDERS. This assessment is used to diagnose young children under the age of six years who are not yet using phrase speech. It is a semi-structured assessment of play, interaction, and social communication and takes about 30 to 60 minutes for a trained clinician to administer. The ADOS may be useful as part of an initial assessment in diagnosing young children with possible autism, but extensive training is needed to learn how to administer it. It is a combination of several earlier research instruments:

- the autism diagnostic observation schedule (intended for adults and children with language skills at a minimum of the three-year-old level)
- another version with additional items developed for verbally fluent, high-functioning adolescents and adults
- a pre-linguistic version intended for children with limited or no language

Autism Screening Instrument for Educational Planning–Second Edition (ASIEP-2)   A screening test, appropriate for age 18 months through adulthood, designed to help professionals identify individuals with autism and to provide information needed to develop appropriate educational plans. This instrument also helps professionals develop appropriate instructional plans in accordance with P.L. 94-142. It can also be used to distinguish between autism and other disorders.

The scale looks at five aspects of behavior, which together provide a clear picture of the individual's functional abilities and instructional needs. It includes five subtests:

- *AUTISM BEHAVIOR CHECKLIST:* sensory, relating, body concept, language, and social self-help behaviors
- *sample of vocal behavior:* spontaneous verbal behavior
- *interaction assessment:* social interaction based on observable behaviors
- *educational assessment:* language performance and communicative abilities through signed or verbal responses
- *prognosis of learning rate*

The entire test can be given by a school psychologist or experienced teacher of autistic children in one and a half to two hours. Results can be plotted on a summary profile to allow the examiner to compare the child's performance to patterns expected for autistic children and for children with other handicaps. This provides a systematic way to assess children who are difficult to test and treat.

autism spectrum disorders (ASD)   A relatively new term that encompasses autism and similar disorders that is gradually replacing the term pervasive developmental disorders. This group of disorders is characterized by varying degrees of problems with communication skills, social interactions, and restricted, repetitive and stereotyped patterns of behavior. The autism spectrum disorders include

- ASPERGER'S SYNDROME, which tends to include milder symptoms
- AUTISTIC DISORDER, which is typically a more severe disorder
- PERVASIVE DEVELOPMENTAL DISORDER–NOT OTHERWISE SPECIFIED, a condition with very minor symptoms or symptoms that otherwise do not meet the specific criteria for other autism spectrum disorders.

Two other rare, very severe disorders that are included in the autism spectrum disorders are RETT DISORDER and CHILDHOOD DISINTEGRATIVE DISORDER. (More recently, many experts tend to exclude Rett disorder from the autism spectrum disorders.)

In 1943 Dr. Leo KANNER of the Johns Hopkins Hospital introduced the term "early infantile autism" after studying a group of 11 children with unusual symptoms. At the same time, German scientist Dr. Hans ASPERGER described a milder form of the disorder that became known as Asperger's syndrome. These two disorders were the first of the five ASDs to be identified.

The ASDs are more common in children than are some better-known disorders such as diabetes, spina bifida, or DOWN SYNDROME. Prevalence studies in the United States, the United Kingdom, Europe, and Asia suggest that ASD occurs in from two to six out of every 1,000 children.

Symptoms and Diagnostic Path
Parents are usually the first to notice unusual behaviors in their child. In some cases, the baby seems

"different" from birth, unresponsive to people or focusing intently on one item for long periods of time. In other cases, symptoms do not appear until after the first one or two years of life. In most cases, the problems in communication and social skills become more noticeable as the child lags further behind other children the same age. Some other children start off well enough. Oftentimes between 12 and 36 months old, the differences in the way they react to people and other unusual behaviors become apparent. The existence of an autism spectrum disorder may be suspected if the child

- does not babble, point, or make meaningful gestures by one year of age
- does not speak one word by 16 months
- does not combine two words by two years
- does not respond to name
- loses language or social skills

Some other indicators include

- poor eye contact
- lack of ability to play appropriately with toys
- excessive ordering of toys or other objects
- attachment to one particular toy or object
- does not smile in response to other's smiling
- apparent hearing problems

The first signs of an autism spectrum disorder also can appear in children who seemed to have been developing normally. Parents are usually correct about noticing developmental problems, such as when an engaging, babbling toddler suddenly becomes silent, withdrawn, aloof, or indifferent to social overtures.

Pediatricians, family physicians, daycare providers, teachers, and parents may initially dismiss signs of ASD, optimistically thinking the child is just a little slow and will "catch up." Although early intervention has a dramatic impact on reducing symptoms and increasing a child's ability to grow and learn new skills, it is estimated that only 50 percent of children are diagnosed before kindergarten.

All children with ASD demonstrate mild to severe deficits in social interaction and in verbal and nonverbal communication, as well as repetitive behaviors or interests. In addition, they may have unusual responses to sensory experiences, such as certain sounds or the way objects look. Each child will display communication, social, and behavioral patterns that are individual but fit into the overall diagnosis of ASD.

Some parents report the change as being sudden, and that their children start to reject people, act strangely, and lose language and social skills they had previously acquired. In other cases, there is a plateau, or leveling, of progress so that the difference between the child with autism and other children the same age becomes more noticeable.

Social symptoms Healthy children are social beings, and early in life they will gaze at people, turn toward voices, grasp a finger, and smile. In contrast, most children with ASD seem to have problems interacting with others in their environment—even their mother or father. Even in the first few months of life, some avoid eye contact and seem indifferent to other people, preferring to be alone. They may resist attention or passively accept hugs; as they get older, they seldom seek comfort or respond to parents' displays of anger or affection in a normal way.

This does not mean that children with ASD are not attached to their parents; rather, their expression of this attachment is unusual and difficult to interpret. To parents, it may seem as if their child does not care about them at all.

Children with ASD also are slower in learning to interpret what others are thinking and feeling, failing to understand subtle social cues such as smiles or grimaces. Without the ability to interpret gestures and facial expressions, the social world appears confusing to these children.

Moreover, many people with ASD have trouble seeing things from another person's perspective, which makes it hard or impossible for them to predict or understand other people's actions. Many people with ASD have trouble regulating their emotions, which results in "immature" behavior such as crying or laughing in situations that are out of context or displaying verbal outbursts that seem inappropriate to those around them.

Individuals with ASD can be disruptive and physically aggressive at times, which can make social relationships more difficult. They may lose control when angry, frustrated, or in a strange or overwhelming environment. They may break things, attack others, or hurt themselves, bang their heads, pull their hair, or bite their arms.

Communication problems   Some children diagnosed with ASD remain mute throughout their lives; others may be delayed but eventually develop language as late as age five to nine years. Some children may learn to use communication systems such as pictures or AMERICAN SIGN LANGUAGE.

Those who do speak often use language in unusual ways, some using only single words, others repeating the same phrase over and over. Some children with ASD parrot what they hear (ECHOLALIA).

Some children who are only mildly affected may have only slight delays in language, or even precocious language and unusually large vocabularies, but have trouble keeping up their end of a conversation, although they often carry on a monologue on a favorite subject.

Many of these children also have trouble understanding body language, tone of voice, or phrases, so that they are unable to interpret sarcasm, for example. Body language of children with ASD also may be hard to interpret, since facial expressions, movements, and gestures rarely match what they are saying. Their tone of voice also fails to reflect their feelings, and is often described as high-pitched, sing-song, or flat and robotic. On the other hand, some children with ASD have fairly good language skills and speak like little adults, failing to pick up on the way their peers speak or adjusting their manner of speech to fit their audience.

Without meaningful gestures or the language to ask for things, people with ASD may scream or grab what they want, and may have a limited understanding of what others need. As they grow up, they can become increasingly aware of their difficulties in understanding others and in being understood, and as a result, may become anxious or depressed.

Repetitive behaviors   Although children with ASD usually appear physically normal and have good muscle control, they may exhibit odd repetitive motions ranging from subtle to extreme. Some children and older individuals spend a lot of time repeatedly flapping their arms, pacing, or walking on their toes, while others suddenly freeze in position. Children can spend hours lining up their dolls in a certain way instead of using them for pretend play; if a toy gets moved, the child may be tremendously upset. This is because some children with ASD need absolute consistency in their environment, so that a slight change in any routine can be extremely disturbing.

Repetitive behavior sometimes takes the form of a persistent, intense preoccupation. For example, the child might be obsessed with learning all about dinosaurs, train schedules, or clocks. Often there is great interest in numbers, symbols, or science topics.

Sensory problems   Sensory information helps people learn from what they see, feel, or hear. When sensory input is faulty, the child's experiences of the world can be confusing. Many children with ASD are painfully aware of and sensitive to certain sounds, textures, tastes, and smells. Some children find the feel of clothes touching their skin to be almost unbearable; others cannot tolerate certain sounds, such as a ringing telephone or the vacuum cleaner. In children with ASD, the brain seems unable to balance the senses appropriately.

On the other hand, some children with ASD are oblivious to extreme cold or pain, so that if such a child breaks a leg, he may not cry—yet a light touch may make the same child scream with alarm.

Mental retardation   Many children with ASD have some degree of thinking impairment in certain areas. A child with ASD may do well on visual skills tests, but score poorly on language subtests.

Seizures   One in four children with ASD develops seizures, often starting either in early childhood or adolescence. Seizures, which are caused by abnormal electrical activity in the brain, can produce a temporary loss of consciousness, a body convulsion, unusual movements, or staring spells.

An electroencephalogram (EEG, a recording of the electric currents in the brain) can help confirm the seizure's presence. In most cases, seizures can be controlled by anticonvulsants.

Diagnosis   While half of all children with one of the autism spectrum disorders are not diagnosed until age four to six, it is possible to diagnose the disorders in a child as early as 18 months old. Since the earlier the condition is identified the earlier treatment can begin and the better the prognosis for the child, early diagnosis is critically important. A good diagnosis can identify whether a child does not have an autism spectrum disorder; if one of the five spectrum disorders does exist, the evaluation can determine the seriousness of the problem, and place the child "on the autism spectrum."

Because there are no medical tests for the autism spectrum disorders, a diagnosis must be based on observing the person's communication, behavior, and developmental levels. Even in very early childhood, parents can begin to observe their child to make sure certain developmental milestones are reached. For example, a two-year-old should be able to point to an object when named, use two- to four-word phrases, and follow simple instructions, according to the U.S. Centers for Disease Control and Prevention. A three-year-old should be able to imitate adults and playmates, play make-believe with dolls, and use pronouns or plural words. Parents might want to check with a pediatrician if their children have not mastered these skills.

Since the five disorders included in the autism spectrum disorders occur on a continuum of symptoms, a careful diagnosis is needed.

- Children who may have some symptoms of the autistic disorders, but do not have enough to be diagnosed with the classical form may be diagnosed with pervasive developmental disorder–not otherwise specified (PDD-NOS).

- Individuals who exhibit autistic behavior but who have well-developed language skills may be diagnosed with Asperger's syndrome—a mild form of autism.

- Children who have the classic symptoms of inability to communicate, form relationships with others, and respond appropriately to the environment might be diagnosed with autistic disorder (autism).

- Children who appear normal in their first several years but then lose skills and begin showing autistic behavior may be diagnosed with childhood disintegrative disorder (CDD).

- A chromosomal analysis can rule out the genetic disease Rett disorder.

Customarily, an expert diagnostic team has the responsibility of thoroughly evaluating the child, assessing the child's unique strengths and weaknesses, and determining a formal diagnosis. The team will then meet with the parents to explain the results of the evaluation.

The diagnosis of an autistic spectrum disorder typically requires a two-stage process. The first stage is a developmental screening during an annual "well child" check-up, followed by a comprehensive evaluation by a multidisciplinary team. During the well-child visit, the pediatrician should observe the child and note appropriate developmental milestones, noting how the child behaves, interacts, and communicates with a parent in the examining room.

Several screening instruments have been developed to quickly gather information about a child's social and communicative development within medical settings. Among them are the CHECKLIST FOR AUTISM IN TODDLERS (CHAT), the MODIFIED CHECKLIST FOR AUTISM IN TODDLERS (M-CHAT), and the Screening Tool for Autism in Two-Year-Olds (STAT). Some screening instruments rely solely on parent responses to a questionnaire, and some rely on a combination of parent report and observation. Important items on these tests that appear to differentiate children with autism from other groups before the age of two include pointing and pretend play.

It is important to remember that screening instruments simply assess the need for referral for a possible diagnosis of an autism spectrum disorder. They cannot be used alone to diagnose the condition. In addition, these screening methods may not identify children with mild autism or high-functioning autism or ASPERGER'S SYNDROME.

For children with milder suspected autism, the Autism Spectrum Screening Questionnaire (ASSQ), the Australian Scale for Asperger's Syndrome, and the most recent CHILDHOOD ASPERGER SYNDROME TEST (CAST), can reliably identify school-age children with Asperger's syndrome or higher functioning autism. The SOCIAL COMMUNICATION QUESTIONNAIRE (SCQ) can be used for children four years of age and older. These tools concentrate on social and behavioral impairments in children without significant language delay.

If after the screening process or during a routine well-child checkup the pediatrician suspects autism or a condition on the autism spectrum, he or she will refer the parents for further formal diagnostic testing to either a developmental pediatrician or a pediatric neurologist, a psychiatrist or psychologist, or to a special team including a NEUROLOGIST, PSYCHOLOGIST, speech language therapist.

Because autism spectrum disorders are so complex and may involve other neurological problems, a comprehensive evaluation should include neurologic and genetic assessment, in addition to in-depth cognitive and language testing. Also, tests developed specifically for diagnosing autism are often used, including the AUTISM DIAGNOSIS INTERVIEW–REVISED (ADI-R) and the AUTISM DIAGNOSTIC OBSERVATION SCALE (ADOS). The ADI-R is a structured interview that covers more than 100 items and is conducted with a caregiver and evaluates four aspects of the child's behavior: the child's communication skills, social interaction, repetitive behaviors, and age-of-onset symptoms. The ADOS is a semi-structured behavioral observation that evaluates communicative and social behaviors that are often delayed, abnormal, or absent in children with ASD.

Still another test for children over age two is the CHILDHOOD AUTISM RATING SCALE (CARS), which helps evaluate the child's body movements, adaptation to change, listening response, verbal communication, and relationships. In this test, the examiner observes the child and obtains information from the parents. The child's behavior is rated on a scale based on deviation from the typical behavior of children of the same age.

Specific diagnostic categories have changed over the years as research progresses and as new editions of the *Diagnostic and Statistical Manual (DSM)* have been issued. Some frequently used criteria include

- absence or impairment of imaginative and social play
- impaired ability to make friends with peers
- impaired ability to initiate or sustain a conversation with others
- stereotyped, repetitive, or unusual use of language

- restricted patterns of interests that are abnormal in intensity or focus
- apparently inflexible adherence to specific routines or rituals
- preoccupation with parts of objects

Ruling out other conditions   Any child with a developmental delay should have a number of other tests to rule out certain disorders, because many of the behaviors associated with autism spectrum disorders are similar to other conditions. A comprehensive hearing evaluation should be done to rule out hearing loss as the cause of abnormal language development; although some hearing loss can occur along with ASD, some children with ASD may be incorrectly thought to have hearing problems. Lead screening is essential for children who often put things in their mouths. Blood tests can rule out metabolic disorders that affect amino acids and lipids in the blood, and a chromosomal analysis can rule out genetic disorders such as FRAGILE X SYNDROME (another genetic disorder causing mental impairment). An electroencephalogram (EEG) can rule out a seizure disorder, and magnetic resonance imaging (MRI) can rule out brain disorders.

Complicating disorders   Because some people with an autism spectrum disorder also may have a behavior disorder, problems with hearing, mental retardation, or eccentric behavior, part of the diagnosis will include not just in identifying the autism condition, but also other complicating disorders.

Treatment Options and Outlook

While ASD cannot be cured, there are many ways to help these children. Each state guarantees special education and related services; the INDIVIDUALS WITH DISABILITIES EDUCATION ACT (IDEA) is a federal program that assures a free public education for children with diagnosed learning deficits. The school district pays for all necessary services, including services by a speech therapist, occupational therapist, school psychologist, social worker, school nurse, or aide. By law, the public schools must prepare and carry out a set of instruction goals, or specific skills to be addressed, for every child in a SPECIAL EDUCATION program. The list of goals is known as the child's INDIVIDUALIZED EDUCATION PROGRAM (IEP).

This IEP is an agreement between the school and the family on the child's goals.

If a child is under three years of age and has special needs, he or she should be eligible for an early intervention program available in every state. The services provided are written into an INDIVIDUALIZED FAMILY SERVICE PLAN (IFSP) that is reviewed at least once every six months. The plan will describe services that will be provided to the child but will also describe services for parents to help them in daily activities with their child and for siblings to help them adjust to having a brother or sister with ASD.

There is no single best treatment for every child with ASD, but almost all experts agree that early intervention is critical. Most experts also agree that most individuals with ASD respond well to highly structured, specialized programs.

Among the many methods available for treatment and education of people with autism, APPLIED BEHAVIOR ANALYSIS (ABA) has become widely accepted as an effective treatment. After 30 years of research, applied behavioral methods appear to help reduce inappropriate behavior and increase communication, learning, and appropriate social behavior in children with ASD. The basic research done by Ivar Lovaas and his colleagues at the University of California, Los Angeles, show that an intensive, one-on-one child-teacher interaction for 40 hours a week provides a foundation for other educators and researchers to help those with ASD attain their potential. The goal of this type of behavioral management is to reinforce desirable behaviors and reduce undesirable ones.

An effective treatment program will build on the child's interests, offer a predictable schedule, teach tasks as a series of simple steps, actively engage the child's attention in highly structured activities, and regularly reinforce behavior.

Parental involvement is also an important part of treatment success. In ABA, parents work with teachers and therapists to identify the behaviors to be changed and the skills to be taught. Because experts now realize that parents are the child's earliest teachers, more programs are beginning to train parents to continue the therapy at home.

Instruction should start as soon as the ASD has been diagnosed. Effective programs teach early communication and social interaction skills. In children younger than three, instruction usually occurs at home or a child care center, including interventions that target specific problems in learning, language, imitation, attention, motivation, compliance, and initiative of interaction. Included are behavioral methods, communication, occupational and physical therapy along with social play interventions.

Children older than three usually receive a school-based, individualized, special education, either in a segregated class with other ASD children or in an integrated class with children without disabilities for at least part of the day. All should provide a structure that will help the children learn social skills and functional communication. Teachers often involve the parents, giving useful advice in how to help their child use the skills or behaviors learned at school when they are at home.

In elementary school, the child should receive help in any skill area that is delayed and be encouraged to grow in his or her areas of strength. Ideally, the curriculum should be adapted to the individual child's needs. Many schools today have an inclusion program in which the child is in a regular classroom for most of the day, with special instruction for a part of the day. This instruction should include such skills as learning how to act in social situations and in making friends. Although higher-functioning children may be able to handle academic work, they too need help to learn social skills and organize tasks and avoid distractions.

During middle and high school years, instruction will begin to include practical matters such as community living, and recreational activities, and include work experience, using public transportation, and learning skills that will eventually be important in living independently. While some ASD behaviors improve during the teenage years, others may get worse. Increased autistic or aggressive behavior may be one way some teens express their newfound tension and confusion. At an age when most teenagers are concerned with popularity, grades, and social skills, teens with autism may realize they are different from their peers. Unlike their classmates, they may not have friends, they may not date, or they may have more problems planning for a career. For some, the sadness that comes with such realization motivates them to learn new behaviors and acquire better social skills.

Medications Medications are often used to treat behavioral problems common in people with ASD, such as aggression, self-injurious behavior, and severe tantrums. Many of these medications are prescribed "off-label," which means they have not been approved by the government for use in children with autism; the doctor can legally prescribe this medicine if he or she feels it is appropriate. Because a child with ASD may not respond to medications in the same way as normal children, it is important that parents work with a physician who has experience with autism.

Antipsychotic medications, many of which work by reducing the activity of the neurotransmitter dopamine, have been used to treat severe behavioral problems. Among the older, typical antipsychotics, HALOPERIDOL (Haldol) was more effective than a placebo in treating serious behavioral problems. However, haloperidol also can have side effects, such as sedation, muscle stiffness, and abnormal movements. Placebo-controlled studies of the newer atypical antipsychotics are being conducted on children with autism. The first such study was on RISPERIDONE (Risperdal); results showed that risperidone was effective and well tolerated for treating severe behavioral problems in children with autism. The most common side effects were increased appetite, weight gain, and sedation. Further long-term studies are needed to determine any long-term side effects. Other atypical antipsychotics that have been studied recently with encouraging results are olanzapine (Zyprexa) and ziprasidone (Geodon). Ziprasidone has not been associated with significant weight gain.

Seizures occur in one in four people with ASD, most often in those who also have significant mental impairment. They are treated with one or more of the anticonvulsants. These include such medications as carbamazepine (Tegretol), lamotrigine (Lamictal), topiramate (Topamax), and valproic acid (Depakote). Although medication usually reduces the number of seizures, it cannot always eliminate them.

Stimulant medications such as methylphenidate (Ritalin) also have been prescribed for children with autism in order to decrease impulsivity and hyperactivity in higher functioning children. Several other medications have been used to treat these symptoms, including antidepressants, naltrexone, lithium, and some of the benzodiazepines such as diazepam (Valium) and lorazepam (Ativan). The safety and efficacy of these medications in children with autism has not been proven.

Controversial treatments There are a number of controversial treatments for ASD. To be accepted as a proven treatment, the treatment should undergo randomized, double-blind clinical trials that compare treatment and no treatment.

Some of the controversial interventions that have been reported as possibly helpful to some children but whose success or safety has not been proven include dietary interventions, vitamin B6, and SECRETIN.

Dietary interventions are based on the idea that food allergies may cause symptoms of ASD and a lack of a specific vitamin or mineral may worsen some symptoms. If parents decide to try a special diet for a given period of time, they should be sure that the child's nutritional status is measured carefully. A diet that some parents have reported to be helpful to their autistic child is a gluten-free, casein-free diet. Gluten is a casein-like substance that is found in the seeds of various cereal plants—wheat, oat, rye, and barley. Casein is the principal protein in milk. Since gluten and milk are found in many of the foods we eat, following a gluten-free, casein-free diet is difficult.

A supplement that some parents believe is beneficial for an autistic child is vitamin B_6, taken with magnesium (which makes the vitamin more effective). The result of research studies is inconclusive; some children appear to respond positively, some negatively, some not at all or very little.

In the search for treatment for autism, there has been discussion in the last few years about the use of secretin, a substance approved by the Food and Drug Administration (FDA) for a single dose normally given to aid in diagnosis of a gastrointestinal problem. Anecdotal reports suggested improvement in autism symptoms, including improved sleep patterns, eye contact, language skills, and alertness. However, multiple clinical trials conducted in the last few years have found no significant improvements in symptoms between patients who received secretin and those who received a placebo, and this treatment is not recommended by the American Academy of Pediatrics.

Adults with ASD

Some adults with ASD, especially those with high-functioning autism or with Asperger's syndrome, are able to work successfully, although communication and social problems often cause problems. These individuals will continue to need encouragement and support in living an independent life. Many others with ASD can work in sheltered workshops under the supervision of managers trained in working with persons with disabilities. A nurturing environment at home, at school, and later in job training and at work, helps persons with ASD continue to learn and to develop throughout their lives.

In most states, the public schools' responsibility for providing services ends when a person with ASD reaches the age of 22. The family is then faced with the challenge of finding living arrangements and employment to match the particular needs of their adult child, as well as the programs and facilities that can provide support services to achieve these goals.

Living arrangements for the adult with ASD

Some adults with ASD are able to live entirely on their own, while others can live semi-independently in their own homes or apartments if they have help with solving major problems, such as personal finances or dealing with government agencies.

Government funds are available for families who choose to have their adult child with ASD live at home, including Supplemental Security Income (SSI), Social Security Disability Insurance (SSDI), Medicaid waivers, and others.

Some families open their homes to provide long-term care to unrelated adults with disabilities. A home that teaches self-care and housekeeping skills and arranges leisure activities is called a "skill-development" home.

Persons with ASD often live in group homes or apartments staffed by professionals who help the individuals with basic needs, such as meal preparation, housekeeping, and personal care. Higher functioning persons may be able to live in a home or apartment where staff visit only a few times a week. These persons generally prepare their own meals, go to work, and conduct other daily activities on their own.

Although the trend in recent decades has been to avoid placing individuals with ASD into long-term-care institutions, this alternative is still available for those who need intensive, constant supervision.

ASD Research

There are many studies now being conducted into the possible cause and treatment of ASD.

Thimerosal In the past few years some parents and some experts have suggested a link between autism and a mercury-based preservative called thimerosal used as a preservative in the measles-mumps-rubella (MMR) vaccine. Although mercury is no longer used in childhood vaccines in the United States, some parents still have concerns about vaccinations. Many large-scale studies have failed to show a link between thimerosal and autism. A panel from the Institute of Medicine is examining these studies, including a large Danish study that concluded that there was no causal relationship between childhood vaccination using thimerosal-containing vaccines and the development of an autism spectrum disorder, and a U.S. study looking at exposure to mercury, lead, and other heavy metals.

Biologic basis of ASD As new brain imaging tools are developed—including computed tomography (CT), positron emission tomography (PET), single photon emission computed tomography (SPECT), and magnetic resonance imaging (MRI)—study of the structure and the functioning of the brain is possible.

Postmortem and MRI studies have shown that many major brain structures are implicated in ASD, including the cerebellum, cerebral cortex, limbic system, corpus callosum, basal ganglia, and brain stem. Other research is focusing on the role of neurotransmitters such as serotonin, dopamine, and epinephrine.

Genetics Evidence points to genetic factors playing a prominent role in ASD, although not all experts agree as to the specific hereditary aspects. Twin and family studies have suggested an underlying genetic vulnerability to ASD. The Autism Genetic Resource Exchange, a project initiated by the Cure Autism Now Foundation and the government, is recruiting genetic samples from several hundred families to further study a possible hereditary basis to ASD.

Autism Tissue Program A national outreach program, directed toward people with autism and their healthy family members, that coordinates the donation of human brain tissue for research into AUTISM SPECTRUM DISORDERS.

Because of the strong suggestion of a hereditary link to autism and the development of advanced techniques to measure gene expression in single neurons, all members of families in which one or more members has autism are encouraged to donate brain tissue. Researchers also need brain tissue from "normal controls" (people who are neither autistic nor related to people with autism) to compare to tissue from affected individuals and their families.

After a death, brain tissue recovery is coordinated nationally by the Autism Tissue Program and by the Harvard Brain Tissue Resource Center, which pays for the costs of tissue recovery. In the event of a death, the next-of-kin contacts the program, and the brain bank will arrange for the donation to be carried out by a pathologist in the patient's area, in the nearest hospital equipped for the procedure. If death has occurred in a hospital, tissue retrieval is usually completed within a few hours and the body is then released to the funeral home for care. If death occurs elsewhere, the body must be transported by the funeral home staff to a local hospital for tissue recovery. The associates at the brain bank work with funeral directors, medical examiners, and pathologists to ensure that the family's requests are fulfilled. The body is treated with respect and compassion by the physicians and scientists involved in this process as tissue is recovered and prepared according to a strict protocol and transferred to the brain bank. Brain and tissue recovery does not interfere with having an open casket or with other traditional religious funeral arrangements. Because many donor families are very much interested in autism research, the next of kin receive updates on research progress.

When they receive brain tissue from a patient with autism, researchers are able to study autism at a cellular and molecular level, checking out particular pathways and even looking at the individual neurons of the brain to help understand both normal and abnormal neurodevelopment. What scientists learn about brain development can be applied to day-to-day educational programs to make the most of the brain's capacity to change. What scientists learn about molecules and neurotransmitters in the brain can lead to new medications, and a better understanding of autism genetics increases the ability to diagnose autism and assess the risks of inheritance.

The Autism Tissue Program is a joint effort of the Autism Society of America Foundation, the National Alliance for Autism Research, and the M.I.N.D. (Medical Investigation of Neurodevelopmental Disorders) Institute at the University of California, Davis.

autistic celebrity family members There are many well-known celebrities who have chosen to write or speak about their autistic family members, including:

- Richard Burton (actor): daughter with his first wife
- William Christopher (Father Mulcahy on the TV show M*A*S*H): son Ned
- Will Clark (baseball player): son
- Myron Cope (Pittsburgh sportscaster): son
- Tom Henke (Toronto baseball pitcher): son
- Audrey Flack (sculptor, photographer): adult child with autism
- Doug Flutie (football player): son Doug, Jr.
- Stephen J. Gould (scientist/writer): son Jesse
- Merton Hanks (football player): daughter Milan
- Scott Mellanby (hockey player): son
- Joe Mantegna (actor): daughter
- Dan Marino (football player): son
- Wynton and Bradford Marsalis (jazz/classical musicians): brother
- Mark McEwen (CBS-TV Morning News weatherman): brother Sean
- Barbara Roberts (former Governor of Oregon): adult child with autism

- Tracy Rowlett (Dallas anchor): son
- Jonathan Shestak (movie producer): son Dov
- Beverly Sills (opera singer): son Bucky
- Phoebe Snow (singer): daughter
- Sylvester Stallone (movie actor): son Seargeoh
- BJ Surhoff (Baltimore baseball player): son Mason
- David Tomlinson (actor who starred in *Mary Poppins, Bedknobs and Broomsticks, The Love Bug,* etc.): son

autistic disorder A severe developmental disorder known popularly as *autism* that affects a person's ability to communicate, form relationships with others, and respond appropriately to the environment. Autistic disorder is a spectrum disorder, which means that its symptoms and characteristics can appear in a wide variety of combinations, from mild to severe. It is one of five related disorders known collectively as the AUTISM SPECTRUM DISORDERS (ASDs). Left untreated, many children with autistic disorder will not develop effective social skills and may not learn to communicate or behave appropriately. Very few individuals recover completely without any intervention.

Autistic disorder is a "developmental disorder," which means that its symptoms usually appear during the first three years of childhood and continue throughout life. Although autistic disorder is defined by a certain set of behaviors, children and adults can exhibit any combination of behavior in any degree of severity. Two children with the same diagnosis can act very differently from each other and have varying skills. Every person with autistic disorder is an individual, with a unique personality and combination of characteristics. Some individuals who are only mildly affected may experience just slight delays in language but have more trouble with social interactions, such as problems starting or maintaining a conversation. The communication style of a person with autistic disorder is often described as one of talking "at" others, using a monologue on a favorite subject that continues despite attempts by others to interject comments.

Most children with this condition look perfectly normal but may spend their time engaged in puzzling and disturbing behaviors that are markedly different from those of typical children. Children with autistic disorder usually do not engage in social play or games with their peers. Unusual behaviors, such as rocking, HAND FLAPPING, or even self-injurious behavior may be evident in some cases. The child may stare into space for hours, throw uncontrollable tantrums, show no interest in people (including his or her parents) and pursue strange, repetitive activities with no apparent purpose. He or she may seem to live in a world of his or her own. Some autistic individuals are remarkably gifted in certain areas, such as music or mathematics.

The result of a neurological disorder that affects the functioning of the brain, autistic disorder has been estimated to occur in as many as one in 500 people. Its prevalence rate makes it one of the most common developmental disabilities, four times more common in boys than girls and not related to race, ethnic origin, family income, lifestyle, or education.

There appears to have been a rapid increase in the number of children diagnosed with autistic disorder, especially in California, which has an accurate and systematic centralized reporting system of all diagnoses of this disorder. The California data show that incidence of autistic disorder appears to be rising rapidly, from one per 2,500 in 1970 to one per 285 in 1999. Similar results have been reported for other states by the U.S. Department of Education. Whereas autism once accounted for 3 percent of all developmental disabilities in California, it now accounts for 45 percent of all new developmental disabilities. Other countries report similar increases.

Experts disagree as to whether—and why—there has been a dramatic increase in autistic disorder over the past two decades; some insist the increase is simply due to better diagnosis, while others argue that the increase is an actual boost in numbers. Still others believe that because there may be more than one cause, there could be more than one reason for the increase. Today, experts are concerned not only about autistic disorder but about all five disorders on the autism spectrum. These cases encompass a greater range of symptoms, including those with only mild symptoms. It is possible that many of today's children with autistic disorder used to be identified as something else, such as learning disabled or mentally retarded. Other children might have been labeled eccentric or unusual but not disabled.

For example, children with Asperger's syndrome fall under the autism spectrum disorder label, even though Asperger's syndrome symptoms tend to be more subtle than full-blown autistic disorder. Other children with even milder symptoms might be diagnosed as PERVASIVE DEVELOPMENTAL DISORDER–NOT OTHERWISE SPECIFIED (PDD-NOS). This category includes a large group of children with less striking impairments in their social and communicative behavior and/or less pronounced repetitive behavior or narrow interests than have children with autistic disorder. There are many more of these children than those who are diagnosed with the more classic autistic disorder.

Autistic disorder is one of five related disorders as defined by the American Psychiatric Association in its diagnostic manual (*Diagnostic and Statistical Manual [DSM-IV-TR]*), known collectively as autism spectrum disorders. Sometimes the term *autism* is used to describe autistic disorder and sometimes it is used to describe all five ASDs, including autistic disorder, Asperger's syndrome, and PDD-NOS. Two other, far more rare conditions also included in the spectrum are RETT DISORDER and CHILDHOOD DISINTEGRATIVE DISORDER.

Causes

Autistic disorder affects the normal development of the brain. Although a single specific cause of the disorder is not known, current research links autistic disorder to biological or neurological differences in the brain. The disorder has been associated with maternal German measles infection, phenylketonuria (an inherited disorder of metabolism), tuberous sclerosis (an inherited disease of the nervous system and skin), lack of oxygen at birth, encephalitis, and infantile spasms.

It is neither a mental illness nor a behavior problem, and it is not caused by bad parenting. No known psychological factors in the development of the child have been shown to cause autistic disor-

der, and neither family income, education, or lifestyle affect the risk of developing the problem.

Heredity   Genetics appears to play an important role in the development of some cases of autistic disorder. In many families, there seems to be a pattern of autistic disorder or related disabilities, which suggests a genetic basis to the disorder. In the general population, the disorder affects up to 0.2 percent of children, but the risk of having a second child with autistic disorder increases more than 50 times—to 10 to 20 percent. An identical twin of a child with autistic disorder is far more likely to have the same condition than a fraternal twin or another sibling. In addition, many studies have identified various thinking disabilities in siblings of children with autistic disorder.

However, at this time no one gene has been directly linked to autistic disorder, and studies trying to identify specific genes associated with the disorder have been inconclusive. Scientists think that the genetic basis is complex and probably involves several combinations of at least 20 or more genes. This is in contrast to other disorders, such as FRAGILE X SYNDROME or Rett disorder, in which single genes have been identified.

Immune system disorder   Some studies have suggested that individuals with autistic disorder may have weakened immune systems. In fact, some experts believe autism may be due, in part, to an autoimmune system disorder. Some believe that in some children, the immune system is weakened either due to faulty genes or environmental insult (such as exposure to certain chemicals), which may predispose the child to autism. Exposure to an additional environmental toxin may then trigger autistic disorder.

Vaccinations   Although genetics play an important role in autistic disorder, environmental factors also may be involved. The possible role of vaccinations, many of which were added to the vaccination schedule in the 1980s and are typically administered to children between ages one and two, is a matter of considerable controversy. Prior to 1990, about two-thirds of children with autistic disorder displayed symptoms at an early age, and only one-third initially appeared to be developing appropriately, regressing some time after age one. Starting in the 1990s, the trend has reversed—fewer than one-third are evidence of early-onset symptoms and two-thirds develop symptoms in their second year.

The concept of a link between autism and vaccines is decidedly controversial. Some experts believe that the measles-mumps-rubella (MMR) combination vaccine is implicated in autistic disorder in some children, pointing to evidence of measles virus detected in the gut, spinal fluid, and blood. They also note that the incidence of autistic disorder began rising significantly when the MMR was introduced in the United States in 1978 and in the United Kingdom 10 years later.

Some experts also suspect thimerosal, a mercury-based preservative in childhood vaccines, may be linked to autistic disorder. The number of vaccines given to children has risen over the last two decades, and many of those vaccines contained thimerosal. These experts believe that the symptoms of mercury poisoning in children are very similar to the symptoms of autistic disorder. In response to these concerns, manufacturers of children's vaccines have removed thimerosal from almost all vaccines administered to children.

On the other hand, the National Institute of Child Health and Human Development (NICHD) argues there has been no conclusive scientific evidence that any part of a vaccine or any combination of vaccines causes autistic disorder. The NICHD also points out that no conclusive data exist that show that any type of preservative (such as thimerosal) used during the manufacture of vaccines plays any role in causing autistic disorder.

In 2001, the Institute of Medicine (IOM) and the American Academy of Pediatrics (AAP) released findings from their separate reviews of the available evidence on a possible link between vaccines and autism. Both groups independently found that existing evidence does not support such a connection.

Still, research continues into the link between autistic disorder and vaccines, including research into the effects of thimerosal on the immune system.

The National Immunization Program at the Centers for Disease Control and Prevention (CDC), along with the AAP and the American Academy of Family Physicians, suggests that physicians follow the recommended childhood immunization schedule that is published every year. Physicians are advised to take careful family histories of all their patients to bring to light any factors that might influence their recommendations about the timing of vaccinations. Some researchers and physicians have recommended an alternative vaccine schedule that recommends delaying some vaccinations and separating the measles, mumps, and rubella vaccinations.

Environmental problems Some of the environmental factors that may play a role in the development of autistic disorder include

- *Oral antibiotics:* Excessive use may cause intestinal problems, such as yeast/bacterial overgrowth, and prevent mercury excretion, although research in this area is controversial.

- *Prenatal exposure to mercury:* Pregnant women who eat seafood high in mercury (such as swordfish or tuna) could be exposing their unborn children to toxic levels.

- *Essential minerals:* Lack of zinc, magnesium, iodine, lithium, and potassium may lead to problems.

- *Pesticides and other environmental toxins.*

Symptoms and Diagnostic Path

Symptoms of autistic disorder vary greatly depending on the developmental level and chronological age of the individual. Some parents report that their child seemed "different" at birth; these children are considered to have *early-onset autistic disorder.* Other parents report that their child seemed to develop normally and then suddenly experienced a major regression, usually between 12 and 24 months of age. These children are diagnosed with *late-onset* or *regressive autistic disorder.* Although some researchers argue that this late-onset regression could not be real, or that the autistic disorder was simply unnoticed by the child's parents, many parents insist that their children had completely normal speech, behavior, and social skills until some time between age one and two.

In any case, whenever it appears, autistic disorder significantly impairs a child's ability to communicate and socialize with others. While severity and symptoms vary according to age, the disorder is significant and sustained. Children with autistic disorder demonstrate little interest in friends or social interactions, often failing to develop verbal and nonverbal communication skills. Typically, these children function at a low intellectual level; most experience mild to severe mental retardation. However, this is by no means true for all individuals with autistic disorder. The condition may be accompanied by average or strong abilities in an isolated area.

During the course of childhood and adolescence, children with this condition nevertheless usually make some developmental gains. Those who show improvement in language and intellectual ability have the best overall prognosis. Although some individuals with autistic disorder are able to live with some measure of partial independence in adulthood, very few are able to live entirely on their own.

The disorder makes it hard for children to communicate with others and relate to the outside world. There may be repeated body movements (hand flapping, rocking), lack of or unusual responses to people, attachments to objects, and/or resistance to changes in routines. In some cases, there may be aggressive or self-injurious behavior. Autism may affect a child's range of responses, and their reactions may appear out of context (for example, laughing inappropriately). Often these children have difficulty maintaining EYE CONTACT, and some use peripheral vision rather than looking directly at others. Often touching or being close to others may be upsetting to a person with autism. Because they may experience sensory information in an unusual way, people with autism sometimes may feel anxiety, fear, and confusion.

There are several specific symptoms from a list in the *DSM-IV-TR* related to these difficulties that children must show in order to meet the criteria for autistic disorder (see below).

Initial warning signs   There are a number of warning signs that parents or teachers may notice that may indicate autistic disorder, in three basic areas: behavior, communication, and social skills.

Behavior

- obsession with objects, interests, or routines
- inappropriate or unusual play with toys
- repetitive body movements or unusual body postures

- attachment to unusual objects
- unusual visual interests
- insensitivity or hypersensitivity to pain, temperature, taste, touch, smell, sounds, light, and so on

Social

- abnormal eye contact
- not noticing when name is called
- preferring to be alone
- ignoring others
- limited imitation (not waving hello or good-bye)
- not initiating social games, such as patty-cake or peekaboo
- little interest in being held
- lack of attention
- limited pointing or gestures

Communication

- echolalia (repeating words or phrases)
- no babbling by 12 months
- no single words by 16 months
- no two-word spontaneous phrases by 24 months
- peculiar use of language
- lack of pretend play
- failure to attract attention
- no use of early forms of communication

While half of all children with autism are not diagnosed until ages four to six, it is possible to diagnose a child as early as age 18 months. Since the earlier the condition is identified the earlier treatment can begin and the better the prognosis for the child, early diagnosis is critically important. A good diagnosis can identify whether a child does not have autism; if autism does exist, the evaluation can determine the seriousness of the problem and place the child "on the autism spectrum."

Because there are no medical tests for autism, a diagnosis must be based on observing the person's communication, behavior, and developmental levels. Even in very early childhood, parents can begin to observe their child to make sure certain developmental milestones are reached. For example, a two-year-old should be able to point to an object when named, use two- to four-word phrases, and follow simple instructions, according to the CDC. A three-year-old should be able to imitate adults and playmates, play make-believe with dolls, and use pronouns or plural words. Parents might want to check with a pediatrician if their children have not mastered these skills.

The diagnosis of autism typically requires a two-stage process. The first stage is a developmental screening during an annual "well-child" checkup, followed by a comprehensive evaluation by a multidisciplinary team. A child's pediatrician should always conduct a developmental screening at every well-baby and well-child visit throughout the preschool years. During the well-child visit, the pediatrician should observe the child and look for appropriate developmental milestones, noting how the child behaves, interacts, and communicates with a parent in the examining room. The doctor should ask questions related to normal development, such as about the child's verbal and gestural language and whether the child holds up objects for a parent to see. The doctor should evaluate a child for autistic disorder if he or she

- does not babble, coo, point, wave, or grasp by 12 months of age
- does not say single words by 16 months of age
- does not say two-word phrases independently (rather than just repeating what someone else says) by 24 months of age
- loses any language or social skill at any age

Several SCREENING INSTRUMENTS FOR AUTISM have been developed to quickly gather information about a child's social and communicative development within medical settings. Among them are the CHECKLIST FOR AUTISM IN TODDLERS (CHAT), the MODIFIED CHECKLIST FOR AUTISM IN TODDLERS (M-CHAT), and the Screening Tool for Autism in Two-Year-Olds (STAT). Some screening instruments rely solely on parent responses to a questionnaire, and some rely on a combination of parent report and observation. Important items on these tests that appear to differentiate children with autism from other groups before the age of two include pointing and pretend play.

It is important to remember that screening instruments simply assess the need for referral for a possible diagnosis of autism; they cannot be used alone to diagnose the condition. In addition, these screening methods may not identify children with mild autism, high-functioning autism, or Asperger's syndrome.

For children with milder suspected autism, the Autism Spectrum Screening Questionnaire (ASSQ), the Australian Scale for Asperger's Syndrome, and the most recent CHILDHOOD ASPERGER SYNDROME TEST (CAST), can reliably identify school-age children with Asperger's syndrome or higher functioning autism. The SOCIAL COMMUNICATION QUESTIONNAIRE (SCQ) can be used for children four years of age and older. These tools concentrate on social and behavioral impairments in children without significant language delay.

If after the screening process or during a routine well-child checkup the pediatrician suspects autism or a condition on the autism spectrum, he or she will refer the parents to either a developmental pediatrician or a pediatric neurologist, a psychiatrist or psychologist, or to a special team including a NEUROLOGIST, PSYCHOLOGIST, and speech language therapist for further formal diagnostic testing. The specialists will rule out other disorders and use assessments specific to autistic disorder.

Diagnosis is made by taking a developmental history and observing behavior. Because autism is a complex disorder that may involve other neurological problems, a comprehensive evaluation should include neurologic and genetic assessment, along with in-depth cognitive and language testing.

In addition, tests developed specifically for diagnosing autism are often used, including the AUTISM DIAGNOSIS INTERVIEW–REVISED (ADI-R) AND THE AUTISM DIAGNOSTIC OBSERVATION SCALE (ADOS). The ADI-R is a structured interview that covers more than 100 items and is conducted with a caregiver. It evaluates four aspects of the child's behavior: the child's communication skills, social interaction, repetitive behaviors, and age-of-onset symptoms. The ADOS is a semi-structured behavioral observation that evaluates communicative

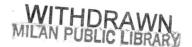

and social behaviors that are often delayed, abnormal, or absent in children with ASD.

Still another test for children over age two is the CHILDHOOD AUTISM RATING SCALE (CARS), which helps evaluate the child's body movements, adaptation to change, listening response, verbal communication, and relationships. In this test, the examiner observes the child and obtains information from the parents. The child's behavior is rated on a scale based on deviation from the typical behavior of children of the same age.

It may not be possible to definitively diagnose autistic disorder or confirm suspected cases in children until the age of three (or sometimes not until four), when the typical behavior becomes more obvious. In some cases, however, the diagnosis may be suspected in the first year of life.

Diagnostic categories have changed over the years as research progresses and as new editions of the American Psychiatric Association's *Diagnostic and Statistical Manual* have been issued. In general, to be diagnosed with autistic disorder, the person must have symptoms that belong to the three main areas of core features—impairment in language, impairment in social interactions, and the presence of repetitive stereotype behaviors or interests. For a diagnosis of autism, a physician will identify specific symptoms from a list in the *DSM-IV-TR* related to these difficulties. A child must show at least some of these symptoms in order to meet the criteria for autistic disorder, some of which include

Problems with social skills, including

- unresponsiveness to people
- lack of attachment to parents or caretakers
- rigid or flaccid muscle tone while being held; resisting being held or cuddled
- little or no interest in human contact
- lack of attachment to parents or caretakers
- lack of response to name
- not smiling (not looking at others)
- avoiding eye contact
- lack of imaginative play
- lack of stranger anxiety

- inability to make friends
- playing alone
- lack of separation anxiety
- unprovoked aggression toward others

Communication problems

- impaired speech or language onset in childhood
- language impairment
- meaningless repetition of words or phrases
- appears deaf sometimes
- inability to maintain conversation
- unusual language
- refusal to speak
- mixing up pronouns

Behavior problems

- self-destructive behavior
- bizarre or repetitive behavior patterns, such as uncontrollable head banging, screaming fits, arm flapping
- lines things up
- very distressed by minor changes in the environment
- overreaction or under-reaction to sensory stimulus
- delayed mental and social skills
- inflexibility
- adherence to routines
- unusual or severely restricted activities
- rocking, hand flapping, hair twirling
- reduced or increased sensitivity to pain or temperature
- tantrums
- regression
- self-mutiliation

Autistic disorder vs. autism spectrum disorders Because autism is considered to be one of five related conditions collectively known as "autism spectrum disorders," it is important to correctly place the child's symptoms on the autism continuum. Some children who may have some symptoms of autism but who do not have enough to be diagnosed with the classical form of the disorder, may be diagnosed with pervasive developmental disorder–not otherwise specified (PDD-NOS). Some who exhibit autistic behavior but who have well-developed language skills may be diagnosed with Asperger's syndrome. Children who appear normal in their first several years but then lose skills and begin showing autistic behavior may be diagnosed with CHILDHOOD DISINTEGRATIVE DISORDER. A chromosomal analysis can rule out RETT DISORDER, a rare sex-linked genetic disorder characterized by inadequate brain growth, seizures, and other neurological problems and part of the spectrum of autism disorders. Autism in itself is diagnosed as autistic disorder.

Ruling out other conditions Because some people with autism also may have a behavior disorder, problems with hearing, mental retardation, or eccentric behavior, part of the diagnosis will consist not only in identifying autism or AUTISM SPECTRUM DISORDERS, but also other complicating disorders. It is, therefore, important to distinguish autistic disorder from other conditions, because early identification is required for an effective treatment program.

Any child with a developmental delay should have a number of other tests to rule out these disorders. A comprehensive hearing evaluation should be done to rule out hearing loss as the cause of abnormal language development. Although some hearing loss can occur along with autism, some children with autism may be incorrectly thought to have hearing problems. Lead screening is essential for children who often put things in their mouths. Blood tests can rule out metabolic disorders that affect amino acids and lipids in the blood, and a chromosomal analysis can rule out genetic disorders such as FRAGILE X SYNDROME. An electroencephalogram (EEG) can rule out a seizure disorder, and magnetic resonance imaging (MRI) can rule out brain disorders.

Customarily, an expert diagnostic team has the responsibility of thoroughly evaluating the child, assessing the child's unique strengths and weaknesses and determining a formal diagnosis. The team will then meet with the parents to explain the results of the evaluation.

Treatment Options and Outlook

While there is no cure for the brain abnormalities that cause autistic disorder, children can learn skills, coping mechanisms, and strategies to ease various symptoms. Intensive, appropriate early intervention greatly improves the outcome for most young children. Most programs will build on the interests of the child, teach functional skills in a highly structured manner using behavioral techniques, follow a consistent schedule of activities, and include visual cues.

Some symptoms may lessen as the child ages and others may disappear altogether; with appropriate treatment, many problem behaviors can be changed so that the person may appear to no longer have autistic disorder. However, most patients continue to show some residual symptoms to some degree throughout their entire lives.

Preschool programs While various preschool models may differ, all emphasize early, appropriate, and intensive educational interventions for young children. Each state guarantees special education and related services. The INDIVIDUALS WITH DISABILITIES EDUCATION ACT (IDEA), P.L. 108-77, and Individuals with Disabilities Education Improvement Act 17 (2004) are federal programs that assure a free appropriate public education for children with autism. Each child is entitled to these services from age three through high school, or until age 21, whichever comes first.

In children younger than three, instruction usually occurs at home or a child care-center, including interventions that target specific problems in learning, language, imitation, attention, motivation, compliance, and initiative of interaction. Effective programs teach early communication and social interaction skills. Included are behavioral methods, communication, occupational and physical therapy, in addition to social play interventions.

While various preschool models may differ, all emphasize early, appropriate, and intensive educational interventions for young children. Other common aspects of treatment may include

• use of techniques from the field of applied behavior analysis

- individualized treatment goals based on the child's unique strengths and weaknesses
- focus on functional communication, such as teaching the child to ask for things he or she wants (using spoken language, sign language, or picture communication)
- initial use of one-on-one instruction until the child is able to benefit from group instruction
- ample opportunities for repetition and rehearsal of new skills
- some degree of inclusion with typically developing children
- activities that build on the interests of the child
- extensive use of visual cues to accompany instruction
- dealing with problem behaviors by trying to understand why a child is acting this way
- structured activities
- extensive staff training
- parent-training to ensure generalization of skills to environments outside of the treatment setting
- strategies for transitioning between activities
- follow up to ensure successful carryover of skills at conclusion of early intervention program

Treatment is most successful when geared toward the individual's particular needs. An experienced specialist or team should design the individualized program, which may include treatments from various fields.

In addition to a preschool program, children with autistic disorder should be trained in functional living skills at the earliest possible age. Learning to cross a street, to buy something in a store, or ask for help are critical skills and may be hard even for average people. Training is aimed at boosting a child's independence and providing opportunity for personal choice and freedom.

Education Studies show that individuals with autistic disorder respond well to a highly structured, specialized education program tailored to the individual's needs. A well-designed early intervention program typically addresses functional communication, social interaction skills, preacademic skills, adaptive behavior, and play. In addition, intervention programs should have a clear mechanism to eliminate any problem behaviors. Techniques from the field of applied behavior analysis are recommended by many experts. Initially, most young children with autistic disorder require a small ratio of children to adults to ensure effective intervention. Ideally, this should include some opportunities for one-to-one instruction.

The laws state that children must be taught in the least restrictive environment, appropriate for the individual child. This statement does not mean that each child must be placed in a regular classroom. Instead, the laws mean that the teaching environment should be designed to meet a child's learning needs, while minimizing restrictions on the child's access to typical learning experiences and interactions. Educating children with autistic disorder often includes a combination of one-to-one, small group, and regular classroom instruction.

To qualify for special education services, the child must meet specific criteria as outlined by federal and state guidelines. Parents can contact a local school principal or special-education coordinator to learn how to have a child assessed to see if he or she qualifies for services under these laws. Educational programs for students with autism should focus on improving communication, social, academic, behavioral, and daily living skills. Behavior and communication problems that interfere with learning sometimes require the assistance of a knowledgeable professional in the autism field who helps to implement a plan that can be carried out at home and school.

The school district pays for all necessary services, including services by a speech therapist, occupational therapist, school psychologist, social worker, school nurse, or aide. By law, the public schools must prepare and carry out a set of instruction goals, or specific skills, for every child in a SPECIAL EDUCATION program. The list of skills is known as the child's INDIVIDUALIZED EDUCATION PROGRAM (IEP). This IEP is an agreement between the school and the family on the child's goals. The special-services team should evaluate and reevaluate each child on a regular basis to see how the child is doing and whether any changes are needed in the IEP.

A child under three years of age with autism should be eligible for an early-intervention program available in every state. The services provided are then written into an INDIVIDUALIZED FAMILY SERVICE PLAN (IFSP) that is reviewed at least once every six months. The plan will describe services that will be provided to the child but will also describe services for parents, to help them in daily activities with their child, and for siblings, to help them adjust to having a brother or sister with autism.

Children older than three usually do best with school-based,/individualized/special/education, either in a segregated class with other children with autism, or in an integrated class with children without disabilities for at least part of the day. All should provide a structure that will help the children learn social skills and functional communication. Teachers often involve the parents, giving useful advice in how to help their child use the skills or behaviors learned at school when they are at home.

After the preschool years, more severely impaired children may continue to require a structured, intensive education and behavior program with a one-on-one teacher to student ratio. However, children with fewer impairments may do well in a normal education environment with appropriate support and accommodations.

In elementary school, the child should receive help in any skill area that is delayed and be encouraged to grow in his or her areas of strength. The classroom environment should be structured so that the program is consistent and predictable. Students with autism learn better and are less confused when information is presented visually as well as verbally. Interaction with nondisabled peers is also important, for these students provide models of appropriate language, social, and behavior skills. To overcome frequent problems in generalizing skills learned at school, it is very important to develop programs with parents, so that learning activities, experiences, and approaches can be carried over into the home and community. Ideally, the curriculum should be adapted to the individual child's needs. Many schools today have an inclusion program in which the child is in a regular classroom for most of the day, with special instruction for a part of the day. This instruction should include such skills as learning how to act in social situations

and in making friends. Although higher functioning children may be able to handle academic work, they, too, need help to organize tasks and avoid distractions. During middle and high school years, instruction will begin to include practical matters such as work, community living, and recreational activities, and include work experience, using public transportation, and learning skills that will be important in community living. While some autistic behaviors improve during the teenage years, others may get worse. Increased autistic or aggressive behavior may be one way some teens express their newfound tension and confusion. At an age when most teenagers are concerned with popularity, grades, and social skills, teens with autism may realize they are different from their peers. Unlike their classmates, they may not have friends, they may not date, or they may not be planning a career. For some, the sadness that comes with such realization motivates them to learn new behaviors and acquire better social skills.

Treatment is most successful when geared toward the individual's particular needs. An experienced specialist or team should design the individualized program, which may include APPLIED BEHAVIOR ANALYSIS, DISCRETE TRIAL TRAINING, OCCUPATIONAL THERAPY, PHYSICAL THERAPY, speech language therapy, and medication. Other, more controversial treatments may include SENSORY INTEGRATION, dietary interventions, vitamins and supplements, music therapy, VISION THERAPY, or AUDITORY INTEGRATION TRAINING.

Behavioral techniques Most autism experts agree that behavioral interventions involving one-on-one interactions are usually beneficial and can sometimes have very positive results in children with autistic disorder. A number of behavioral modification therapists have been used effectively in children with autistic disorder to improve symptoms of inappropriate, repetitive, and aggressive behavior and to provide autistic patients with skills they need to function. Most types of behavior therapy are based on the theory that rewarded behavior is more likely to be repeated than behavior that is ignored.

Behavioral interventions should involve a substantial amount of time each week, between 20 to 40 hours, depending on whether the child is in school. These methods focus on prompting as much as necessary to achieve a high level of success, with a gradual fading of prompts, and must include proper training of therapists and ongoing supervision. Effective behavior therapy also involves regular team meetings to maintain consistency between therapists and check for problems. It is most important that therapists keep the sessions fun for children, in order to maintain their interest and motivation. These comprehensive behavioral treatment programs show promise in helping children with autism learn the skills they need to develop and interact with the world, and many new approaches are being designed and tested, some of which focus on reshaping a child's learning environment, while others seek to match treatment to a child's individual needs.

In general, behavior management therapy works to reinforce wanted behaviors and reduce unwanted behaviors. At the same time, these methods also suggest what caregivers should do before or between episodes of problem behaviors and what to do during or after these episodes. Typically, behavior modification involves highly structured, skill-oriented activities based on a patient's needs and interests that requires intense, one-on-one training with a therapist and extensive involvement of the caregiver (usually the parent).

Applied behavioral analysis (ABA). This is the most well researched of all behavioral treatment methods for autistic disorder. In this approach developed by autism expert Ivar Lovaas and his colleagues at the University of California at Los Angeles (UCLA), therapists work intensely, one-on-one, with a child for 20 to 40 hours a week. Children are taught skills in a simple step-by-step manner, such as teaching colors one at a time. The sessions usually begin with formal, structured drills, such as learning to point to a color when its name is given, and then, after some time, there is a shift towards generalizing skills to other situations and environments. The goal of this type of behavioral management is to reinforce desirable behaviors and reduce undesirable ones.

ABA programs are most effective when started before age five, although they can be helpful with older children. ABA programs are especially effective in teaching nonverbal children how to talk. Parents are also encouraged to learn ABA tech-

niques; qualified behavior consultants often hold workshops on how to provide ABA therapy.

In one study published by Dr. Lovaas at UCLA, trained graduate students spent two years of intensive, 40-hour-a-week behavioral intervention working with 19 young autistic children ranging from 35 to 41 months of age. Almost half of the children improved so much that they became indistinguishable from typical children, and these children went on to lead fairly normal lives. Of the other half, most had significant improvements; a few did not improve very much.

Several other types of training are based on the principles of ABA, including discrete trial training (DTT), which has been shown in multiple studies to significantly improve symptoms among children with autistic disorder. This type of teaching breaks a learning task into tiny components, uses positive reinforcement to teach each part in isolation, and provides the child with the level of repetition and rehearsal necessary to acquire each subskill. However, well-designed ABA programs should not exclusively use DTT. Rather, they should incorporate other ABA techniques, such as methods of generalizing skills to the natural environment.

Relationship development intervention (RDI) is a new method that focuses on teaching children with autistic disorder specifically how to develop relationships, first with their parents and later with their peers. It directly addresses the development of social skills and friendships.

TEACCH This commonly used intervention program, developed from the field of special education, is called the Treatment and Education of Autistic and Related Communication Handicapped Children (TEACCH). This method emphasizes the use of a structured environment using one-on-one teaching in classrooms that provide visual cues on how to complete tasks. TEACCH also encourages children to be more independent by teaching them to use newly mastered skills in less-structured environments, such as mainstream classrooms. Classrooms using TEACCH components incorporate visual cues, a high level of structure and routine, and other environmental accommodations to maximize a child's success.

This program was developed at the University of North Carolina/Chapel Hill in 1971 by developmental psychologist Eric Schopler to provide a structured learning environment for children with autism as a way of improving their strengths and independence. The multidisciplinary program involves the family and community in an intensive treatment regimen—five hours a day, five days a week—in a TEACCH classroom.

Floor time This type of treatment involves an informal play session between a child and a partner, which uses interactive experiences to enable a child to move along to the next developmental stage. Floor time was developed by psychiatrist Stanley Greenspan, M.D., as part of his Developmental Individual Difference Relationship-Based Model (DIR)—an alternative to the behaviorism approach based more on relationships. Floor time lets a child be the boss. During floor time, parents should do what their child wants to do, playing eye-to-eye with the child, allowing him or her to take the lead as parents try to open and close as many "circles of communication" as possible.

Social skills training People with high-functioning autistic disorder can benefit from special training in understanding the unwritten social rules and body language signals that people use in social interaction and conversation. Social "scripting" can be used to teach appropriate responses and prepare the individual for transitions. In very young children, they may be in the form of photographs or pictures.

Relationship development intervention (RDI) is a new method that teaches children with autistic disorder specifically how to develop relationships, first with their parents and later with their peers. It directly addresses the development of social skills and friendships.

Speech-language therapy The field of speech-language pathology offers numerous approaches to improve a child's language, which is one of the primary problems in autistic disorder. Speech-language therapists can help people with autism improve their general ability to communicate and interact with others effectively, as well as develop their speech and language skills. Therapists may teach nonverbal ways of communicating (such as sign language) and may improve social skills that involve communicating with others to initiate language development in young children with

the disorder. They may also help people to better use words and sentences and to improve rate and rhythm of speech and conversation.

This type of treatment may help many autistic children, especially if it is integrated with other home and school programs. This works particularly well in children with autistic disorder who also have APRAXIA, a phonological disorder, or other language-specific difficulties. Sign language or a pictorial exchange communication method may be very helpful in developing speech in autistic individuals.

Some speech-language pathologists provide AUDITORY INTEGRATION TRAINING (AIT), which involves listening to processed music for a total of 10 hours (two half-hour sessions per day, over a period of 10 to 12 days). This controversial research has been inconclusive, although anecdotal reports suggest that AIT improves auditory processing, decreases or eliminates sound sensitivity, and reduces behavioral problems in some autistic children. The American Academy of Pediatrics also discourages the use of AIT, citing the lack of any empirical evidence that it is effective.

Computer-based auditory interventions help children who have delays in language and have difficulty discriminating speech sounds. However, research into these interventions has primarily been conducted with children with dyslexia rather than autistic disorder and has mainly been conducted by the company producing the program.

Picture exchange communication systems (PECS) This type of treatment helps people with autism communicate using pictures that represent ideas, activities, or items. The patient is able to convey requests, needs, and desires to others by handing them a picture.

Physical and occupational therapy Often, children with autism have limited gross and fine motor skills, so physical therapy can be helpful in these cases. Physical therapy is used to improve problems with gross motor skills, such as walking, running, and climbing stairs. Although these skills are typically not impaired in children with autistic disorder, a physical therapist should be included if a child with autistic disorder also has other disabilities, such as cerebral palsy.

Occupational therapists can help people with autism find ways to adjust tasks and conditions that match their needs and abilities. Such help may include finding a specially designed computer mouse and keyboard to ease communication or identifying skills that build on a person's interests and individual capabilities.

Because many autistic individuals have mild to severe sensory problems, some experts believe they may respond to sensory integration training as taught by occupational thearpists. The field of occupational therapy offers strategies to improve problems with fine motor and adaptive skills, such as dressing, eating, and writing, that are sometimes seen in children with autistic disorder. For example, these children may be either over- or undersensitive to sound, sight, smell, touch, and taste. This is a type of behavior modification that focuses primarily on stimulating the senses of motion/ balance, touch, and joints and ligaments (proprioception). In an attempt to address these difficulties, some occupational therapists use a controversial treatment called sensory integration therapy (SIT), which focuses primarily on stimulating these senses. Sensory integration therapists teach techniques to provide a "sensory diet" for children by touching their skin, dressing them in specially weighted vests, swaddling, providing deep-pressure squeezes, swinging, and so on.

While many experts believe there is no sound research supporting SIT, repeated exposure to various forms of sensory input may desensitize children with autistic disorder, allowing them to better tolerate specific stimuli that previously caused distress. However, although sensory integration therapy techniques are common in some school settings, the American Association of School Psychologists does not recommend their use, and the National Academy of Sciences cites the lack of any sound scientific evidence for this intervention.

Medication   Although there are no medications specifically designed to treat autism, there are many psychiatric medications used to treat specific symptoms often found in autism, such as aggression, self-injury, anxiety, depression, obsessive-compulsive disorder, and attention deficit hyperactivity disorder (ADHD). These medications generally work by altering the level of neurotransmitters in the brain.

Medication can improve the behavior of a person with autism. Health-care providers often use medications to deal with a specific behavior, such as reducing self-injurious behavior. As these symptoms are minimized, the person with autism can focus on other things, including learning and communication. Some of these medications have serious risks involved with their use; others may make symptoms worse at first or may take several weeks to become effective. Not every medication helps every person with symptoms of autism.

Health care providers usually prescribe medications on a trial basis, to see if they help. A child's health-care provider may have to try different dosages or different combinations of medications to find the most effective plan. Families, caregivers, and health-care providers need to work together to make sure that medications are working and that the overall medication plan is safe.

Use of any one particular medication is typically based on a specialized physician's (such as a psychiatrist, developmental-pediatrician, or pediatric neurologist) evaluation of the patient's symptoms. Dosages need to be adjusted differently for each person, and one medication may be ineffective or have negative effects, while others are helpful. For some classes of drugs the doses that successfully ease symptoms may be much lower for those with autistic disorder than for healthy people.

Psychiatric medications are widely used to treat the symptoms of autistic disorder, and they can be beneficial to many older children and adults. However, there are concerns over their use, and there is relatively little research on their effects in children with autistic disorder. There are almost no studies on the long-term effects, especially for the newer medications, and there is a concern that their long-term use in children may affect their development. Because these drugs treat the symptoms, but not the underlying biomedical causes of autism, it is important to balance risk versus benefit.

Antidepressants are used to treat depression, obsessive-compulsive behavior, and anxiety that may appear in people with autism. In addition, these drugs may reduce the frequency and intensity of repetitive behavior; ease irritability, tantrums, and aggression; and improve eye contact and responsiveness. In particular, selective serotonin reuptake inhibitors (SSRIs) are the newest group of antidepressants that treat problems such as obsessive-compulsive behaviors and anxiety, resulting from an imbalance in one of the body's chemical systems that are sometimes present in autism. These medications may reduce the frequency and intensity of repetitive behaviors; decrease irritability, tantrums, and aggressive behavior; and improve eye contact. SSRIs include fluvoxamine (Luvox), fluoxetine (Prozac), and bupropion (Wellbutrin). Tricyclics are another type of antidepressant used to treat depression and obsessive-compulsive behaviors. Although these drugs tend to cause more side effects than the SSRIs, sometimes they are more effective for certain people.

Antipsychotic medications may help control hyperactivity, behavioral problems, withdrawal, and aggression sometimes experienced by people with autism by affecting the brain of the person taking them. Antipsychotics include clozapine (Clozaril), RISPERIDONE (Risperdal), olanzapine (Zyprexa), and quetiapine (Seroquel). Use of this group of drugs is the most widely studied treatment for autism. In some people with ASDs, these drugs may decrease hyperactivity, reduce stereotyped behaviors, and minimize withdrawal and aggression.

Benzodiazepines can be used to treat behavioral problems, panic, and anxiety sometimes found in people with autism. Benzodiazepines include diazepam (Valium), lorazepam (Ativan), and alprazolam (Xanax). Discontinuing these drugs after long-term use may cause withdrawal symptoms.

Biomedical intervention Biomedical intervention typically refers to a variety of controversial treatments, including numerous vitamins and nutritional supplements, special dietary interventions that restrict certain types of foods, agents designed to remove heavy metals from the body, medications that treat yeast or fungi, and medications whose use in children with autism has not been thoroughly investigated. These treatments are often used by doctors who focus on a biomedical explanation of autistic disorder.

The DEFEAT AUTISM NOW! (DAN!) Program features nutritional support, diet changes, and detoxification aimed at addressing core problems of autism rather than symptoms. Some of the major interventions suggested by DAN! practitioners include

- nutritional supplements, including certain vitamins, minerals, amino acids, and essential fatty acids
- special diets totally free of gluten (from wheat, barley, rye, and possibly oats) and free of dairy (milk, ice cream, yogurt, and so on)
- testing for hidden food allergies, and avoidance of allergenic foods
- treatment of intestinal yeast overgrowth
- detoxification of heavy metals

While the use of dietary modifications and supplements to treat autism is controversial, changing the diet or adding vitamin supplements may improve digestion and eliminate food intolerances or allergies, which may contribute to behavioral problems in autistic patients.

Studies have found high levels of proteins from wheat, oats and rye (gluten), and casein (protein in dairy products) byproducts in patients with autism, suggesting that the incomplete breakdown or excessive absorption of these substances may affect brain function. However, cutting out food containing gluten and casein may cause side effects and should not be done without the advice of a health-care practitioner. Nevertheless, eliminating dietary gluten/casein for some children has immediate and startling effects obvious to their parents within hours or days. Children who seem to respond most dramatically to the removal of dairy have a history of ear infections, inconsolable crying, poor sleeping patterns, and excessive craving of milk and dairy foods. Gluten intolerance is generally indicated by loose stools and/or a craving for bread and pasta.

Because this is a relatively harmless intervention, some experts suggest it should be attempted as soon as possible after a diagnosis to see if a child does respond. If so, further exploration into biochemical treatment is recommended.

Some studies have suggested that vitamin B, magnesium, and cod liver oil supplements may improve behavior, eye contact, attention span, and learning in patients with autism. Vitamin C may improve depression and ease symptoms in patients with autism.

Vision therapy   More recently, some optometrists have become involved in the treatment of autistic disorder. Referred to as "developmental optometrists," they offer controversial vision therapy, including techniques such as prisms, special lenses, and vision exercises. Pediatricians and ophthalmologists typically discourage vision therapy, citing lack of any research.

Supplemental therapy   Additional supplemental therapies include music therapy, art therapy, and animal therapy. Some children with autistic disorder do seem to respond to these treatments, although they should be considered a supplementary intervention rather than a primary mode of treatment.

Contrary to popular belief, many children and adults with autism can make eye contact and can show affection and demonstrate a variety of other emotions in varying degrees. Like other children, they respond to their environment in both positive and negative ways. Although there is no "typical" type of person with autism, children with autism can learn and function productively and improve with appropriate education and treatment.

With appropriate treatment, some behaviors associated with autistic disorder may lessen over time. Although communication and social problems will continue in some form throughout life, difficulties in other areas may improve with age, education, or diminished stress level. Many individuals with autistic disorder enjoy their lives and contribute to their community in a meaningful way, as they learn to compensate for and cope with their disability.

Some adults with autistic disorder live and work independently in the community, and can drive a car, earn a college degree, and even get married. Some may only need some support for particularly stressful experiences, while others require a great deal of support from family and professionals.

Adults with autism may live in a variety of residential settings, ranging from an independent home or apartment to group homes, supervised apartment settings, other family members or more structured residential care. More and more support groups for adults with autism are appearing, and many individuals are forming their own networks to share information, support each other, and speak for themselves.

Individuals with autistic disorder are providing valuable insight into the challenges of this disability by publishing articles and books and appearing on TV to discuss their lives and disabilities. The prognosis for individuals depends on the degree of their disabilities and on the level of therapy they receive.

See also ACHENBACH CHILDHOOD BEHAVIOR CHECKLIST; AUTISM BEHAVIOR CHECKLIST; AUTISM DIAGNOSTIC INTERVIEW–REVISED.

autistic savant   An individual with AUTISTIC DISORDER who displays unusual aptitude for one or more specific skills, such as math calculations, musical ability or superior memory for particular facts. In the past, individuals with these exceptional skills were called *idiot savants,* but this pejorative description was changed after a 1978 article in *Psychology Today,* when Dr. Bernard Rimland introduced the term "autistic savant." Other experts prefer the term "savant syndrome," because individuals with other developmental disorders besides autism also can have savant skills.

About 10 percent of all people with autistic disorder are savants, but only about 1 percent of people with other developmental disorders, including those with mental retardation, have savant skills. Since other developmental disabilities are much more common than autistic disorder, however, about half of those with savant syndrome have autistic disorder, and the other half have some other form of developmental disability, mental retardation, or brain injury or disease. Thus, not all savants are autistic, and not all autistic persons are savants.

The most common types of savant abilities are called "splinter skills," and include behaviors such as obsessive preoccupation with and memorization of material such as sports trivia, license plate numbers, maps, historical facts, or odd things such as airplane motor sounds. "Talented savants" are those who have musical, artistic, mathematical, or other special skills, usually within one area. "Prodigious savants" have a very rare ability in which their special skill is so outstanding that it would be spectacular even if it were to occur in a nonhandicapped person. There are fewer than 50 prodigious savants in the world today who would meet this high standard.

Savant skills are usually limited to certain areas of expertise: music, art, quick calculation or other mathematical skills, calendar calculating, and mechanical/spatial skills. Calendar calculating appears to be an ability developed almost exclusively among savants.

Music is the most common savant skill, usually involving an ability to play the piano by ear or sing with perfect pitch. Although musical performance skills are most typical, some savants are outstanding composers, usually linked to performance ability. In fact, the triple syndrome of mental disability, blindness, and musical genius has occurred with an unusual frequency during the past 100 years.

The next most common savant skill is artistic talent (often in the form of painting, drawing, or sculpting). Extremely fast calculating or other mathematical skills, such as the ability to figure out multi-digit prime numbers despite being unable to perform even the most basic adding or subtracting, is also common.

Mechanical ability (especially repairing intricate machines) or unusual spatial skills such as intricate map and route memorizing are seen somewhat less frequently.

Calendar calculating is common among savants, particularly considering how rare this obscure ability is in the general population. Beyond being able to name the day of the week that a date will occur on in any particular year, calendar calculating includes being able to name all the years in the next 100 in which Easter will fall on March 23, for example, or all the years in the next 20 when July 4 will fall on a Tuesday.

Autistic savants occasionally may display other skills, including the ability to easily learn a variety of foreign languages or other unusual language skills, exquisite smell or touch discrimination, perfect appreciation of passing time without access to a clock face, or profound knowledge in a specific field, such as neurophysiology, statistics, or history.

While always controversial, there have been some reports that a few savants appear to demonstrate extrasensory perception skills.

Typically, one of these unique skills appears in each person with savant syndrome, although sometimes one person may experience multiple skills. No matter what type of skill, it is always combined with prodigious memory.

The reason some autistic individuals have savant abilities is not known, but the syndrome occurs four to six times more often in boys than girls. This is probably due to the fact that autistic disorder likewise has the same disproportionate male/female ratio.

The condition can be congenital (genetic or inborn), or can be acquired later in childhood, or even in adults, but the extraordinary skills are always linked with an incredible memory of a special type—extremely deep but very, very narrow.

autoimmune system disorder An increasing number of studies have found that individuals with autism may have problems with their immune systems. Some scientists describe autism as an autoimmune system disorder.

Some experts believe that autism may occur when a person's immune system is compromised due to inherited abnormal genes, exposure to chemicals, or both; born with this predisposition, exposure to an additional environmental insult could then lead to autism.

aversive techniques A behavioral method that uses unpleasant punishment to decrease or eliminate problem behaviors. Aversive methods are primarily used to treat only severe self-injurious behavior and should only be used when nonaversive techniques have been unsuccessful. Aversive techniques may be used when individuals cause extreme harm to themselves, such as biting or hitting themselves or banging their heads hard enough to cause tissue damage. Because punishment techniques are often less successful than reinforcement strategies, aversive techniques are typically combined with positive reinforcement of alternative desired behavior.

basic skills Fundamental abilities necessary to function on a daily basis. The mastery of basic skills is necessary to progress to higher levels of achievement. These abilities include self-care activities, such as using the toilet, dressing, grooming, eating, cooking and cleaning. Academically, basic skills include speaking, spelling, reading, writing, and arithmetic.

behavioral therapy A goal-oriented, generally short-term method using in treating autistic individuals. This type of therapy can help people change the way they act, feel, or think when dealing with particular troublesome circumstances. Behavior therapists usually focus on the current situation, rather than the past.

Types of behavioral therapy used to treat people with autism include APPLIED BEHAVIORAL ANALYSIS (ABA), and DISCRETE TRIAL TRAINING (DTT).

The method arouses controversy in cases in which punishment and aversives are used to decrease self-destructive behaviors.

behavior modification The systematic application of reinforcers (rewards) and/or punishments as a way of reducing or eliminating problem behavior, or to teach people new skills or responses. Behavior modification is based on the idea that since all behavior is learned, with appropriate treatment it also can be *unlearned* by using positive or negative consequences. Many autism experts believe that the most appropriate education for children with autism includes early, intensive behavior modification therapy.

Behavior modification is used by psychologists, social workers, teachers, and other professionals to change an individual's reaction to a situation. There are two major approaches to behavior modification, one based on the work of the late psychologist B. F. Skinner, the other based on the work of psychologist Albert Bandura.

Skinner believed that all behavior is learned by interacting with the environment, and that bad behavior is learned the same way normal behavior is learned. Skinner believed that rewarded behavior is likely to be repeated, and punished behavior is likely to be avoided. Therefore, a behavior modification program should establish a program that rewards specific desired behaviors.

Bandura's approach emphasizes learning through imitation, believing that a person can learn to avoid an unpleasant situation without experiencing it. Individuals can also learn new skills by watching and imitating others. Bandura emphasized the effectiveness of role models who speak and act consistently, and this applies especially to young children.

Behavioral modification programs for children with autism are based on training the child to behave in a more appropriate and socially accepted manner. This typically consists of an immediate correction of any aberrant behavior. Many of the most difficult behaviors, if dealt with early, may become controlled; if neglected, these behaviors can lead to wild, impulsive, uncontrollable behavior that may require institutionalization. Modeling specific social skills or strategies, communication patterns, and other positive behavior is especially important for children with autism, who require specific direct instruction as well as consistent modeling.

benzodiazepines A class of drugs such as diazepam (Valium), lorazepam (Ativan), and alprazolam

(Xanax) that may be used to treat behavioral problems in people with autism.

Side Effects

Side effects include drowsiness, fatigue, lack of muscle coordination (ataxia), and dizziness. Discontinuing these drugs after long-term use may cause withdrawal symptoms including abdominal and muscle pain, convulsions and tremors, insomnia, sweating, or vomiting.

Bérard, Guy   A French ear, nose, and throat doctor who developed an auditory training program (Bérard AIT) in the early 1950s. His idea was to train the brain to identify the important sounds coming into the ear and ignore the secondary noises.

Bérard learned about an auditory stimulation intervention called the Audio-Psycho-Phonology approach (or the TOMATIS METHOD), which was developed by the late Dr. Alfred Tomatis. Bérard worked with Tomatis for a short period of time, eventually leaving because he felt the Tomatis method was inefficient and incorrectly focused on the emotional aspects of hearing.

See also BÉRARD AUDITORY INTEGRATION TRAINING.

Bérard Auditory Integration Training (Bérard AIT or AIT)   A controversial treatment program for people with autism that involves listening to processed music for a total of 10 hours (two half-hour sessions per day, over a period of 10 to 12 days). The experimental program uses sound and tone variations fused into classical music to unravel problems common to people with autism. Each special compact disc features a gradual change in the peaks and pitch of sound filtered through the music. The goal is to hit "receptor points" within the ear. However, there are no documented studies that show a decrease in behavior problems.

Guy Bérard, a French ear, nose and throat doctor, first developed the program in the early 1950s as a way of training the brain to identify the important sounds coming into the ear and ignore the secondary noises. In his research, Dr. Bérard observed that many of those suffering from some forms of neurological disorders appeared to have very sensitive, or hyperacoustic, hearing. Often misdiagnosed as autistic, he believed that many children with learning disabilities are trapped in a world of hypersensitivity to sound, confusing brain stimuli, and frequency imbalances between the right and left ear. He believes that exercising the middle-ear mechanism by using modulated and filtered music may produce improvement in patients with a wide variety of learning and speaking problems.

It is not clear what the minimum age should be to receive AIT, but current recommendations set the minimum age at three years. If the child is an appropriate candidate, the only behavioral requirement is that he or she accepts headphones. Each client starts with a behavioral profile and audiogram, together with counseling before and after the sessions over a course of 10 days. Although the program typically involves listening to processed music for a total of 10 hours (two half-hour sessions per day, over a period of 10 to 12 days), at some AIT clinics, it is acceptable to have a one- or two-day break after five days of listening. During the listening sessions, the person listens to processed music. That is, the AIT sound amplifier attenuates low and high frequencies at random from the compact discs and then sends this modified music through headphones to the listener. This random selection of frequencies is termed *modulation*. Follow-up profiles of each participant are made to judge behavioral changes.

Activities can be done during and after the 10 days of AIT to help the individual integrate and adjust to the changes derived from AIT. Many practitioners recommend participation in sensory integration activities even during the 10-day period of AIT and in the following weeks to help reduce any irritability and hyperactivity that may occur and may help reorganize the system more quickly.

Bettelheim, Bruno (1903–1990)   A controversial child psychologist who believed that the symptoms of autistic children were caused by a cold unloving mother and an absent father and that the lack of early emotional stimulation damaged the central nervous systems of these children.

Bettelheim received his doctoral degree in philosophy in 1938 from the University of Vienna, and was subsequently imprisoned in Dachau and Buchenwald during the Nazi occupation of Austria. After emigrating to the United States in 1939, he taught psychology at the University of Chicago from 1944 to 1973 and directed the Chicago-based Orthogenic School for children with emotional problems, placing special emphasis on the treatment of autism.

Although untrained in analysis, Bettelheim considered himself a Freudian fundamentalist who, in spite of overwhelming evidence to the contrary, was convinced that autism had no organic basis but that it was caused by parents who hated their children.

He believed the only way to treat autism was to separate the autistic child from his parents (a process he called "parent-ectomies"). Bettelheim then advocated nurturing the children with positive experiences until they felt comfortable enough to stop being autistic. After his death, however, several of the children in his school accused him of abusive treatment, and his detractors charged that much of his educational background was invented.

Although his theories on autism have been discredited, he did write several well-known books on child development, including *The Informed Heart* (1960), *The Empty Fortress* (1967), and *The Uses of Enchantment* (1976). A depressed individual for most of his life, Bettelheim died by suicide in 1990, six years after his second wife died of cancer.

body language Physical movements that express emotion and modify communication. People with AUTISTIC DISORDER have a very hard time deciphering the body language of others, which interferes with their social skills and communication. At the same time, it can be difficult to understand the body language of a person with autism. Most people smile, for example, when talking about things they enjoy, or shrug when a question cannot be answered. But the facial expressions, movements, and gestures of people with autism may not match what they are saying. Their tone of voice also may fail to reflect their feelings.

Boston Higashi school An international program serving children and young adults with autism based upon the tenets of DAILY LIFE THERAPY

developed by the late Dr. Kiyo Kitahara of Tokyo, Japan. Dr. Kitahara's method provides children with systematic education through group dynamics and a combined program of academics and technology, arts, music, and physical education. The goal of this educational approach is for individuals to achieve social independence and dignity and to benefit from and contribute to society. The school also tries to promote autism education and research through the Higashi Institute for Professional Development.

brain The brain is the major organ of the human nervous system, part of a complex network of nerve cells and fibers responsible for controlling all the processes in the body and the main orchestrator of thought, speech, emotion, and memory. Sensations from nerves extending from the central nervous system to every other part of the body are received, sorted, and interpreted by the brain.

The brain is split into two halves, known as the left and the right hemispheres. They are separated by a groove called the corpus callosum, a closely-packed bundle of fibers that connect the right and left sides and allow the two hemispheres to communicate. Although the two halves look identical, in fact they are specialized to perform different functions, and they control different parts of the body.

The left side of the brain controls movements in the right side of the body, and the right brain controls the left side. This is because the nerves to each side of the body cross over at the top of the spinal cord. Although the two hemispheres are linked by the corpus callosum and share information, one half of the brain is always considered "dominant." Right-handed people almost always have a dominant left hemisphere. Left-handed people probably have a dominant right hemisphere. In addition, each half of the brain specializes in certain areas. The right hemisphere controls visual-spatial skills such as painting, music, and creative activities, recognizing faces, shapes, and patterns, and judging size and distance. It is also considered to be the seat of imagination, emotion, and insight. The left hemisphere is the center of speaking, reading, writing, and understanding language, and many aspects of mathematics, such as performing calculations. It is considered to be the logical, problem-solving side of the brain.

On each side of the brain are three main areas: the extension of the spinal cord deep within the brain called the brain stem; the CEREBELLUM; and the cerebrum.

The brain stem controls basic body functions like heart rate and breathing that are responsible for life and typically operates without any conscious control. It serves as a relay station, passing messages between various parts of the body and the cerebral cortex. It is made up of the midbrain, the medulla, and the pons. Right behind the brain stem is the small, apricot-sized cerebellum, responsible for controlling coordination and balance and for fine-tuning a person's motor activity, body movements, and the muscles used in speaking. The largest area of the brain is the cerebrum, whose four sections completely wrap around the midbrain. It is this area that handles conscious and complicated jobs like thinking, speaking, and reading.

The gray outer surface of the cerebrum, as wrinkled as a walnut, is the CEREBRAL CORTEX. It is in the cortex that sensory messages are received and interpreted, and where all the brain's orders are sent. The cerebral cortex is responsible for the higher mental functions, general movement perception, and behavioral reactions—all areas that may cause problems for people with autism. While its wrinkled surface does not take up much space within the skull, if it were flattened out the cerebral cortex would cover an average office desk.

Deep within the brain, in front of the brain stem, are a variety of structures of crucial importance in maintaining body functions, including the thalamus, hypothalamus, pituitary gland and basal ganglia. The basal ganglia is a gray mass deep in the cerebral hemisphere that serves as a connection between the cerebrum and cerebellum. It also helps regulate automatic movements.

The four lobes of the brain are broad surface regions in each hemisphere that are named for the bones of the skull lying above them: the frontal, parietal, temporal, and occipital lobes. The frontal lobe is considered to be the seat of a person's personality and the critical area for thought. Within the parietal lobe are areas that control the sensations of pain, itching, heat, and cold. It is the occipital lobe's job to interpret what a person sees. The temporal lobe contains the auditory cortex, which is responsible for hearing.

See also BRAIN AND AUTISM.

brain and autism   Scientists have only recently been able to study the brains of patients with autism with the emergence of new brain imaging tools, including computed tomography (CT), positron emission tomography (PET), single photon emission computed tomography (SPECT), and magnetic resonance imaging (MRI).

Postmortem and MRI studies have shown that many major brain structures are implicated in autism, including the cerebellum, CEREBRAL CORTEX, limbic system, corpus callosum, basal ganglia, and brain stem. The cerebral cortex is responsible for the higher mental functions, general movement perception, and behavioral reactions—all areas that may cause problems for people with autism. Other research is focusing on the role of neurotransmitters such as serotonin, dopamine, and epinephrine.

Recent neuroimaging studies have shown that a contributing cause for autism may be abnormal brain development beginning in the infant's first months. This "growth dysregulation hypothesis" holds that the anatomical abnormalities seen in autism are caused by genetic defects in brain growth factors. It is possible that sudden, rapid head growth in an infant may be an early warning signal that will lead to early diagnosis and effective biological intervention or possible prevention of autism.

See also BRAIN.

case history A record of a person's family, health, developmental, educational, psychological, and social experiences. Typically, the creation of a case history involves the analysis of records as well as interviews with parents, teachers, and the individual. Case histories are an important component of assessment in all cases of learning or psychological difficulty.

Center for the Study of Autism A center in Salem, Oregon, that provides information about autism to parents and professionals, and conducts research on the efficacy of various therapeutic interventions. The center collaborates extensively with the Autism Research Institute in San Diego, California.

For contact information, see APPENDIX I.

cerebellum A prominent hindbrain structure important for coordinating and integrating motor activity.

cerebral cortex The most complex area of the brain, the cerebral cortex is the convoluted covering of the two hemispheres also known as gray matter. The body's control and information processing center, it is organized into four lobes: frontal, parietal, occipital, and temporal, each concerned with different functions.

It is divided into two equal halves (or spheres) called hemispheres. The left hemisphere processes information logically; for example, it helps a person read, speak, and write language or compute an equation. The right hemisphere is responsible for more processing of spatial information, such as recognizing a friend's face or appreciating a piece of artwork.

Because the brain carries out many different functions, its cells are also specialized. Different types of neurons are distributed across different layers in the cortex in arrangements that characterize the several areas of the hemispheres, each one with its own functions.

The cerebral cortex represents in humans a highly developed structure concerned with the most familiar functions associated with the human brain, including intelligence and personality, interpretation of sensory impulses, movement, and the ability to plan and organize. Its distinctive shape arose during evolution as the volume of the cortex increased more rapidly than the cranial volume, so that the entire brain structure folded in onto itself.

Checklist for Autism in Toddlers (CHAT) A screening checklist used by general practitioners at the 18-month well-baby visit to identify children at risk for social-communication disorders such as autism. CHAT is based on the well-known behavioral characteristics of autism, and provides an inexpensive, quick, and easy-to-administer screening method. The test is a preliminary screening method whose results suggest either that autism is unlikely or possible (requiring further evaluation).

The CHAT, which was first published in 1992, takes only about five to ten minutes to administer and score. The short screening measure consists of two sections: the first nine items are questionnaire items filled out by parents, and the last five are observations made by a primary health care worker. Key items assess behaviors that, if absent at 18 months, put a child at risk for a social-communication disorder. These behaviors include joint attention, including "pointing to show," "gaze-monitoring" (such as looking in the direction a parent is looking) and pretend play (such as pretending to pour a beverage from a toy teapot).

There are five key items; children who fail all five key items have a high risk of developing autism; children who fail two items have a medium risk of developing autism. Any child who fails the CHAT should be screened again about a month later so that children who are just slightly delayed are given time to catch up. Any child who fails the CHAT for a second time should be referred to a specialist clinic for diagnosis.

If a child passes the CHAT the first time, no further testing is required, but passing the CHAT does not guarantee that a child will never develop a social-communication problem of some type. If the CHAT suggests autism is unlikely, it is still important to assess the at-risk child for other developmental or medical problems and continue regular periodic surveillance for problems.

chelation   A series of intravenous infusions containing a synthetic amino acid (EDTA) that will bind with metals and create a compound that can be excreted in the urine. Because some experts believe that autism may be linked with excess mercury or other metals, in theory once these metals are removed, their toxic effects are eliminated, and the individual with autism should begin to show improvement.

While chelation therapy has generated a great deal of publicity within the autism community, the overwhelming opinion of the traditional medical community is that it is an unproven therapy that should be avoided. Chelation is a controversial treatment for individuals with autism, with potential adverse effects.

It is not illegal for a physician to prescribe chelation therapy to treat autism, but without valid research studies, any treatment that has not been properly researched should be undertaken with a degree of skepticism.

Child Behavior Checklist   A type of behavioral questionnaire that contains a list of behavioral problems that are rated by the parent as "not true," "somewhat true," or "very true." Children are compared with others of the same age on anxiety, depression, hyperactivity, and so on. Because it is helpful on any behavior checklist to obtain input from teachers and parents, teacher forms are also available. Because each teacher and parent is likely to see the student from a different perspective, the best overall view of the child's behavior is obtained by comparing many different viewpoints.

Childhood Asperger Syndrome Test (CAST)   A preliminary screening for ASPERGER'S SYNDROME developed in the United Kingdom. Most Asperger's syndrome and high-functioning autism screening tools are designed for use with older children, and are used to differentiate these disorders from other AUTISM SPECTRUM DISORDERS or other developmental disorders such as MENTAL RETARDATION and language delays. Assessments for Asperger's concentrate on social and behavioral impairment in children four years of age and older—individuals who usually develop without significant language delay. These tests are quite different from assessments designed to be used to screen very young children, highlighting more social/conversational and behavioral concerns.

childhood autism rating scale (CARS)   A widely-used standardized test specifically designed to help diagnose autism with children as young as two years of age. It also can provide information about a child's ability level and learning style, and is used as a diagnostic tool for placing a child on the autistic spectrum.

The test was published in 1980 by Dr. Eric Schopler at the University of North Carolina and is intended to be a direct observational tool used by a trained clinician. It takes about 20 to 30 minutes to administer, and rates a child in 15 areas on a scale up to four, yielding a total up to 60.

The 15 items of the CARS include

- relationships with people
- imitation
- affect
- use of body

- relation to nonhuman objects
- adaptation to environmental change
- visual responsiveness
- auditory responsiveness
- near receptor responsiveness
- anxiety reaction
- verbal communication
- nonverbal communication
- activity level
- intellectual functioning
- general impression

A score of 15–29 is considered "non-autistic," a score of 30–36 is considered "autistic," and a score of 37–60 is considered "severely autistic."

The CARS may be useful as part of the assessment of children with possible autism in early intervention programs, preschool developmental programs, and developmental diagnostic centers. Most experts agree it seems to be practical and well researched, despite the limited research on its use in children under three years of age and the lack of separate norms for individuals of different ages.

Because it gives a symptom severity rating, the CARS may be useful for periodic monitoring of children with autism and for assessing long-term outcomes. It is very important that professionals using the CARS have experience in assessing children with autism and have adequate training in administering and interpreting the CARS.

CARS can help collect consistent information to help estimate the prevalence of autism and assess functional outcomes, especially if tied to other information about interventions and service delivery.

childhood disintegrative disorder (CDD) A rare yet serious condition in which a child older than age three stops developing normally and regresses to a much lower level of functioning, typically after a serious illness, such as an infection of the brain and nervous system. The disorder is associated with seizures and is more common in boys. Patients with the condition usually require lifelong care.

CDD was first described in 1908, many years before autism, but it has only recently been officially recognized. This condition resembles autism and appears only after a relatively prolonged period of clearly normal development (usually two to four years).

Although apparently rare, experts believe the condition probably has often been incorrectly diagnosed. Fewer than two children per 100,000 with AUTISM SPECTRUM DISORDER could be classified as having CDD.

Several different patterns of this condition have been identified. CDD may begin slowly or relentlessly. There may be progressive deterioration, developmental plateaus with little subsequent improvement, or—much less often—marked improvement.

The cause of childhood disintegrative disorder is unknown, but it has been linked to neurological problems.

Symptoms and Diagnostic Path
CDD occurs most often in boys, with symptoms typically appearing between ages three and four. Until this time, patients develop appropriate skills in communication and social relationships for their age. In fact, it is this long period of normal development before regression that helps differentiate CDD from AUSTIC DISORDER or RETT DISORDER.

Symptoms include extensive and pronounced losses in motor, language, and social skills, including loss of expressive or receptive language, nonverbal behavior, and play. In addition, the child develops difficulties in social interaction (failing to develop friendships and being unable to start or sustain a conversation) and begins performing repetitive behaviors similar to those that occur in children with autism. Quite often the child gradually deteriorates to a severely retarded level.

Once regression begins, the loss of skills such as vocabulary are more dramatic in CDD than they are in classical autism. CDD also is often accompanied by loss of bowel and bladder control, seizures, and a very low IQ.

A doctor makes the diagnosis based on the symptoms and by ruling out both childhood schizophrenia and other pervasive developmental disorder such as autistic disorder. The most important signs of CDD are previously normal development through age three to four and then, over a few months, a gradual loss of previously established abilities. Generally, the diagnosis is made with a loss of functioning in at least two areas, such as language, motor, or social skills.

Treatment Options and Outlook

Childhood disintegrative disorder cannot be specifically treated or cured, and most children, particularly those who are severely retarded, need lifelong care. Unfortunately, the prognosis for this disorder is limited. The loss of functioning will likely be permanent. However, to some degree, behaviors can be modified. The available data suggest that generally the prognosis for this condition is worse than that for autism.

child psychiatrist   A physician who specializes in the diagnosis and treatment of disorders of thinking, feeling, or behavior that affect children, adolescents, and their families. Child psychiatrists can prescribe medication.

To become a child psychiatrist, the student must complete four years of medical school, at least three years of residency training in medicine, neurology, and general psychiatry with adults, and two years of training in psychiatric work with children, adolescents, and their families in an accredited residency in child and adolescent psychiatry.

After completing medical school, graduates must pass a licensing test given by the board of medical examiners for the state in which they want to work. Psychiatrists must then take and pass the certifying examination given by the Board of Psychiatry and Neurology. (In order to be board-certified in child and adolescent psychiatry, a candidate must first be board-certified in general psychiatry.)

Children's Health Act of 2000   A law enacted in November 2000 that includes a lengthy list of provisions to improve the health of America's children, including establishment of the National Center on Birth Defects and Developmental Disabilities; legislation to improve newborn screening, boost autism research and pediatric research in general; and authorization of a national surveillance program designed to monitor maternal and infant health.

Autism Research and Surveillance

The act authorizes the expansion of federal research on autism. It establishes three regional centers, recognized for their excellence by the Centers for Disease Control and Prevention (CDC), to analyze information on autism and pervasive developmental disabilities, combining clinical and basic research in autism. The act increases spending on autism research from $15 million to more than $50 million per year for five years, and also provides a national physician awareness program. Additionally, it calls for establishing a program to provide information on autism to health professionals and the general public, and establishes a committee to coordinate all autism-related activities within the government.

The Children's Health Act of 2000 was responsible for the creation of the Interagency Autism Coordinating Committee (IACC), a committee that includes the directors of five NIH institutes—the National Institute of Mental Health, the National Institute of Neurological Disorders and Stroke, the National Institute on Deafness and Other Communication Disorders (NIDCD), the National Institute of Child Health and Human Development (NICHD), and the National Institute of Environmental Health Sciences (NIEHS)—as well as representatives from the Health Resource Services Administration, the National Center on Birth Defects and Developmental Disabilities (a part of the Centers for Disease Control), the Agency for Toxic Substances and Disease Registry, the Substance Abuse and Mental Health Services Administration, the Administration on Developmental Disabilities, the Centers for Medicare and Medicaid Services, the U.S. Food and Drug Administration, and the U.S. Department of Education.

The Committee, instructed by Congress to develop a 10-year agenda for autism research, introduced the plan at the first Autism Summit Conference in November 2003. The plan indicates priorities for research for years one to three, years four to six, and years seven to 10.

The five NIH institutes of the IACC have established the Studies to Advance Autism Research and Treatment (STAART) Network, composed of eight centers that will support research in the fields of developmental neurobiology, genetics, and psychopharmacology. Each center is pursuing its own particular mix of studies, but there also will be multi-site clinical trials within the STAART network. The STAART centers are located at University of North Carolina–Chapel Hill, Yale University, University of Washington, University of California–Los Angeles, Mount Sinai Medical School, Kennedy Krieger Institute, Boston University, and the University of Rochester.

A data coordination center will analyze the data generated by both the STAART network and the Collaborative Programs of Excellence in Autism (CPEA). This latter program, funded by the NICHD and the NIDCD Network on the Neurobiology and Genetics of Autism, consists of 10 sites. The CPEA is at present studying the world's largest group of well-diagnosed individuals with autism characterized by genetic and developmental profiles. The CPEA centers are located at Boston University, University of California–Davis, University of California–Irvine, UCLA, Yale, University of Washington, University of Rochester, University of Texas, University of Pittsburgh, and the University of Utah.

The NIEHS has programs at the Center for Childhood Neurotoxicology and Assessment, University of Medicine & Dentistry, and the Center for the Study of Environmental Factors in the Etiology of Autism, University of California–Davis.

child study committee A group of school members who review and decide plans of action for students. Typically, a student is referred to the child study committee because of concerns about school performance, either academic or behavioral. The committee usually consists of at least three people, including the school principal or a delegate, the teacher or teachers, and a special educator or school counselor. It also may include a school psychologist, speech/language pathologist, and/or other specialist.

citalopram An antidepressant drug that in proper dosages may be safe and well tolerated in treating children and adolescents with AUSTISM SPECTRUM DISORDERS (ASDs). Citalopram also may be appropriate for children and adolescents who have not responded adequately to other antidepressants of this type, especially for easing symptoms overlapping with obsessive-compulsive disorder, other anxiety disorders, or other mood disorders. However, controlled studies with larger numbers of children and adolescents with ASDs are necessary to more conclusively determine the safety and usefulness of this drug in treating ASD symptoms.

Citalopram belongs to a class of drugs called selective serotonin reuptake inhibitors (SSRIs)—such as Prozac—traditionally prescribed for depression. The SSRIs also have been shown to significantly improve some behavior problems associated with ASDs such as AUTISTIC DISORDER and ASPERGER'S SYNDROME.

In the nerve cell, serotonin sends messages to help regulate mood; SSRIs can boost the level of serotonin in people with abnormal levels of this chemical, which can ease depression and symptoms of PDDs.

Side Effects
Mild side effects might include headache, sedation, or agitation, which are not usually severe enough to make people stop taking the medication.

Clemons, Alonzo Prodigious AUTISTIC SAVANT who is a gifted sculptor living in Boulder, Colorado.

A head injury during childhood damaged his brain, changing the way he thought, learned, and communicated, but also triggering a fascination with modeling materials and a tremendous drive to sculpt. Even in situations where he did not have access to modeling clay, his determination to make models of animals was so strong that he found materials in his environment that he could use for sculpting.

Soon he was molding clay into amazingly detailed animal figures that he had never seen—yet Alonzo could not even feed himself or tie his shoes. Alonzo can see a fleeting image on a television screen of any animal and in less than 20 minutes sculpt a perfect replica of that animal in three-dimensional accuracy. The wax animal is correct in each and every detail—every fiber and muscle.

For more than 20 years he practiced his art in obscurity, until the early 1980s when the movie *Rain Man,* starring Dustin Hoffman as an autistic man with remarkable memory skills, brought international media attention to a phenomenon known as the SAVANT SYNDROME.

His world premier at the Driscol Gallery in Aspen, Colorado, featured 30 of Alonzo's bronze sculptures, portraying the progression from a rough and primitive style to smooth and elegant fine art. Critics believe his greatest work so far is a sculpture entitled "Three Frolicking Foals." The life-sized sculpture took just three weeks for Alonzo to create. Since his 1986 premiere exhibit, Alonzo continues to sculpt and move out into the world; he lives in his own apartment in Boulder, and he has a part-time job as housekeeper in Boulder at the YMCA. When not busy with those duties, he works out with weights and other equipment; he has shared his weight-lifting skills in the Special Olympics competition.

Gifted Hands, Inc. is now the official representative and contact point for information about Alonzo and his works.

clinical observation   The study and analysis of a child's behavior and performance in a clinical setting. This observation may involve analysis of behaviors during testing, mood and behavior during a clinical interview, or the observations of behavior in more open-ended assessment contexts, such as play in the case of young children. Clinical observation is an important component of assessment for autism.

clomipramine (Anafranil)   A tricyclic antidepressant sometimes used to treat people with autism. Although it has shown some positive effects in treating some of the behavior problems typical of autism, this compound is not prescribed often to patients with autism because it is often not well tolerated.

clonazepam (Klonopin)   A benzodiazepine drug used to treat epilepsy and other convulsive disorders, ease anxiety, and sometimes help individuals with autistic disorder who also have serious behavioral disturbances such as aggression or self-injury.

Clonazepam acts by influencing the action of the neurotransmitter GABA (gamma-aminobutyric acid), a chemical that ferries messages between brain nerve cells; GABA inhibits the transmission of nerve signals, thereby reducing nervous excitation.

With daily use for as briefly as four weeks, patients may develop tolerance so that larger doses of the drug are needed to achieve the same beneficial effects. Suddenly discontinuing the use of a medication such as clonazepam may cause hyperexcitability, which can lead to serious withdrawal symptoms such as convulsions, depression, hallucinations, restlessness, and sleeping problems.

clonidine (Catapres)   A drug that may be used to help manage behavior and induce sleep in patients with autism. The drug directly affects the brain by mimicking the action of an adrenaline-like chemical, which in turn triggers a drop in levels of other adrenaline-like chemicals in the brain (noradrenaline and serotonin). Because several studies have linked autism with neurochemical problems like this, drugs that act directly on these brain systems, such as clonidine, appear to decrease at least some of the aggressive, obsessive-compulsive, and self-stimulating behaviors associated with autism, according to controlled studies.

Unfortunately, there are no completely effective, reliable drugs for the primary symptoms of autism (such as problems with social situations, communication, language, and empathy). What drugs often can do is ease some of the secondary problems of autism, such as aggression, self-injury, agitation, mood instability, and hyperactivity.

There have not been many large-scale, controlled studies, but individual reports and small studies suggest that a variety of drugs may help at least some patients. In one small study, clonidine seemed to produce a calming effect in many of the nine patients, which improved their ability to interact socially and reduced inattention and repetitive behaviors. Patients had better social relationships and sensory responses, as measured by the REAL LIFE RATING SCALE, but no significant improvement in language and specific sensory motor behavior.

Side Effects

The most common side effect is low blood pressure, which could trigger a fainting episode if the person is anemic or gets tired or hot. Extra care should be used when combining this drug with another that also lowers blood pressure. Because of this blood pressure-lowering capability, patients who stop taking clonidine must do so slowly to avoid a spike in blood pressure; typically, the drug is slowly decreased over a two-week period.

In addition, patients taking clonidine were very tired and sedated during the first two weeks of treatment. (The sedation that this drug produces is often the reason this drug is prescribed, especially for autistic individuals with trouble falling asleep.)

Less common side effects include dry mouth, confusion, and depression.

cluster   An unusually large number of occurrences of a disease or condition in one place. In early 1999, an autism cluster was reported in Brick Township, New Jersey. The U.S. Centers for Disease Control and Prevention (CDC) and the Agency for Toxic Substance and Disease Registry responded to local calls for investigation after it was discovered that the town had about 40 cases among 6,000 children. An average occurrence would be about 20.4 cases per 6,000. In the suburban town of Granite Bay, California, about 30 miles east of Sacramento, 22 of the 2,930 children enrolled in grades K-6 are autistic. One would expect a typical incidence of just 10.2 cases in 3,000 children.

New Jersey parents attributed the cases of autism to the water and to a nearby landfill, but federal investigators never identified any pollutants. In Granite Bay, there seemed to be nothing that would indicate a problem. Some Brick Township officials counter that the numbers may be skewed because some families with autistic children moved to Brick for the school district's highly regarded program, one of the first in the state.

cognitive ability   A general term that refers to the broad cluster of mental skills involved in learning, thinking, and processing information.

Examples of cognitive abilities include memory, attention, language development, comprehension, production, problem-solving, critical analysis, and concept formation.

Although it is possible to generalize about the overall cognitive ability of a child, it is far more important and valuable to understand the ways in which specific cognitive functions interact and depend on one another and to assess strengths and difficulties in a more specific fashion.

Collaborative Programs of Excellence in Autism (CPEAs)   Programs that link 129 scientists from 23 universities in the United States, Canada, Britain, and five other countries with more than 2,000 families of people with autism. The CPEAs were originally included in an international Network on the Neurobiology and Genetics of Autism begun in 1997 by the National Institute of Child Health and Human Development (NICHD), in collaboration with the National Institute on Deafness and Other Communication Disorders (NIDCD). The CPEAs were designed to conduct research into possible causes of autism, including genetic, immunological, and environmental factors. In 2002, the NICHD and NIDCD renewed funding for the CPEA Network through 2007

Each site is studying a unique aspect of autism, but core information collected by CPEA sites in their individual studies can be combined and used to study broader research questions that no project could address alone. This shared data set may allow scientists to find similarities and differences among people with autism and their families that would not be possible through a single study. In fact, as a result of the CPEAs, researchers have now assembled a database on the genetics and outward characteristics of the largest group of well-diagnosed persons with autism in the world.

Currently, the CPEA Network sites in the United States include the following:

Boston University   Studies of social-communicative abilities in autism, language delays and problems in autism; and brain pathology underlying social-communicative and language impairments in autism, using structural and functional magnetic resonance imaging.

University of California, Davis Imitation and motor function in autism; measurement, predictors, course, causes, and external validity of regression in autism; and a longitudinal study of the developmental course of autism.

University of California, Los Angeles How social communication, and language deficits in autism start and develop; follow-up and extension of certain treatments for autism; phenotype and genotype in inversion and duplication of chromosome 15; and neuroimaging and deficits in social communication in autism.

University of Pittsburgh Organizing information into concepts in persons with high-functioning autism and Asperger's syndrome; visual perception and visual processing in persons with high-functioning autism and Asperger's syndrome; sensory, motor, and executive problems in persons with high-functioning autism and Asperger's syndrome; and functional brain imaging of language and cognition in persons with high-functioning autism and Asperger's syndrome. This research is done in conjunction with Carnegie-Mellon University and the University of Illinois, Chicago.

University of Rochester Medical Center Animal models and mechanisms of injury in autism; behaviors that distinguish autism from other disorders; and mutations in genes involved in early development and influences on gene function. This research is done in conjunction with the University of Rochester Medical Center's Departments of Pediatrics and Neurology, the Hospital for Sick Children (Toronto), Cornell Medical College, and the U.S. Environmental Protection Agency.

University of Utah Genetics and genetic susceptibility of autism; brain development; and serotonin function and immune system functioning in autism.

University of Washington The relationships between the brain and behavior in autism; language problems characteristic of autism; early diagnosis of autism and resulting outcomes; neuroimaging studies of autism; and the genetics of autism.

Yale University Genetics of persons with autism; the genetics of persons with autism and Asperger's syndrome, their families, and family members with related disorders; changes to the nervous system in autism; behavior problems, epilepsy, and puberty in adolescents with autism; and regression studies that seek to define the phenomena, predict outcomes, and evaluate medical factors that may play a role, such as vaccines, seizures, and prenatal conditions. This research is done in conjunction with the University of Michigan, the University of Chicago, and Harvard University.

Affiliated Programs

Two sites that are not currently CPEAs are affiliated with the Network.

University of California, Irvine Genes involved in autism; and brain structure and regression in autism.

University of Texas Health Science Center at Houston Development of communication and social behavior and its relationship to brain function in autism; abnormalities in brain structure related to autism; and animal studies of brain structure, injury, and behavior.

communication delay Speech and language patterns that develop at a slower pace than would be typically expected.

communication disorders A wide variety of problems in using speech and understanding language, including use of written, spoken, or symbol system affecting the function, form, and/or content of language. Autism is considered to be a communication disorder. Other communication disorders related to the AUTISM SPECTRUM DISORDERS include EXPRESSIVE LANGUAGE disorder, mixed receptive-expressive language disorder, phonological disorder, and dyspraxia.

The communication problems of people with autism vary, depending upon the person's intellectual and social development. Some may be unable to speak, and others may have rich vocabularies and are able to talk about many topics in great depth. Most people with autism have little or no problem with pronunciation; instead, most have problems effectively using language or have problems with word and sentence meaning, intonation, and rhythm.

Symptoms and Diagnostic Path

Those people with autism who *can* speak often say meaningless things. For example, an autistic individual may repeatedly count from one to ten or repeat scripted dialogue from a favorite video or things previously heard (called ECHOLALIA). One form of echolalia is called immediate echolalia, in which an autistic individual repeats whatever is said to him instead of answering the question. In delayed echolalia, an individual may say, "Do you want something to drink?" whenever he or she is asking for a drink, or may repeat phrases out of context.

Other communication problems involve using stock phrases, such as, "My name is Susan" to begin a conversation even with close friends or family. Some people simply repeat monologues or entire segments of commercials or shows they have heard on TV.

Some very bright autistic individuals may be able to speak in depth about topics in which they are interested, such as stop signs or railroads, but are unable to engage in an interactive conversation on those topics.

Many autistic individuals do not make eye contact, have poor attention spans, and do not use gestures either as a primary means of communication (such as with AMERICAN SIGN LANGUAGE) or to assist verbal communication (such as pointing to an object they want).

Some autistic individuals speak in a high-pitched voice or use robot-like speech and are often unresponsive to the speech of others. They may not respond to their own names. As a result, some autistic individuals are mistakenly diagnosed with a hearing problem.

The correct use of pronouns also may be a problem for autistic individuals. For example, if asked, "Are you wearing blue jeans today?" the individual may answer, "You are wearing blue jeans today," instead of, "Yes, I'm wearing blue jeans."

Of course, not all autistic individuals have impaired communication. Many do develop possibly uneven speech and language skills to some degree, although not to a normal ability level. For example, vocabulary development in areas of interest may be accelerated, and many individuals have good memories for recent information. Some people with autism may be able to read words well before the age of five but may not be able to under-

stand what is read. Others have musical talents or advanced ability to count and perform mathematical calculations. Approximately 10 percent show "savant" skills or detailed abilities in specific areas such as calendar calculation, musical ability, or math.

Treatment Options and Outlook

If a communication disorder is suspected, the child's physician will usually refer the child to a variety of specialists, including a speech-language pathologist, who performs a comprehensive evaluation of the child's ability to communicate and then designs and administers treatment.

There is not one general treatment method that improves communication in all individuals with autism. The best treatment begins early, during the preschool years, and is individually tailored, targeting both behavior and communication and involving parents or primary caregivers. The goal of therapy is to improve useful communication.

For some, working on verbal communication is a realistic goal; for others who are unable to reliably echo words or sounds said by others, functional communication is best obtained via gestures or using pictures. Sometimes teaching these forms facilitates the development of spoken speech. Some individuals with autism may remain dependent upon nonvocal forms of communication. Gestural communication may include informal gestures, such as pointing at desired things, shaking, or nodding one's hand. Alternatively, some individuals learn more complex communication using American Sign Language. Picture forms of communication may include pointing to symbols (such as a picture board) or a more complex system, such as Picture Exchange Communication System (PECS). The decision to use sign versus a pictural form of communication with nonvocal individuals usually depends on whether their motor imitation skills are stronger than their visual discrimination skills (in which case teaching gestures may be easier) or the reverse (in which case PECS or a similar system may be more successful).

Treatment should include periodic in-depth evaluations provided by an individual with special training in the evaluation and treatment of speech and language disorders, such as a speech-language pathologist. Psychologists and behavioral analysts also may work with the person to reduce unwanted behaviors that may interfere with the development of communication skills.

No medications have been found to specifically help communication in autistic individuals.

communications notebook A notebook sent with a student (typically a special education student or young student) to and from school by which parents and teachers maintain frequent, possibly daily, communication. Typically, this notebook details information about the student's behavior or progress during the day.

community care facility (CCF) A nonprofit health facility that provides 24-hour nonmedical residential care to children and adults with DEVELOPMENTAL DISABILITIES (such as autism) who are in need of personal services, supervision, and/or assistance essential for self-protection or to help with the ACTIVITIES OF DAILY LIVING.

confidential file In relation to SPECIAL EDUCATION, a confidential file is a limited access file maintained by the school that contains evaluations and any other information related to special education placement. Parents have the right to know the information contained in a confidential file and to have copies of any materials.

Connors Parent/Teacher Rating Scales–Revised These two types of behavioral questionnaires are checklists—one for parents, one for teachers—on which they can rate a variety of behavior problems on a four-point scale. Several versions of this scale are available; the 48-item parent scale and the 39-item teacher scale are both standardized. Because many of the items on the hyperactivity scale involve acting out and other annoying behaviors, this scale may not identify the child who exhibits attention deficits and HYPERACTIVITY but who is well socialized. Behavioral characteristics include

- antisocial activity
- anxiety
- conduct disorder
- disorganization
- hyperactivity
- learning problems
- obsessiveness
- psychosomatic ailments
- restlessness

In this version, the "Hyperactivity Index" had been renamed the Connors Global Index. It is included on the forms for teachers and parents.

constipation Difficulty or inability to have a bowel movement. Many children with autism have chronic constipation and/or diarrhea. (Diarrhea may actually be due to constipation—that is, only liquid is able to leak past a constipated stool mass in the intestine). Manual probing often fails to find an impaction. An endoscopy may be the only way to check for this problem. Consultation with a pediatric gastroenterologist is required.

controversies in autism Because autism is such a complex and poorly understood condition, there are many controversies surrounding ideas about its cause and treatment.

Autism as Disability
Well-adapted autistic people and autistic people who can function independently argue that rather than considering autism a disability, it might better be considered a different kind of personality. Critics argue that some severely autistic people cannot live independently and need constant supervision during the course of their lives.

Controversial Causes of Autism
Most experts agree that there appears to be some type of brain problem underlying autism, with a likely strong genetic component, and that there may be some type of interaction with environmental factors. However, beyond that basic consensus,

experts disagree about many of the more specific causes of autism. Among some of the more controversial theories of autism are

- vaccinations
- food allergies
- mineral or vitamin deficiencies
- immune system problems
- YEAST overgrowth
- oral antibiotics
- prenatal exposure to mercury or other toxic substances
- pesticides and environmental toxins
- prenatal or birth trauma

Generally, experts agree that some individuals appear to have a genetic predisposition for autism and believe that there may be some type of interaction with environmental factors.

Treatment Controversies

There are several well-developed and widely used approaches to the treatment of autism, including basic behavioral approaches and lots of one-on-one FLOOR TIME. Beyond that basic philosophy, there are a host of specific treatments. Each of these methods have their own supporters and critics, and universal agreement on the most effective treatments has not been reached. Some approaches that are considered to be more controversial by at least some experts include

- SENSORY INTEGRATION therapy
- AUDITORY INTEGRATION TRAINING
- dietary interventions
- mineral and vitamin supplements
- visual treaments and IRLEN LENSES
- FACILITATED COMMUNICATION

Aversives to Manage Behavior

While it is important to deal with atypical behaviors that can be dangerous, the risk of aversives is the fact that they can be misused. Generally, AVERSIVE TECHNIQUES should be the treatment of last resort used to address very severe behavior problems that,

if untreated, may cause harm to the patient or others. Some people with autism engage in dangerous behaviors (such as repeatedly striking their head with enough force to cause injury). Some would be able to function more freely in society if they are taught how to manage their own behavior, and some people believe these benefits are worth the use of aversives.

Critics argue that aversive methods are never helpful, and that if such methods are allowed, aversives will be abused and that someone, somewhere could overuse the methods. Critics also insist that other methods achieve the goals as well or better.

corporal punishment Any intervention designed to or likely to cause physical pain with intention to stop or change behavior. In the United States, the most typical form of school corporal punishment is the striking of a student's buttocks with a wooden paddle by a school authority because the student disobeyed a rule. More than half of all states ban the use of corporal punishment in schools because of its harmful physical, educational, psychological, and social effects on students. In states where it is allowed, many school boards voluntarily prohibit it. Still, almost a half million children are being hit each year in public schools, a disproportionate number being minority children and children with disabilities.

The use of corporal punishment has been declining in U.S. schools because of waning public acceptance, increased litigation against school boards and educators, and legal bans. Corporal punishment is a technique that can easily be abused and lead to physical injuries.

Most experts agree that corporal punishment contributes to the cycle of child abuse and pro-violence attitudes of youth by teaching that it is an acceptable way of controlling the behavior of others. While discipline is important, effective alternatives are available to help students develop self-discipline. Such alterntives include programs and strategies for changing student behavior, for changing school or classroom environments, and for educating and supporting teachers and parents. Alternatives for changing student behavior include, but are not limited to

- helping students achieve academic success by identifying academic and behavioral problems and strengths
- behavioral contracting
- positive reinforcement of appropriate behavior
- individual and group counseling
- disciplinary consequences that are meaningful to students and have an instructional or reflection component
- social skills training

cow's milk allergy   See ALLERGY TO COW'S MILK.

craniosacral therapy   An alternative treatment for children with AUTISTIC DISORDER that involves a gentle hands-on approach. Proponents claim that the therapy helps improve central nervous system function, dissolve the effects of stress, and strengthen the immune system.

During the hour-long treatment, the osteopathic physician places the hands on the patient's neck, feet, jaws, and sacrum, identifying areas of restriction, compression, or tension through the body, which may in turn be impeding function of organs, muscles, nerves, blood vessels, and body tissues.

Treatment is generally soothing, comforting and pleasant and creates a sense of ease, calmness, and well-being. Babies can be treated while cradled in the mother's arms or while asleep.

The treatment was developed at the beginning of the 20th century by osteopathic physician Wil-liam Sutherland and further developed by osteo-path John E. Upledger in the 1970s.

cross-categorical   A system for grouping students with disabilities. Cross-categorical grouping places students with different kinds of disabilities into the same instructional setting at the same time.

Crossley, Rosemary   Australian speech therapist and author who developed the method of FACILI-TATED COMMUNICATION. Through intensive work with institutionalized girls and women with severe communication disorders, Crossley discovered a way to support their communication using a combination of keyboards, letterboards, and physical support, usually at the hand, wrist, elbow, or shoulder. The results were considered to be groundbreaking, as the girls and women learned to read and write contrary to all expectations.

However, more recent studies of facilitated communication have shown that the person helping the autistic individual actually inadvertently directs the communication. The American Psychological Association and the American Academy of Pediatrics both issued a policy statement calling the method discredited and noting there is no scientifically demonstrated support for the method.

cumulative file   The general file containing all the educational records and information maintained for any child enrolled in school. Parents have a legal right to inspect the file and have copies of any information contained in it.

daily life therapy A type of treatment for autism combining physical education, art, music, and academics with development of communication and daily living skills to promote social independence, imported from Japan in 1987. The therapy, which is taught at the BOSTON HIGASHI SCHOOL, is an educational approach designed to foster independence for children who tend to be socially isolated; it is not a specific therapeutic treatment for children with autism but an educational methodology for all children.

"Seikatsu Ryouhou" was developed by the late Dr. Kiyo Kitahara nearly 38 years ago, based on her experience teaching an autistic child in her regular kindergarten class. Recognizing that children with autism tend to be socially isolated, developmentally delicate, and often anxious, sensitive, and fragile, Kitahara developed a unique educational approach to address these characteristics. Her educational philosophy is characterized by respect and love, offering a set of practices intended to dilute, rather than exaggerate, the autistic child's sense of deficit and difference. This educational holistic approach is based on bonding between child and teacher and is not designed as a set of techniques to eliminate the behaviors of autistic children.

The primary focus of this therapy is to stabilize emotions by strengthening independent living and self-esteem. Children learn to dress themselves, to eat properly, and to use the bathroom independently. Through the mastery of self-care skills, children develop self-confidence and are encouraged to try other adaptive skills.

Kitahara also believed that the key to social development was extensive physical exercise that would release endorphins as natural inhibitors of anxiety and reduce aggression, self-stimulatory behavior, and hyperactivity, as well as increase on-task behavior and minimize periods of wakefulness at night. Through physical education, children gain control of their bodies and consequently of their behavior. Children learn to ride the unicycle, to roller-skate, and to master the balance disk and various Higashi exercises. Through play and physical education, children develop self-control and learn to cooperate and coordinate activities and exercises with other children.

Instruction is another important part of daily life therapy, focusing on a whole language approach to language arts. The whole language approach is an educational philosophy that describes language learning as a natural outgrowth of a process integrating speaking, listening, reading, and writing. The whole language approach emphasizes that reading is closely linked to spoken language, so students are exposed to language-rich classrooms to help make them better readers and writers. Instruction is also given in mathematics and social sciences, with special attention to a child's own interests. Special subjects, including art and music, can help develop creativity, enabling autistic children to express themselves through painting, drawing, and musical performance. Elementary children at Higashi learn to play the keyboard harmonica and the violin. The alto recorder is taught to middle school and high school students, some of whom also participate in a jazz band. Children learn age-appropriate songs, and are encouraged to vocalize sounds or words to the music.

Aversive measures, punishment, medication, or time-out procedures are never used to change behavior. Neither psychotropic medication or medication for behavior control is used. Instead, the method emphasizes concentration on the child's strengths rather than the undesirable behavior.

Kitahara was convinced that autistic children must be given age-appropriate activities and intellectual stimulation and that they can express feelings and harbor academic potential similar to those of more typical children.

Modeling and imitating peers helps each child develop appropriate behaviors and encourages interaction between students. Clear directions for correct posture and eye contact are emphasized, and verbal and physical prompts are given for alternate, incompatible behaviors. Consistency and follow-through by all staff members clarifies expectations, sets limits, and provides redirection. Verbal and nonverbal cues are given in a concise, uniform way, creating a predictable and secure environment for the students.

The curriculum emphasizes social relationships, and many opportunities to practice skills are provided throughout the day and are integrated into a predictable and structured routine.

Initial guidance focuses on reducing the child's exclusivity of food choices and improving sleeping patterns—both of which are important in normalizing family life.

From early childhood, all students are given chores and responsibilities; careers and functional academics are emphasized for middle school and high school students in order to promote independence. Students at Boston Higashi participate in a variety of vocational activities including clerical, custodial, and food service to enable them to develop good work habits and learn to work independently. Employment education is practiced in both the school and community work settings and is always set in the actual work environment rather than the classroom.

Daily life therapy stresses that education should be conducted in an environment of normality. In the Tokyo program, the format is a mixed educational setting with children of all types of ability; in the Boston program, some children are included in mainstream classrooms with typical age peers. The goal of Boston Higashi School is lifelong inclusion in the community.

DAN!   See DEFEAT AUTISM NOW!

DeBlois, Tony (1975–) A prodigious musical savant who is blind and autistic with a spectacular musical gift, who specializes in jazz. The Randolph, Massachusetts, native was born prematurely (one lb. ¾ oz.), and began playing the piano at age two, when his mother bought him a $10 chord organ at a garage sale.

Within weeks, he was tapping out a few notes from "Twinkle, Twinkle, Little Star," and by age three, he played harmony to Lawrence Welk. At five, the year he began piano lessons and was diagnosed as autistic, his mother began to use music to influence his behavior. When DeBlois answered a question correctly, she would play his favorite song ("Dueling Banjos").

As with all autistic savants, DeBlois has severe deficits in addition to his gifts, especially in motor skills. He was taught how to play the violin because the motion would teach him how to brush his teeth and was given lessons on the drum because the motion helped him learn to brush his hair. It was not until he was 26 that he learned how to manipulate the buttons on his pajamas and, a year later, the small buttons on his tuxedo. He was slow in verbal skills and at 16 was still unable to carry on a conversation.

He enrolled at the Perkins School for the Blind in Massachusetts, but the only type of music he was able to study there was classical. In order to study jazz piano, he enrolled in jazz classes at the Rivers School, a private preparatory school in Weston. When the prestigious Berklee College of Music in Boston asked Rivers to select one of its students for a $1,000 scholarship to Berklee, Rivers chose DeBlois. Impressed with the boy's work during the summer session, Berklee invited him to return full time. DeBlois graduated magna cum laude from the Berklee College of Music, in Boston, on Mother's Day, 1996.

Even among savants, his skill is remarkable. Most musical savants have an incredible ability to duplicate what they hear. What distinguishes DeBlois is his capacity to improvise, especially in jazz. And while most musical savants are limited to a specific instrument (typically the piano), DeBlois has learned many instruments and plays them well.

Besides piano, DeBlois plays as many as 20 other musical instruments, 12 of them proficiently, including organ, harmonica, guitar, harpsichord,

English handbells, violin, banjo, drums, trumpet, saxophone, clarinet, ukulele, mandolin, and flute. Although his special emphasis is in jazz, he also plays many other musical styles ranging from country to classic. He can sing in German, French, Spanish, and Taiwanese, among other languages.

When not playing musical instruments, he enjoys swimming, exercise equipment, the computer, and ballroom dancing.

DeBlois was the subject of the 1997 CBS TV movie *Journey of the Heart,* inspired by actual events in his life. He has appeared on a variety of TV and radio shows exploring the SAVANT SYNDROME, received a number of awards, including the Foundation for Exceptional Children's "Yes, I Can" Award, and has performed in concert in Singapore, Taiwan, and Ireland.

Defeat Autism Now! (DAN!) A treatment approach for autism that features nutritional support, diet changes, and detoxification aimed at addressing core problems of autism rather than symptoms. Some of the major interventions suggested by DAN! practitioners include

- nutritional supplements, including certain vitamins, minerals, amino acids, and essential fatty acids
- special diets totally free of gluten (from wheat, barley, rye, and possibly oats) and free of dairy (milk, ice cream, yogurt, and so on)
- testing for hidden food allergies, and avoidance of allergenic foods
- treatment of intestinal bacterial/yeast overgrowth
- detoxification of heavy metals

desipramine (Norpramin, Pertofrane) A tricyclic antidepressant used in some patients with autism to treat hyperactivity, inattention, and impulsivity.

Side Effects

Common side effects include upset stomach, drowsiness, weakness or tiredness, excitement or anxiety, insomnia, nightmares, dry mouth, sensitivity to sunlight, and appetite or weight changes.

Less common side effects include constipation, difficulty with or frequent urination, blurred vision, changes in sex drive or ability, and excessive sweating. Rarely, severe side effects may include jaw, neck, and back muscle spasms, slow or difficult speech, shuffling walk, persistent fine tremor or inability to sit still, fever, difficulty breathing or swallowing, severe skin rash, yellowing of the skin or eyes, or irregular heartbeat.

developmental disability A legal term used to describe an entire group of conditions that challenge a person's ability to learn and function independently. The term was coined in the 1970s for the purpose of policy planning and federal funding, and government programs addressing these disabilities became the first agencies to use the term.

Although eventually the term "developmental disability" often was used interchangeably with "MENTAL RETARDATION," the legal definition of "developmental disability" includes AUTISTIC DISORDER as well as cerebral palsy, epilepsy, and mental retardation. A developmental disability must occur before age 21 in order to meet the federal definition and qualify a person for special education services, Supplemental Security Income, and Medicaid.

Many governmental and insurance regulations note a difference between services for developmental disabilities and those for mental illness.

developmental expressive language disorder A disorder in which a child has lower-than-normal proficiency for his or her age in using language, such as with vocabulary, the production of complex sentences, and recall of words.

developmentally appropriate practice (DAP) A set of guidelines ensuring that educational programs are appropriate for each child's age and developmental stage. The guidelines were recommended by the National Association for the Education of Young Children (NAEYC) in the early 1990s, requiring that early education programs be child-centered and child-directed, with little effort to explicitly teach specific skills.

Developmentally appropriate practice has been debated by special educators who believe that early intervention and direct skill instruction is essential to help children with learning disabilities address their learning needs. They argue that by refraining from direct teaching, the gap between delayed children's abilities and their same-age peers grows larger rather than narrower.

Dexedrine   See DEXTROAMPHETAMINE.

dextroamphetamine (Dexedrine)   Stimulant medication used to treat people with attention deficit hyperactivity disorder (ADHD) and also sometimes used to treat individuals with autism, especially those with hyperactivity and poor attention span. These drugs work by increasing the person's ability to concentrate and pay attention and by reducing impulsivity and hyperactivity.

Side Effects

Side effects include palpitation, fast heart rate, high blood pressure, overstimulation, restlessness, dizziness, insomnia, high or low mood, tremor, headache, exacerbation of tics, TOURETTE SYNDROME, and psychotic episodes (rare at recommended doses). Other symptoms include dry mouth, unpleasant taste, diarrhea, constipation, and other gastrointestinal disturbances. Appetite and weight loss may also occur, as may impotence or changes in libido.

See also DEXTROAMPHETAMINE/AMPHETAMINE (ADDERALL).

dextroamphetamine/amphetamine (Adderall)   A stimulant medication that may be prescribed for children with autism as a way of increasing focus and decreasing impulsivity and hyperactivity in high-functioning patients. Adderall XR is a long-acting form of this stimulant that can be given just once a day, so that patients do not have to take a dose at noon. Adderall XR usually lasts 10 to 12 hours.

Side Effects

Side effects are often dose related and include appetite loss, insomnia, abdominal pain, high blood pressure, nervousness, and rapid heart beat. The prescribing information for Adderall XR in the United States was revised in August 2004 to add a warning about sudden death and heart risks. Before the update on Adderall XR's prescribing information, the medication already carried the strongest Food and Drug Administration warning, highlighted in a black box, that amphetamines "have a high potential for abuse" and "should be prescribed or dispensed sparingly." Separate warnings on the label caution against use during pregnancy or while breast-feeding.

Diagnostic and Statistical Manual of Mental Disorders–Fourth Edition, Text Revision (DSM-IV-TR)   The basis for all psychiatric classification, this diagnostic manual is published by the American Psychiatric Association (APA) and used by most practicing clinicians and insurance companies in the United States. Organized by categories of disorders, the text also provides diagnostic criteria and associated disorders for each listing. The first edition was published in 1952; the fourth edition was published in 1994, significantly updating and adding listings from previous editions.

The APA continues to update the *DSM* about every decade. The most recent update is the *DSM-IV-TR*; in this update, the most important material remains the same as in the previous version. The only things that have changed substantially are the text accompanying the diagnoses and some parts of the introduction and appendixes.

In order for a diagnosis to be made, the individual's behavior must match the criteria listed for a specific disorder in *DSM-IV-TR*. One criticism of the *DSM* is that there are no separate categories or criteria for the diagnosis of children. While the behavior may be slightly different, which is typically noted, children are essentially diagnosed using the same criteria as are used with adults. In addition, because a diagnosis from the *DSM* is typically required for health insurance coverage, some critics suggest that individuals, particularly children, may be prematurely diagnosed with serious disorders.

The *DSM-IV-TR* can be used for many purposes: as a source of diagnostic information to enhance clinical practice, research, and education; and to communicate diagnostic information to others.

Each revision of the *DSM* is the result of a systematic, comprehensive review of the psychiatric literature, and contains the most up-to-date information available to assist the clinician in making a differential diagnosis.

diarrhea   Many autistic children have chronic diarrhea, which actually may be caused by chronic CONSTIPATION as a result of only liquids that can leak past a constipated stool mass in the intestine. In this case of diarrhea related to constipation, manual probing often fails to find an impaction. An endoscopy may be the only way to check for this problem. Consultation with a pediatric gastroenterologist is required.

dietary interventions   Although most experts agree that autism is not caused by diet, individuals with autism may exhibit low tolerance of or allergies to certain foods or chemicals. While not a specific cause of autism, these food intolerances or allergies may contribute to behavioral problems. Some parents have reported significant changes when specific substances are eliminated from the child's diet.

Individuals with autism may have trouble digesting certain proteins such as gluten or casein. Preliminary research in the United States and England has found higher levels of certain peptides in the urine of children with autism, suggesting their bodies are not completely breaking down peptides from foods that contain gluten (found in the seeds of various cereal plants, such as wheat, oats, barley, and rye) and casein (the principal protein found in milk and dairy products). The incomplete breakdown and the excessive absorption of peptides may disrupt brain function. Professionals and parents conclude that until scientists discover why these proteins are not broken down, removing proteins from the diet is the only way to prevent further brain and gastrointestinal damage.

However, experts caution that it is important not to withdraw gluten or casein food products from a child's diet all at once, which could cause withdrawal symptoms. Eliminating such foods from the diet should therefore be done with the advice of a health care practitioner. Since gluten and casein are found in many common foods, following a gluten-free, casein-free diet is not easy. Parents who are interested in providing this type of diet to their child with autism should consult a gastroenterologist or nutritionist to help design a healthy diet plan.

See also VITAMINS AND AUTISM.

differential diagnosis   A systematic method of diagnosing a disorder that lacks unique symptoms or signs. There are a number of other conditions that may sometimes be confused with autism, which is why a careful diagnostic workup must be performed. Conditions that cause symptoms similar to autism include ASPERGER'S SYNDROME, CHILDHOOD DISINTEGRATIVE DISORDER, RETT DISORDER, PERVASIVE DEVELOPMENT DISORDER–NOT OTHERWISE SPECIFIED (PDD-NOS), childhood psychoses (such as schizophrenia), FRAGILE X SYNDROME, hearing loss, and metabolic disorders.

A number of tests can rule out some of these conditions. For example, blood tests can rule out metabolic disorders that affect amino acids and lipids in the blood, and chromosomal analysis can rule out some genetic disorders. A comprehensive hearing test can rule out deafness as the cause of abnormal language development, while an electroencephalogram (EEG) can rule out a seizure disorder. A magnetic resonance imaging (MRI) scan can rule out brain disorders.

discrete trial training   An instructional method, often used as part of APPLIED BEHAVIOR ANALYSIS (ABA) programs, that is based on principles of learning theory demonstrated to be an effective intervention for autism.

The discrete trial training method is used to control the mass of information and interaction that normally confronts a child with autism so that it can be presented slowly. This control manages learning opportunities so that learning occurs in small steps and skills are more easily mastered by the child. Skills are arranged from simple to complex. In this method, every task given to the child consists of a request to perform a specific action, a response from the child, and a reaction from the therapist. The therapist does not just correct behaviors, but also teaches skills from basics such as toileting and dressing to more involved activities such as social interaction. Discrete trial training is usually used as part of an intensive behavioral therapy approach.

Simple skills must be mastered before new learning opportunities are presented, in which the child then builds upon the mastered skill toward a more complex one. Learning opportunities are presented in a "training trial" format, and each training trial— no matter what the skill being taught— consists of four major components:

1. The teacher or therapist presents a brief, distinctive instruction or question (stimulus).
2. The instruction is followed by a prompt if the child needs one, to elicit the correct response and to make sure the child is successful. Initially, prompts may be complete hand-over-hand assistance, but, gradually, prompts are slowly stopped until the child is able to be independently successful.
3. The child responds either successfully in an independent fashion or with the help of some level of prompting. In some cases of tasks that seem to have been mastered, the child may be allowed to respond incorrectly (response).
4. The teacher or therapist provides an appropriate "consequence" using a process of differential reinforcement: correct responses that are performed independently earn the highest level of reward, which may be an edible treat, a toy, hugs or praise, depending on the child's current level of learning. Partially prompted successful responses may earn less reinforcement. Incorrect responses are usually ignored or corrected.

Discrete trial training begins with two main goals: teaching learning readiness skills, such as sitting in a chair and paying attention, and decreasing behaviors that interfere with learning, such as tantrums and aggression. In addition, the basic rules of social interaction are established. Children are taught how to learn from the environment through the introduction of clear stimulus-response-reward cycles. Once the child has learned to sit quietly and

pay attention, more complex skills such as social behavior and communication can be taught.

Social skills training begins with eye contact, and moves toward imitation, observational learning, expressive affection, and social play. Communication skills usually start with receptive object labels and progress to expressive verbal language, followed by spontaneous communication.

However, discrete trial training is insufficient to teach children to initiate behavior. Therefore, most behavioral programs also include "mand" training. This involves teaching the child to make expressive demands so that the child will learn that functional language results in getting something the child wants. *Mand* is a word coined by B. F. Skinner in his book, *Verbal Behavior*, in which he discussed the different functions of verbal behavior (including nonvocal communication such as sign and picture symbols). For example, he maintains that saying "juice" when one wants a drink of juice (mand) is a very different behavior than saying "juice" after a teacher points to a glass of juice and says: "What is this?" It is yet another skill to say "juice" after a teacher says: "What is something we drink?" Autistic children may learn to say "juice" in response to one situation but not others. Therefore, all functions may need to be specifically taught in the context of natural environmental teaching and discrete trial teaching.

Generalization training then moves the drills into more natural environments. Children with autism often do not spontaneously learn from their environment and some may need to be taught virtually everything they are expected to learn. Therefore, as part of a broader applied behavior analysis intervention, discrete trials target numerous goals and objectives.

As a result, an effective ABA intervention requires many hours of child/therapist sessions—at least 30 (40 are better) hours a week, seven days a week, for at least two years. Young autistic children who received less intensive treatment made some modest gains, but normal or near-normal functioning was achieved reliably only when treatment was provided for 30 to 40 hours a week for at least two years.

However, discrete trial training represents only one of dozens of teaching strategies within the field of ABA. For example, other methods of teaching used within ABA-based programs include PECS (picture exchange communication system), photo activity schedules, chaining, shaping, graduated guidance, and functional communication training.

Division TEACCH   The primary goal of the TEACCH program is to help people with autism to live or work more effectively at home, at school, and in the community by reducing or removing autistic behaviors.

A program began in 1966 at the University of North Carolina as a child research project to provide services to children with autism and their families. Today, TEACCH the acronym for "Treatment and Education of Autistic and related Communication-handicapped Children," provides a wide range of services to a broad spectrum of toddlers, children, adolescents, and their families, including diagnosis and assessment, individualized treatment programs, special education, social skills and job training, and parent training and counseling. TEACCH also maintains an active research program and provides training for professionals.

TEACCH uses many basic principles from the field of ABA, although it does not typically involve the same level of data collection to monitor progress or try to achieve as intensive of an approach as most ABA programs.

dolphin-assisted therapy (DAT)   A controversial therapeutic approach used to increase speech and motor skills in children and adults who have been diagnosed with developmental, physical, and/or emotional disabilities, such as AUTISTIC DISORDER. Those who support this theory believe that when a child with autism interacts with a dolphin, the interaction increases the child's attention span.

Dolphin therapy began in 1978 following research by David Nathanson, Ph.D., a PSYCHOLO-GIST specializing in therapy for children with special needs. Nathanson explained that the key to learning is to increase sensory attention so that increased learning will occur. Children with autism have trouble paying attention, so therefore they have difficulty learning. Nathanson developed a series of carefully controlled experiments using dolphins

and children with Down syndrome, and found that the children learned four times faster when they were rewarded with being in the water with the dolphins. Essentially, this constitutes principles of ABA: when the child performs a desired action, he or she gets to interact with the dolphin.

There are several different programs providing dolphin therapy, including the Full Circle Program at the Clearwater Marine Aquarium in Clearwater, Florida, where, in addition to behavior modification (requesting the child to perform a task and then giving a reward of dolphin time), the program also allows the children to participate in preparing the dolphins' food, feeding them, observing, interacting during training sessions, and giving rubs. With the new skills that the children learn in the program, the therapists claim that the children develop positive self-esteem and empowerment in all areas of their lives.

Another program offered by the Human Dolphin Institute in Panama City Beach, Florida, focuses on child empowerment, in which children are introduced to wild dolphins. This interaction is said to empower children by enhancing their intellectual, emotional, and physical well-being and improving learning abilities and communication skills. Aside from actual contact with the dolphins, this program also includes swimming and snorkeling lessons, proper etiquette during dolphin encounters, ocean field trips, expressive arts (dance, music, breathing, drawing), and helping the children use the newly acquired skills and abilities.

What Critics Say

Critics of DAT argue that dolphin therapy does not help the child with special needs any more than would interaction with any other service animals, such as dogs and horses. Such critics say that time spent with any kind and gentle animal can break through the child's barrier and provide successful results.

Some proponents of DAT counter that when a dolphin interacts with a human, it triggers a greater harmony between the left and right sides of the human brain, which they believe is caused by the dolphin's sonar (the ability to transmit sound waves to locate objects in front of them). Further, the medical director of Convimar at Mexico City's Aragon

Aquarium claims that dolphins seem to be able to sense problem areas in the brains of children using their sonar. They somehow see the damage and emit the appropriate frequency to help heal them. Mexican experts at the aquarium claim that 90 percent of clients show significant improvement.

However, critics counter that it is unlikely that dolphins could target any particular area of a person's brain with sonar. Any success with the dolphin experiments could be more likely caused by the opportunity to interact with dolphins, which they say could probably be replicated by giving the patients a puppy.

Most programs are five to six days long, and the cost can range anywhere from $2,000 to $6,000. Although dolphin-assisted therapy may help those children who respond positively to animals, it is not a miracle cure and parents should be cautious about any organization that claims otherwise.

Most experts believe there is no scientific evidence at all that using dolphins is helpful.

Down syndrome   As many as 10 percent of children diagnosed with Down syndrome also have autism. Although experts believe that autism only rarely occurs in children with Down syndrome, it may be more common in those persons with Down syndrome who also show superimposed behavioral problems.

However, many dual diagnoses may go undiagnosed, since many doctors are unaware that the two conditions may coexist. Autism is a much more complicated condition to diagnose than is Down syndrome; there are no blood tests, genetic markers, facial features, or other characteristics that apply to all autistic persons. Instead, the diagnosis is subjective, based on observations of certain behaviors. At the same time, diagnosis and treatment of autism is much more critical than for Down syndrome, because without early detection and intervention, the autistic person's life may be much more limited than would that of a person with Down syndrome.

Most infants with Down syndrome have fewer problems with social and emotional development, smiling when talked to at two months of age, smiling spontaneously at three months, and recognizing parents at three and a half months; each of

these milestones show only about a one-month delay. However, some studies do suggest that smiling and laughing may be slightly less intense than for healthy babies.

Babies with Down syndrome begin to enjoy patty-cake and peekaboo games at about 11 months, which is about three months later than for healthy babies. Studies in the second year of life show the babies to be skilled in social communication—warm, cuddly, and normally responsive to physical contact, unlike babies with autism. This normal emotional responsiveness continues into adult life, and as studies of teenagers have shown, it develops into proper empathy, making the person with Down syndrome a sensitive and socially aware person.

A child with Down syndrome suspected of having a complicating behavior disorder such as autism will not show these normal behaviors in the social and emotional areas. Some of the primary behavior that may suggest the possibility of autism in a child with Down syndrome include

- extreme isolation: The child does not relate to people normally and prefers to be left alone, refusing to join in group play with other children. Unlike children with Down syndrome, who are very lovable and huggable, the autistic child does not want to be held.

- anxious obsessive desire for the preservation of sameness: Any differences in daily routines can cause a breakdown.

- lack of eye contact: Autistic persons may not often make eye contact but will look away or stare through others.

- stereotypical movement: repetitive movements, such as flapping hands or waving a toy back and forth

Because some of the above characteristics (especially stereotyped behaviors) are normal for a child with Down syndrome, the diagnosis of autism is more difficult in these children. There are a number of reasons why cases of autism in children with Down syndrome are not reported.

One problem is that autism must be diagnosed before age three. One reason is that parents of a young child with Down syndrome tend to be concerned with its possible medical complications; developmental delays are expected, so it does not occur to parents or professionals to consider autism. Only when the child becomes older may it become clear that autism is also present.

Duane syndrome   A rare disorder that causes unusual eye movement problems and that sometimes occurs in people with autism. The gene that is involved with Duane Syndrome (HOXD1 gene) also has been linked to autism.

Although the condition was originally thought to be due to fibrosis of one of the eye muscles, today experts have realized that it is caused by lack of development of the control center of the sixth nerve in the brain. Interestingly, most of these patients do not have double vision when looking to the side.

Symptoms and Diagnostic Path

This disorder, present at birth, is characterized by a limited ability to move the eye inward toward the nose, outward toward the ear, or in both directions. In addition, when the affected eye moves inward toward the nose, the eyeball retracts and the eye opening narrows. In some cases, when the eye attempts to look inward, it moves upward or downward.

Treatment Options and Outlook

Surgery should not be performed unless there is a cosmetic problem when looking straight ahead. A simpler solution is to wear special glasses with prisms to eliminate the head turn.

dyspraxia   See APRAXIA.

early childhood assessment Testing that identifies early developmental and learning problems in preschool and primary grade children. Early childhood assessment practices allow for accurate and fair identification of the developmental needs of infants, preschoolers, and young children.

Sound early childhood assessment should involve a multidisciplinary team, including school psychologists with specialized training in the assessment of the young child who view behavior and development from a longitudinal perspective.

Early assessment of potential problems is essential because of a child's broad and rapid development. Intervention services for any psychological and developmental problems are essential and cost-effective.

Standardized assessment procedures should be used with great caution in educational decision-making because such tools are inherently less accurate when used with young children. Multidisciplinary team assessments must include multiple sources of information, multiple approaches to assessment, and multiple settings in order to yield a comprehensive understanding of children's skills and needs. Therefore, assessments should center on the child in the family system and home environment, both substantial influences on the development of young children.

early intervention program A program designed to identify and provide intervention for infants and young children who are developmentally delayed and at high risk for school failure. The purpose of this type of program is to help prevent problems as the child matures.

These programs address the needs of young children from birth to the beginning of school, with a collaborative effort from parents and medical, social services, and educational professionals. The pre-academic skills that may need help include self concept, fine and gross motor skills, awareness of sounds, visual discrimination, communication and language development, thinking skills, and social skills. Nationally recognized early intervention programs include Project Head Start and Reading Recovery.

See also INDIVIDUALIZED FAMILY SERVICE PROGRAM.

echolalia Mechanical repetition of words or phrases, sometimes hours after the words are heard. Echolalia is one of the classic signs of autism, in which the person will repeat a word with the same intonation as the person who said it originally, yet will not seem to understand what he is repeating. Sometimes the repetition will feature just an echoed word; other autistics will mimic whole sentences or even conversations, even using convincing accents and the voices of other people.

Immediate echolalia is a type of repetition in which an autistic individual repeats whatever is said to him instead of answering the question. In delayed echolalia, an individual may reply, "Do you want something to drink?" any time he or she is asking for a drink. Alternatively, delayed echolalia may occur as scripted repetition of dialogue from a video or conversation that is totally out of context.

educational consultant A term used to describe a range of individuals with varying backgrounds and areas of expertise regarding education. For example, some educational consultants may specialize in college placement, while others may provide testing and specialize in primary or secondary school placement or consultation. An educational consultant may or may not have a background in learning disabilities or autism. Consultants who specialize in special education should have a background in assessment.

An educational consultant may provide counseling to help student and family choose a school, college, or other program that will foster academic and social growth. Educational consultants can provide a student and family with individual attention, firsthand knowledge of hundreds of educational opportunities, and the time to explore all of the options. Consultants may specialize in college admission, boarding school, summer programs, troubled teens, international students or learning disabilities.

educational evaluation An educational evaluation is typically part of the process of defining an INDIVIDUALIZED EDUCATION PROGRAM (IEP). Educational evaluation may involve administration of standardized academic tests, assessment of performance in different academic areas, and observation of classroom performance. To be effective, evaluation should encompass a number of different types of measures and involve the entire range of academic skill areas.

See also INDEPENDENT EDUCATION EVALUATION.

Education for All Handicapped Children Act of 1975 (PL 94-142) This significant legislation, renamed the INDIVIDUALS WITH DISABILITIES EDUCATION ACT in 1990, requires the provision of a free and appropriate public education to children with disabilities such as autism.

education for autistic children Early intervention programs are available for children younger than age three; for children over age three, there are preschool and school programs available. Parents should contact their local school district for information on their local programs.

In some cases, a separate program for special needs children may be best, but for higher-functioning children, integration into a regular school setting may be more appropriate, provided that there is enough support (a part- or full-time aide, or other accommodations as needed).

Parents of an autistic child should consult with their child's teacher and school specialists on an INDIVIDUAL EDUCATION PROGRAM (IEP), which outlines in great detail the child's educational program. Additionally, meeting with the child's classmates and/or their parents can be helpful in encouraging other students to interact positively with the autistic child. In some states, home therapy programs (such as APPLIED BEHAVIOR ANALYSIS and SPEECH THERAPY) may be funded by the school district, rather than through the state. However, it may take considerable effort to convince the school district to provide those services. In other states there is no option other than private pay to fund a home therapy program.

electroencephalogram (EEG) A graphic record of the electrical activity at the surface of the brain. An EEG can be used to differentiate autism from other disorders with similar symptoms. An EEG reading is obtained by attaching small electrodes to the scalp, which allows the regular electrical potential of the brain to be amplified and recorded in graphic form by an electroencephalograph.

Characteristic changes in type and frequency of the waves during both awake and asleep states can provide different information about the brain and how it is functioning.

eligibility The criteria for whether a student with autism is eligible for special education services or not is determined by the INDIVIDUALIZED EDUCATION PROGRAM team. The team should consider qualitative and quantitative information from the assessment process.

Many states continue to determine eligibility as learning disabled by a discrepancy formula, which is a mathematical equation that shows a significant discrepancy between a student's achievement (achievement test scores) and potential (IQ score).

However, recent studies discourage the practice of determining eligibility solely on discrepancy of test scores, and encourage the consideration of other significant factors such as observations and the experiences of teachers and parents.

See also INTELLIGENCE QUOTIENT.

emotional and behavioral disorder (EBD) A condition in which behavioral or emotional responses of a child interfere with performance in self care, social relationships, personal adjustment, academic progress, classroom behavior, or work adjustment. Early identification and intervention for students with emotional and/or behavioral problems is essential and requires specialized educational programming.

EBD is more than a transient, expected response to stress in the child's environment; the problem persists even with individualized interventions, such as feedback, consultation with parents, and modification of the educational environment.

Symptoms and Diagnostic Path

EBD must be exhibited in at least two different settings, at least one of which is school-related. It can coexist with other handicapping conditions, such as schizophrenia, affective disorders, anxiety disorders, or other disturbances. It is important that the assessment identify both the strengths and needs of the individual and those with whom the student interacts. The assessment should ensure that the child's difficulties are not primarily due to transient developmental or environmental variables, cultural or linguistic differences, or influences of other handicapping conditions. Referral for special services should not be used as a disciplinary action or an effort to resolve conflicts.

The results of the assessment should provide information about:

- *environmental factors:* the relationship between the instructional, social, and community environment and the student's specific problems
- *strengths:* the resources of the student, family, teacher(s), and school setting
- *history:* duration of the difficulties, their relationship to specific developmental or situational stressors, and previous attempts to resolve the difficulties

- *intensity:* how severe the problems are in affecting school achievement, social skills, or interpersonal relationships within the school setting
- *pervasiveness:* the number of settings in which difficulties occur in the school, family, or community
- *persistence:* the extent to which difficulties have continued despite the use of well-planned, empirically-based, and individualized intervention strategies provided within lesser restrictive environments
- *developmental/cultural data:* the extent to which the student's behavior is different from the behavior expected for children of the same age, culture, and ethnic background. Information should be obtained from a variety of sources that can provide data about the child's difficulties across various settings.

The assessment should include information about a child's behavioral and emotional functioning, developmental history, areas of significant impairment in school, adaptive behavior and achievement, impairment outside the school setting in areas such as vocational skills, and social skills or interpersonal relationships. Because biological and neurological factors may contribute to, cause, or trigger problem behaviors, consultation with medical care providers and consideration of relevant student and family medical history is important.

Formal methods for gathering information may include behavior checklists, standardized self-reports, structured interviews, rating scales, and other appropriate assessment techniques. Informal methods, such as behavior observation and analysis of work samples, can also be useful.

Treatment Options and Outlook

Eligibility for services under the category of emotional/behavioral disorders should not automatically imply placement in a categorical special education program. Since emotional and behavioral disorders have many influences, interventions for children with these disorders must be comprehensive. Interventions should be planned by a team that includes the parent, the child, the school psychologist and other teachers, administrators, and community service providers. Intervention plans should take into account the strengths of the child, the family, the child's teachers, and the school.

Most schools exist primarily as an educational setting rather than a treatment setting, so children with significant emotional or behavioral disorders may need treatment outside school.

Individualized academic and curricular interventions Children with emotional or behavioral problems frequently achieve below grade expectations in academic areas. Academic problems often seem less important than a student's behavioral difficulties. Students may benefit from adaptations to the curriculum, alteration of the pace of delivery, improvements to the instructional and organizational ecology, and instruction in learning and study skills.

Consultation with teachers Teachers may benefit from a discussion of the needs of the student and the most effective strategies to help the child improve behavior. Teachers will also benefit from the psychosocial support component of consultation in dealing with the frustration and isolation that often is present when working with children with significant problems.

Consultation and partnership with parents Parents will benefit from consultation directed at understanding their child's difficulties, developing and implementing effective behavior management strategies, and working collaboratively with other caregivers. The parent may also need assistance with negotiating the array of services available in the community.

Individual and group counseling Counseling may help the student more readily improve social skills and school adjustment. Students often need help in dealing with the stress in their environment and understanding responsibility and self-directedness.

Social skills training Students with emotional and behavioral disorders often have problems with social skills, so social skills training in the child's multiple environments is often helpful.

Crisis planning and management Crises should be anticipated and plans for dealing with crises should be a part of the student's intervention plan.

Specialized educational settings By law, children must be provided services in the least restrictive environment that meets the student's academic, psychological, and social needs. Many students' needs can

be effectively addressed through consultation with teachers and parents, short-term counseling, and interventions in the regular classroom setting.

Job and transitional planning Career exploration, pre-vocational and vocational skills development, and transition to the after-high-school world should be included for all adolescents with emotional and behavioral disorders.

emotional/behavioral tests Psychological tests that measure how parents, teachers, and the child rate the child's behavior, attitudes, and feelings at home and at school. They include

- Behavior Assessment System for Children
- Conner's Behavior Rating Scales
- ACHENBACH CHILDHOOD BEHAVIOR CHECKLIST
- Reynolds Child Depression Scale
- Piers Harris Self-Concept Scales
- Differential Test of Conduct and Emotional Problems
- Assessment of Interpersonal Relationships
- Depression and Anxiety in Youth Scale
- Multidimensional Depression Inventory

emotional disturbance Emotional, behavioral, or mental disorders that can interfere with a child's ability to learn. Emotional disturbance is defined under the INDIVIDUALS WITH DISABILITIES EDUCATION ACT.

Experts are not sure what causes emotional disturbance, but various factors such as heredity, brain disorder, diet, stress, and family functioning have been suggested as possible causes. More than 463,172 children and youth with serious emotional disturbances were provided services in the public schools in 1998.

Symptoms and Diagnostic Path
Many children who do not have emotional disturbances may act out occasionally, but when children have serious emotional disturbances these behaviors continue over long periods of time. Some of the characteristics and behaviors seen in children who have emotional disturbances include

- short attention span, impulsiveness
- acting out, fighting
- withdrawal, excessive fear or anxiety
- immaturity (inappropriate crying, temper tantrums, poor coping skills)
- learning difficulties (academically performing below grade level)

Children with the most serious emotional disturbances may experience distorted thinking, excessive anxiety, bizarre behavior, or abnormal mood swings.

Emotional disturbance is a condition exhibiting one or more of the following characteristics over a long period of time and to a severe degree:

- an inability to learn that cannot be explained by intellectual, sensory, or health factors
- an inability to build or maintain satisfactory relationships with other children and teachers
- inappropriate types of behavior or feelings under normal circumstances
- a general unhappiness or depression
- a tendency to develop physical symptoms or fears associated with personal or school problems
- The term includes schizophrenia. The term does not apply to children who are socially maladjusted, unless it is determined that they also have an emotional disturbance

The federal government is currently reviewing the way in which serious emotional disturbance is defined.

Education

Educational programs for students with a serious emotional disturbance need to include attention to mastering academics, developing social skills, and increasing self-awareness, self-esteem, and self-control. Career education (both academic and vocational programs) is also a major part of secondary education and should be a part of every adolescent's transition plan as outlined in his or her INDIVIDUALIZED EDUCATION PROGRAM (IEP).

Students eligible for special education services under the category of "serious emotional distur-

bance" may have IEPs that include psychological or counseling services as a related service. This is an important service and must be provided by a qualified social worker, psychologist, or guidance counselor.

epilepsy A neurological disorder that can lead to convulsions, partial and full loss of consciousness, and "absences" (temporary daydream-like inattention). It occurs more frequently in autistic people and their families than in the general population; in fact, one-third of the population of people with autism have developed seizures in early adult life.

Epsom salts baths A mineral product (hydrated magnesium sulfate) normally dissolved in bathwater to ease achy muscles and smooth rough skin. Epsom salts are named for the mineral waters of Epsom, England, where they have been used since the 1600s. Epsom salts can be used as an alternative source of magnesium and sulfate, since both can be absorbed through the skin.

Some experts believe that children with autism can benefit from daily Epsom salts baths. The theory is that many children with autism lack sulfur in their blood and do not absorb sulfur-based substances well. Some experts believe a lack of sulphur may cause many of the autistic symptoms, and believe that Epsom salts baths are one way to replenish this loss. Epsom salts help sulphation—the process in which enzymes help the body detoxify itself.

Other experts who do not necessarily support the theory do acknowledge that the baths will not hurt the child. (CAUTION: No one should take an Epsom salts bath if he or she has high blood pressure or a heart or kidney condition.)

Low sulfur levels could cause many problems. For example, sulphate is important for detoxification of metals and other toxins, and since boys excrete more sulfur than girls, they may be more susceptible to sulfation problems. Some researchers also found that the ileum of the intestine lacks sulfur, which would lead to a leaky gut. Sulphate also is needed to release pancreatic digestive enzymes; many enzyme levels theoretically would be impaired if sulfur levels were low.

In addition to Epsom salts baths, some doctors recommend magnesium sulfate cream.

The daily Epsom salts bath typically contains one and one-half to two cups of Epsom salts, which is first dissolved in very hot water; the tub is then filled with very warm water. The individual should soak for about 30 minutes or longer; hair can be washed in this water. Children should not drink the bathwater. Children should not rinse off before getting out of the bathtub; they should just dry off and go to bed.

estate planning   Making special long-range financial plans is imperative for parents of an autistic child, who must plan for the social, medical, and financial needs of their autistic offspring. If the child's autism is severe enough to affect mental capability, there is an even greater need to create a special estate plan. Because autism often impairs a person's ability to manage financial affairs while simultaneously increasing financial need, parents must be sure that assets are available after their deaths to help the child while also making sure that the assets are protected from an inability to manage them.

First, parents should realistically assess the child's disability and the prognosis for future development. A professional evaluation of the child's prospects and capability of earning a living and managing financial assets is a good idea. It is always possible to change an estate plan as more information about the child becomes available.

Next, parents should estimate the size of their estate and the prospective living arrangements of the child with autism. These living arrangements will have a tremendous impact on how the estate should be distributed. If parents believe a guardian or conservator is necessary, they need to recommend a potential guardian or conservator in the will.

The parents should analyze the earning potential of the child and consider what government benefits the child is eligible to receive. Support for a person with autism usually comes from state and federal benefits via actual grants (such as Social Security or SUPPLEMENTAL SECURITY INCOME) or support programs such as subsidized housing or a sheltered workshop job.

Some government benefits are not affected by the child's financial resources. For example, Social Security Disability Insurance (SSDI) beneficiaries receive their benefits whether they need the money or not. Regardless of what the parents leave to a son or daughter with a disability, the Social Security payments will still be paid once the person has qualified.

Some government benefits (such as Supplemental Security Income and Medicaid) carry financial eligibility requirements. If a person with autism has too many assets or too much income, no benefits will be paid. Those who are eligible because of low income can become ineligible when they inherit money, property, or other assets. Therefore, a child who receives government benefits with financial eligibility requirements needs to have parents who arrange their estate to minimize loss of benefits.

Finally, some government programs available to individuals with autism charge according to what the person can afford to pay. Many states will charge the autistic individual for program benefits if income is high enough.

Some parents choose to disinherit a child with autism if assets are relatively modest and the child's needs high, which would then force the child to rely on federal and state supports after the parents' death. This is especially helpful if parents wish to help their other children.

Alternatively, parents can leave a child with autism an outright gift, which is the best idea if the child with autism is not going to be receiving government benefits. If mentally competent, the child can hire help with managing the gift, but if the child has a cognitive disability, an outright gift is never a good idea, because this person may not be able to handle the financial responsibilities.

A trust is preferable if parents want to leave a gift to support a child. Alternatively, some parents leave a morally obligated gift to another child. The danger of morally obligated gifts is, of course, that the morally obligated recipient may ignore the wishes of the parents. Morally obligated gifts can be useful when the parents have a modest amount of money and do not expect a lifetime of care for their child with autism, but instead want their healthy children to use some of the inherited money to help their sibling with special needs.

Special Needs Trust

The only reliable method of making sure that the inheritance actually has a chance of reaching a person with a disability when he or she needs it is through the legal device known as a Special Needs Trust (SNT). The SNT can manage resources while maintaining the individual's eligibility for public assistance benefits. The family leaves whatever resources it deems appropriate to the trust, which is managed by a trustee on behalf of the person with the disability. While government agencies recognize SNTs, they have imposed some very stringent rules and regulations upon them, which is why any family thinking about an SNT should consult an experienced attorney—not just one who does general estate planning, but one who is very knowledgeable about SNTs and current government benefit programs.

Special needs trusts are imperative for a child with autism. The provisions can be broad or limiting. For many parents, a trust is the most effective way to help the child, by keeping assets so that they will be available to the child but will not disqualify him or her for government benefits.

The actual cash benefits of government assistance are generally quite small and force the individual to live below the poverty level. This means that if the autistic child is to have any type of meaningful lifestyle, the family or local charities have to provide supplemental assistance. With recent changes in the Social Security Administration, the primary government benefit programs are recognizing that family contributions to the person's well-being can only improve his or her overall quality of life. As long as the family's contributions are supplementary, as opposed to duplicating government benefit programs, they are permitted. Thus, the current government benefit programs do permit the family to provide some supplementary income and resources to the person with a disability. However, the government regulations are very strict, and they are carefully monitored.

One wrong word or phrase can make the difference between an inheritance that really benefits the person with a disability and one that causes the person to lose access to a wide range of needed services and assistance. The Special Needs Trust does not belong to the person with a disability—it is established and administered by someone else.

The person with the disability does not have a trust but is nominated as a beneficiary of the trust and is usually the only one who receives the benefits. The trustee (the manager) is given the absolute discretion to determine when and how much the person should receive.

evaluation   Collecting and analyzing information about a child and administering tests for the purpose of diagnosis or treatment. In educational settings, an evaluation is a required part of a plan for special-education services, usually called an INDIVIDUALIZED EDUCATION PROGRAM (IEP). For the evaluation of DEVELOPMENTAL DISABILITIES or learning disabilities, multiple assessments are required, including intelligence and achievement tests.

A parent can ask the school to test a child, or school staff may ask parents for permission to do an evaluation. If staff members think a child may have a disability and may need special education and related services, they must evaluate the child before providing these services. This evaluation is free to the family.

The group involved in a child's evaluation will include

- at least one of the child's regular-education teachers
- at least one of the child's special-education teachers or service providers
- parents
- a school administrator expert in special-education policies, children with disabilities, the general curriculum, and available resources
- an expert who can interpret the evaluation results and talk about what instruction may be necessary
- individuals (invited by parents or the school) with knowledge or special expertise about the child
- the child, if appropriate
- representatives from other agencies responsible for paying for or providing transition services
- other qualified professionals such as a school psychologist, occupational therapist, speech language therapist, physical therapist, medical specialists

Members of the group will begin by checking the child's school file and recent test scores and conducting interviews with parents and teachers.

Before staffers can go any further, they must ask the parents for permission and describe what tests will be used and any other ways the school will collect information about the child.

Although tests are an important part of an evaluation, they are only a part. The evaluation should also include the observations of professionals who have worked with the child, the child's relevant medical history, and the parents' ideas about the child's experiences, abilities, needs, and behavior.

It is important that the school evaluate a child in all areas of possible disability. For example, the tests should evaluate

- language skills (speaking and understanding)
- thoughts and behavior
- adaptability to change
- school achievement
- intelligence
- movement, thinking, learning, seeing, and hearing function
- job-related and other post-school interests and abilities

Tests must be given in the child's native language or by other means of communication (for example, sign language if the child is deaf). Tests must not be biased, and the tests must be given correctly. Evaluation results will be used to determine if the child has a disability and whether the child is eligible for special education and related services. This decision will also be based on local policies about eligibility for these special services.

Under the INDIVIDUALS WITH DISABILITIES EDUCATION ACT (IDEA), parents have the right to be part of any group that decides a child's eligibility for special-education and related services. The IDEA lists 13 different disability categories under which a child may be eligible for services:

- autism
- deaf-blindness
- deafness

- hearing impairment
- mental retardation
- multiple disabilities
- orthopedic impairment
- other health impairment (such as having limited strength, vitality, or alertness) that affects a child's educational performance
- serious emotional disturbance
- specific learning disability
- speech or language impairment
- traumatic brain injury
- visual impairment, including blindness

Parents have the right to receive a copy of the evaluation report and to receive a copy of the paperwork concerning the child's eligibility for special education.

If the child is eligible for special-education and related services (such as speech-language therapy), parents meet with the school to discuss special educational needs and to create an IEP for the child. The IEP is a written document that parents and school personnel develop together to describe a child's educational program, including special services.

If a child is not eligible for special-education and related services, the school must inform parents in writing and must provide information about an appeal if the parents disagree with this decision. Parents have the right to disagree with the eligibility decision.

expressive language   Language used to communicate meaningful information via vocal, gestural, or symbolic means. Expressive language requires the child to describe things in a unique way, not just repeat what others before had said. Researchers have found that the average child with an AUTISTIC DISORDER today has an IQ of about 50 and that at least 40 percent of them do not develop any expressive language.

eye contact   A form of nonverbal communication often absent in people with AUTISTIC DISORDER. Being able to make eye contact is one of the primary foundations for the development of social skills. Although poor eye contact is probably the most common symptom reported by parents of young children with autism and is often the first and most obvious symptom, not all children with autism have poor eye contact.

Many countries have strong cultural assumptions about eye contact. In the United States, failure to make eye contact is often interpreted as signaling dishonesty, discomfort, impoliteness, inattention, or having something to hide. Direct eye contact is considered to reflect openness, honesty, and politeness.

Even in the first few months of life, many infants diagnosed with autism avoid eye contact. Typically, instead of making eye contact with others, the person with autism will look away or appear to look right through other people.

Some evidence suggests that individuals with autism use different neural circuitry to process faces. What appears to be a simple perceptual task is difficult for individuals with autism. Research is under way to try to understand the differences in the brains of people with autism that explain this difficulty.

Increased eye contact is one of the goals of treatment for autism, and is part of social skills training.

eye-hand coordination   A combination of visual skills and fine motor skills of the hand. Eye-hand coordination is required for many daily activities, such as handwriting, drawing, and typing on a keyboard, dressing (such as buttoning, zipping, and tying shoes), and for many sports, such as throwing and catching in basketball and baseball. The term dysgraphia is used when individuals have poor eye-hand coordination, resulting in poor control of handwriting.

eye-hand-foot coordination   The ability to control and direct movements of feet (and legs) in accordance with visual stimuli. Examples of eye-hand-foot coordinated activities are operating a kick or foot-drive potter's wheel and driving a car.

face recognition Children with AUTISM cannot recognize faces as readily as can typically developing children. While in the past this was wrongly attributed to a supposed inability to recognize faces all at once, researchers now believe that autistic children do appear to process faces all at once, just like other children, although their focus may be a bit more narrowly centered on the region of the mouth.

This suggests that face recognition abnormalities in autism are not fully explained by problems with whole-face processing and that there is an unusual significance of the mouth region when children with autism process information from people's faces. Scientists suggest this may be a result of the autistic child's specific problem with processing facial information from the eyes, or because of an aversion to looking at eyes, so that the mouth takes on greater significance as a primary way of communicating for the autistic child. This is consistent with studies that show children with autism are delayed by several years in spontaneously following shifts of gaze from others and that they depend on vocal cues to establish attention.

It is also possible that autistic impairments in language functioning foster a tendency to pay more attention to mouths so the child can make sense of speech via lip reading, especially when other communicative cues from the eyes are inaccessible.

In nonautistic individuals, when a picture of a face is turned upside down, recognition is severely disrupted, much more so than with inversion of nonface objects. This has been taken as evidence that people typically recognize a face all at once, as an entire unit.

In a Boston University study, researchers studied face recognition first with normal children between nine and 11. In this study, children were asked to look at whole faces and match them to the same or a similar face with only one different feature (eyes, nose, or mouth). The second study assessed children with high-functioning autism or language impairment or delay. In this second study, children saw only one isolated face part (such as the mouth) that was different in the face comparison test, and they were asked to identify the face part that differed in the whole face. Both upright and inverted faces and face parts were shown to all children.

As expected, normal children and children with language delays were better at recognizing face parts represented in the whole face. These children were most accurate at identifying faces based on differences in eyes. The autistic children showed an advantage over typical children in recognizing differences in the mouth, but were far less efficient than normal children at telling differences in faces from the eyes.

facilitated communication (FC) A discredited method of communication in which a "facilitator" supports the hand or arm of the autistic patient while he or she uses a typewriter or computer keyboard, or an alphabet facsimile. The method is based on the idea that the autistic person has an "undisclosed literacy." The facilitator typically pushes against the autistic person's arm and finger ostensibly without affecting key selection, so that the autistic person can push them toward the desired key.

The technique was developed in Australia by Rosemary Crossley for people with severe physical handicaps. In the United States, the center for FC is Syracuse University, which houses the Facilitated Communication Institute. The institute, established in 1992, conducts research, provides training to teach people to become facilitators, hosts seminars and conferences, publishes a quarterly newsletter, and produces and sells materials promoting FC, including a six-part video series.

Since its introduction in the United States in 1990, it has generated a growing tide of controversy. In fact, repeated studies have supported the notion that the "message" is actually coming from the facilitator rather than the autistic individual. Facilitators may be either deliberately faking their role in the process or unconsciously transmitting their impressions of what they believe the autistic person might want to communicate, rather than actually intuiting the unconscious desires of the autistic individuals from slight hand movements.

Tests have not supported the authenticity of facilitated communication, and in 1994 the American Psychological Association (APA) asserted that studies have repeatedly demonstrated the method is not scientifically valid. The American Academy of Pediatrics likewise considers this technique as ineffective.

Because of its supposed ability to give the nonverbal autistic person the ability to communicate, facilitated communication has been used to elicit accusations of abuse. But according to the APA, information obtained as a result of facilitated communication should not be used to confirm or deny allegations of abuse or to make diagnostic or treatment decisions.

"Facilitated communication is a controversial and unproved communicative procedure with no scientifically demonstrated support for its efficacy," according to a 1994 position statement by the APA. While some people passionately believe that facilitated communication has given language to those who could not previously speak, most experts in autism insist that this type of communication is inherently unreliable.

Despite the lack of studies proving it works, and despite evidence of widespread facilitator manipulation, FC is sometimes commonly used in SPECIAL EDUCATION.

Family Educational Rights and Privacy Act (FERPA) This act, also known as the Buckley Amendment, outlines procedures and guidelines for maintaining and disclosing student records. Under this law, parents and students over 18 years of age have the right to review education records within 45 days of their application and to request a change of records that the parent or student believes to be inaccurate or misleading.

Individuals also have the right to request disclosure of records that contain personally identifiable information.

Under the act, such information may also be disclosed without consent to school officials with a legitimate educational interest. (The definition of "school official" includes an individual employed by a school district as an administrator, supervisor, teacher, or support staff member and may also include other individuals performing official functions, such as school board members.)

FERPA is important legislation for parents of children with learning disabilities who seek services under the INDIVIDUALS WITH DISABILITIES EDUCATION ACT because it governs the circumstances under which information related to a child's academic performance and learning needs may be made available to others.

family history An important component of a thorough health assessment. A family history will identify developmental factors, together with family events, dynamics, and other conditions, that may have had an impact on the individual. A family history may also point toward potential genetic links between an individual's condition and those of parents or other family members.

If parents have a child with AUTISM, there is an increased likelihood, estimated at 5 percent to 8 percent, that any children they have in the future will also develop autism. Many studies have identified cognitive disabilities, which sometimes go undetected, in siblings of autistic children. Siblings should be evaluated for possible developmental delays and learning disabilities, such as dyslexia.

See also GENES AND AUTISM; GENETIC MARKER.

fathers Teaching a father how to talk to and play with his autistic child in a home setting can improve communication and increase the number of intelligible words the youngster speaks by more than 50 percent, according to a 2005 study at the

University of Florida, published in the journal *Nursing Research*.

Caring for an autistic child can be a never-ending, difficult job. In most cases care is provided by mothers, leaving many fathers feeling as if they cannot connect with their autistic child, researchers say. During training, fathers learned to initiate play with their children through animated repetition of their children's vocalizations and actions. Fathers were told to resist the temptation to direct their child's play and instead to follow the child's lead.

Researchers were surprised to find that unlike the mothers in a previous study, many fathers actually took the lead in training their spouses and other family members in the techniques they learned.

Researchers believe it is important for both the child's mother and father to be involved in parent training whenever possible. Potential benefits that may follow from a father's participation include increased frequency of interaction and improved quality of interaction between a father and his child with autism, increased treatment time for the child, and support for the child's mother.

Feingold, Ben F. (1900–1982)   Pediatric allergist who developed a special diet, based on eliminating preservatives and artificial dyes and colorings, for children with hyperactivity and behavior problems such as AUTISTIC DISORDER.

Starting his practice of medicine as a pediatrician, Dr. Feingold taught pediatrics at Northwestern University Medical School, and later became chief of pediatrics at Cedars of Lebanon Hospital in Los Angeles. He specialized in child and adult allergies, and he retired at the age of 81 as chief emeritus of the Department of Allergy of Kaiser-Permanente Medical Center in San Francisco.

Dr. Feingold used a diet similar to one developed at the Mayo Clinic to treat skin conditions and asthma related to aspirin sensitivity. The elimination diet excluded aspirin and foods believed to contain salicylate compounds, as well as synthetic colorings and flavorings. When patients dramatically improved, Feingold began to recommend the food plan more widely at the clinic.

Some of the parents of allergic children with hyperactivity reported that not only did their child's allergy symptoms improve, but the child calmed down and was doing better in school. Eventually, Dr. Feingold began to try this regimen (the "K-P diet") on children with behavior problems and autism who had not responded to any other treatment. The results were encouraging and began to appear in newspaper articles.

In 1973, after eight years of clinical research, Dr. Feingold announced his findings at a meeting of the American Medical Association and published articles in various medical journals. His work was greeted with enthusiasm by his colleagues, who had been seeing an alarming increase in the number of children diagnosed as hyperactive. However, others in the food and drug industry disagreed with his conclusions vehemently.

Dr. Feingold's book *Why Your Child Is Hyperactive* was published in 1974, after which the press dubbed his diet the FEINGOLD DIET.

Feingold diet   A special elimination diet popular with parents of individuals with AUTISTIC DISORDER that excludes foods believed to contain salicylate compounds (such as tomatoes, apples, and oranges) as well as synthetic colorings and flavorings and preservatives. This diet is believed by some experts (and many parents) to ease the symptoms of autistic children.

fenfluramine   A drug no longer available that had been considered useful in some, but not all, studies of AUTISTIC DISORDER. The drug had been used primarily to treat hyperactivity, stereotypy, and withdrawal in autistic individuals.

Some people with autism have abnormally high blood levels of the mood-regulating neurotransmitter serotonin, and fenfluramine decreases serotonin concentrations. As a result, well into the 1990s many children and some adults with autism were treated with fenfluramine, which seemed to have had some positive effects on some individuals.

However, in 1997 fenfluramine was taken off the market because of apparent damage to the heart in some patients who were taking it in combination with other drugs to lose weight. As part of the $3.75 billion settlement, the company recommended that those who took fenfluramine as a diet pill should consult their doctors about whether to have the health of their hearts assessed.

floor time An informal play session often used with autistic children that uses interactive experiences to enable a child to move to the next emotional developmental stage. Floor time is an engaging, playful experience between a child and a partner, which facilitates the six stages of emotional development. These stages are the foundations of relationships, communication, and learning. The idea of floor time was developed by psychiatrist Stanley Greenspan, M.D., as part of his DIR (Developmental Individual-Difference Relationship-Based Model). An alternative to the behaviorism approach, DIR is based more on teaching skills.

At its core, floor time involves a parent playing eye-to-eye with a child and letting the child be the boss. The adult cedes control and lives in the child's moment. Ideally, during floor time parents should do what their child wants to do, even if it means playing dollhouse or battleships over and over. Greenspan stresses that effective communication with children is increasingly ignored in daily life. More and more, he says, parents think that being in the same room with a child is the same thing as interacting with that child, no matter how distracted the parent might be.

Greenspan, a clinical professor of psychiatry and pediatrics at George Washington Medical School, began developing floor time in the 1970s. He specializes in early childhood development and outlined his floor time approach in *The Child with Special Needs* in 1998.

His concept is better known among parents with autistic children. About half of the 200 autistic children who received floor time therapy with Greenspan and their parents became fully functioning children, according to one anecdotal study; another 30 percent made substantial progress.

According to Greenspan, floor time focuses on relationships by helping to build emotional capacity, thought processes, and communication, while helping a parent figure out a child's personality and how he thinks. It can build empathy, creativity, warmth, and reflective thinking.

During floor time, parents try to open and close as many "circles of communication" as possible. Another way to think of this is "back-and-forths" or reciprocal exchanges.

There are five steps in floor time:

1. Observe the child
2. Open the circle of communication
3. Follow the child's lead
4. Expand and extend
5. Child closes circle of communication

For example, if the child hugs a doll, the parent asks the doll's name. The child answers, or gives the doll a hug and offers it to the parent for a kiss. This response closes the communication that the parent has opened.

Another example:

1. A child asks for milk.
2. Parent opens the circle of communication by asking more questions: "Do you want chocolate milk or plain milk? Do you want a big glass or a small glass?"
3. If the child has trouble with choices, the parent can make the choices very obvious, asking, "Do you want the milk in a box or in a glass?"
4. Parent then tries to pour the milk before opening the carton. Can the child solve this problem? Comments can help the child process: "Oh, no! Why won't the milk come out?"

Greenspan believed that his floor time approach should begin when a child is a baby or toddler, but it does not have to be restricted to young children.

fluoxetine (Prozac) An antidepressant of the class called selective serotonin reuptake inhibitors (SSRIs). Traditionally prescribed for depression, the SSRIs have also been shown to significantly improve symptoms associated with AUTISTIC DISORDER and ASPERGER'S SYNDROME. Fluoxetine helps to lessen stereotyped behaviors and self-injurious movements with few side effects.

Although there are no psychiatric medications that can directly target autism itself, many antidepressant medications can be used to treat specific symptoms often found in autism, such as aggression, self-injury, anxiety, depression, obsessive-compulsive disorders, and attention deficit hyperactivity disorder (ADHD). In particular, serotonin reuptake inhibitors (SSRI) have been effective in treating depression, obsessive-compulsive behaviors, and anxiety that are sometimes present in autism.

Because researchers have consistently found abnormally high levels of the neurotransmitter serotonin in the blood of a third of individuals with autism, experts suggest that the SSRI drugs that lower serotonin levels could potentially reverse some of the symptoms in autism. Prozac is one drug that has been studied as a possible autism treatment, and studies have shown that they may reduce the frequency and intensity of repetitive behaviors, and may decrease irritability, tantrums, and aggressive behavior. Some children have shown improvements in eye contact and responsiveness.

For some classes of drugs, the doses that can reduce symptoms such as aggression or anxiety are much lower for people with autism than for other patients. For example, the best dose for SSRI drugs such as Prozac may be only one-third of the typical starting dose for depressed patients. Too high a dose in patients with autism may trigger agitation or insomnia.

There is no medical test to determine whether Prozac or another antidepressant medication will work best. Instead, doctors use a "trial and error" approach, as dosages need to be adjusted differently for each person, and one medication may be ineffective or have negative effects while others are helpful.

Side Effects

Mild side effects might include headache, sedation, or agitation, which are not usually severe enough to make people stop taking the medication.

See also FLUVOXAMINE.

fluvoxamine (Luvox)   Antidepressant of the class called selective serotonin reuptake inhibitors (SSRIs). Traditionally prescribed for depression, the SSRIs have also been shown to significantly improve symptoms associated with AUTISTIC DISORDER and ASPERGER'S SYNDROME. Fluvoxamine helps to lessen

STEREOTYPIES and self-injurious movements with few side effects.

Although fluvoxamine is not as popular as FLUOXETINE (Prozac), it causes less agitation and more sedation.

Side Effects

Mild side effects might include headache and sedation, which are not usually severe enough that people stop taking the medication.

folic acid   A B vitamin vital to pregnant women to prevent neural tube defects in unborn children. Folic acid has also been linked to both improving, and causing, autism.

In 1992 the U.S. Food and Drug Administration (FDA) recommended a folic acid intake of 400 mcg per day. But because the FDA worried that women ignored their recommendations, food has been fortified with folic acid since 1998. As a result, neural tube defects have dropped substantially.

Yet some experts expressed concern that folic acid might be related to the increase in autism cases. Part of the problem is that there is no government system in place, through the FDA or any other health organization, to monitor the effects of this supplement.

The food supply did not include folic acid until 1998, and autism rates began to rise substantially before then. Almost no studies have been done to look directly or even indirectly for the adverse effects of elevated folate intakes. There is no solid evidence that folic acid causes a person to be more likely to have autism, but there is no evidence proving it is not in some way responsible, either.

On the other hand, there are many proponents of using large amounts of folic acid as an autism treatment, including the Autism Research Institute founded by Dr. Bernard Rimland.

food allergies   See ALLERGY TO COW'S MILK; FEINGOLD DIET.

fragile X syndrome   A hereditary condition that causes a wide range of mental impairment, from mild learning disabilities to severe MENTAL RETAR-DATION (mostly in boys). The most common inherited form of mental retardation, the condition got its name from the fact that one part of the X chromosome has a defective piece that appears pinched and fragile when seen under a microscope. Also known as Martin-Bell syndrome, marker X syndrome, or Escalante syndrome, fragile X syndrome is associated with a number of physical and behavioral characteristics.

The behavior of some children with fragile X syndrome is quite similar to that of children with autism. Although most children with fragile X syndrome do not have all the characteristics of autism, about 15 percent are diagnosed as autistic. More often, children have "autistic-like" features, such as poor EYE CONTACT, HAND FLAPPING, and poor SOCIAL SKILLS.

The syndrome accounts for approximately 5 percent of mental retardation in boys, but has also been linked to learning disabilities, speech and language disorders, and mathematics and motor disabilities.

The biological cause of fragile X and the pattern of transmission of the disease are complex. Fragile X syndrome is transmitted from parent to child through the DNA in the sperm and eggs. Many inherited diseases (such as sickle cell anemia and hemophilia) are caused by a single error in the genetic code in a person's DNA. Fragile X syndrome, on the other hand, is not caused by a single change in DNA, but by the *multiplication* of part of the genetic information. This is known as a trinucleotide repeat disorder.

In normal children, a section of the DNA in the FMR1 gene is repeated about 30 times. In a child with fragile X, that DNA section repeats about 55 to 200 times. Someone with the full mutation has 200 to 800 repeats.

Because most genes have a very low rate of mutation, most children who inherit a disease have at least one parent who is a carrier for that disease, since new mutations are rare. But the FMR1 gene can be unstable, which leads to frequent mutations. Once the FMR1 gene changes from normal to unstable (called a "permutation"), it is highly likely that it will mutate from one generation to the next. This means that there can be a family with no history of fragile X syndrome in which the condition suddenly appears in a number of offspring.

Symptoms and Diagnostic Path

This syndrome affects individuals in a wide variety of ways. Children with fragile X syndrome are often described as sweet and loving, with a strong desire for social interaction and humorous situations. Some children experience significant challenges, including behavioral problems, while the impact on others is so minor that they will never be diagnosed. Boys and girls experience quite different physical, cognitive, behavioral, sensory, speech, and language problems. In general, however, girls with fragile X either do not have the characteristics seen in boys, or the characteristics show up in a milder form.

The difference is probably due to the fact that girls have two X chromosomes instead of the one that boys carry. This means that girls with fragile X have two sets of instructions for making FMRP (the fragile X mental retardation protein)—one that works and one that does not. Boys with fragile X have only one X chromosome with its nonfunctioning FMR1 (fragile X mental retardation 1) gene. It appears that girls are able to produce enough of the FMRP to fill most of the body's needs, but not all.

Anxiety in both boys and girls manifests itself in various ways. Some children with fragile X have trouble with changes in routine or stressful events such as fire drills. Parents often report that their children stiffen up when angry or upset, becoming rigid and very tense. Crowds and new situations may cause boys to whine, cry, or misbehave so as to get out of the overwhelming situation. Many of the behavior problems of both boys and girls with fragile X syndrome overlap with the conversational problems they have. The poor eye contact and problems in keeping a conversation going cause many social weaknesses. Perseverative speech and self-talk may be symptoms of anxiety.

Many children with fragile X syndrome have some cognitive problems, and their overall potential may be lower than that of their peers and siblings. Children may be both mentally retarded and learning disabled, meaning that their overall IQ is lower than average, but that they have particular weaknesses on specific skills that are above and beyond what would be predicted based on their intelligence. At the same time, they may perhaps demonstrate relative strengths in other areas. Children with fragile X syndrome often have these varying patterns. Thinking skills are also affected by attention deficit hyperactivity disorder (ADHD), seizure disorders, anxiety, speech and language disorders, sensory motor problems, and other issues that may affect test taking and learning.

Many boys, and some girls, are described as mentally retarded. Children with fragile X syndrome progress at a slower developmental pace and with a lower end result than do normally developing children. Disabilities in adapting to the environment refer to delays in life skills, not just academics. However, many children with fragile X achieve more than would be expected based upon an IQ score alone.

Boys Several physical features are commonly associated with fragile X syndrome. Boys with fragile X often have distinctive facial features, connective tissue problems, and enlarged testicles that appear after the onset of puberty. However, none of these features occurs in all boys with fragile X. The primary physical features of fragile X syndrome in boys are long faces and prominent, long ears—characteristics that are more common in boys over age 10. However, long ears are also common among mentally retarded boys who do not have fragile X syndrome. When compared to mentally retarded boys who do not have fragile X syndrome, those with fragile X have a larger head circumference, head breadth, and head length.

Up to 80 percent of boys with fragile X syndrome have delays in their cognitive ability; between 10 and 15 percent of boys tested may have IQs in the borderline or mild mental retardation range. Up to 90 percent of boys with the condition are considered to be distractible and impulsive, with many meeting criteria for diagnosis of attention deficit hyperactivity disorder, which can appear as hyperactive/impulsive subtype, inattentive subtype, or the combined form. These children often may have short attention spans and difficulty staying on task.

Many boys have unusual, stereotypic behaviors, such as hand flapping and chewing on skin,

clothing, or objects, which may be connected to sensory processing problems and anxiety. Sensory processing problems may include tactile defensiveness, sensitivity to sound or light, and poor eye contact. About 90 percent of boys with fragile X syndrome are reported to have some type of sensory defensiveness.

Girls A permutation in the FMR1 gene typically has little or no effect on a girl's behavior and educational ability, but it may affect several facial characteristics, causing, for instance, prominent ears and prominent jaw. Girls with the full mutation may have some of the physical features associated with fragile X boys, including a long face. Some girls with the full mutation have learning disabilities. About 30 percent of girls with the full mutation score above 85 on an IQ test, with the other 70 percent mostly in the borderline or mild mental retardation range.

Girls may show less hyperactivity but still have many symptoms of attention deficit disorder. Girls with the full mutation of the fragile X gene appear to have some behavioral and emotional difficulties. Shyness, anxiety, depression, and difficulties with social contacts are most often mentioned as characteristics of girls with fragile X.

Thirty percent of females with fragile X are condered genetic carriers of the condition. They appear to be more mildly affected, and may experience shyness, anxiety, and panic attacks. Sons of a carrier female have a 38 percent risk of mental retardation; daughters have a 16 percent risk.

In the past, the only laboratory test for fragile X syndrome was a chromosome test, but in 1991 a DNA test (the FMR1 gene test) was introduced as the most accurate way to detect fragile X syndrome. The chromosome test is still available through most labs, however, and is used for a variety of diagnostic purposes.

Treatment Options and Outlook

There is no cure for fragile X syndrome, but there are many treatments that may help the children with the disorder to progress. Early intervention during preschool is important, but to reach full potential, a child may need speech and language therapy, occupational therapy, and physical therapy to help with the physical, behavioral, and cognitive issues typical of the condition. In later school years, SPECIAL EDUCATION programs that fit a child's individual needs can be effective, although children should be integrated into regular education whenever possible. At home, parents can try to provide a regular routine in a calm atmosphere. Medications can help treat symptoms of aggression, seizures, hyperactivity, and short attention span.

The outlook for children with fragile X syndrome is best when the disease is diagnosed early. In most cases, the mental retardation typical of this condition is mild, and people with fragile X syndrome usually have a normal lifespan.

free and appropriate public education   SPECIAL EDUCATION and related services provided at public expense, under public supervision and direction and without charge, to meet the standards of the state's department of education and are based on an INDIVIDUALIZED EDUCATION PROGRAM.

Under Public Law 94-142 and IDEA (the INDIVIDUALS WITH DISABILITIES EDUCATION ACT), children with certain disabilities must be provided with "a free appropriate public education which emphasizes special education and related services. . . ."

Under the act, states are required to ensure that disabled children have equal access to educational services but, states are not expected to provide all of the services that may be required for students to reach their full potential.

See also EDUCATION FOR ALL HANDICAPPED CHILDREN ACT (PL Law 94-142).

friends   Although young children with autism may seem to prefer to be by themselves, one of the most important issues for older children and adults is the development of friendships with peers. It can take a great deal of time and effort for them to develop the social skills needed to interact successfully with other children, but it is important to start early. In addition, bullying in middle and high school can be a major problem for students with autism, and the development of friendships is one of the best ways to prevent this problem.

Friendships can be encouraged informally by inviting other children to the home to play. In school, recess can be a valuable time for teachers to encourage play with other children. Furthermore, time can be set aside in school for formal "play time" involving children with autism and volunteer peers. Typical children usually think that play time is much more fun than regular school, and it can help develop lasting friendships. This is probably one of the most important aspects of a student's INDIVIDUALIZED EDUCATION PROGRAM.

Children with autism often develop friendships through shared interests, such as computers, school clubs, model airplanes, and so on. Parents and teachers should encourage activities that the autistic individual can share with others.

full inclusion   A placement in which a special-education student receives instruction within the regular classroom setting for the entire school day. The student may receive help from a paraprofessional who provides necessary support for the child to be successful.

functional MRI (fMRI)   A type of magnetic resonance imaging (MRI) scanning in which scientists can see what parts of the brain are active while a subject is performing a task, such as solving a math problem. fMRI can highlight which areas of the brain in some individuals with autism are active during various tasks.

gender differences Autism affects about three or four times as many boys as girls, although experts are not sure why. Hans Asperger originally believed that no girls were affected by the syndrome he described in 1944, although clinical evidence later caused him to change his thinking.

In one 1981 study, researchers found that among people with high-functioning autism or ASPERGER'S SYNDROME there were as many as 15 times as many boys as girls. On the other hand, when researchers looked at individuals with learning problems as well as autism, the ratio of boys to girls was closer to 2:1. This suggests that while girls are less likely to develop autism, when they do they are more severely impaired.

Other experts speculate that many girls with Asperger's syndrome are never referred for diagnosis, and so are simply missing from statistics. This could be because the diagnostic criteria for Asperger's syndrome are based on the behavioral characteristics of boys, who are often more noticeably "different" or disruptive than girls with the same underlying deficits. Girls with Asperger's syndrome may be better at hiding their problems in order to fit in with their peers and in general may have a more even profile of SOCIAL SKILLS.

Another hypothesis is based on evidence that in the general population, girls have better verbal and social skills, while boys excel in visuo-spatial tasks. There may be a neurological basis for this, so that autism can be interpreted as exaggeration of "normal" sex differences. But environmental and social factors also may play a part in sex differences in ability, which suggests that the poorer verbal skills of boys may have no direct connection to their higher incidence of autism.

In 1964 autism expert Bernard Rimland pointed out that boys tend to be more susceptible to organic damage than girls, and it is now almost universally accepted that there is an organic cause for autism.

More recently, researchers have suggested a genetic explanation for the differences, which may be located on the X chromosome. Girls inherit two X chromosomes, one from each parent, but boys inherit only one, from their mothers. Therefore, it could be that the X chromosome girls inherit from their fathers contains an imprinted gene which "protects" the carrier from autism, thus making girls less likely to develop the condition than boys. This theory has been used to support Asperger's view that autism and Asperger's syndrome are at the extreme end of a spectrum of behaviors normally associated with "maleness."

Researchers have outlined several possible ways that the autism gene could be transmitted on the sex-linked X chromosome. However, researchers are still a long way from identifying a simple genetic cause for autism. It is likely that several genes on different chromosomes will be found to be associated with autism, which means that the idea that autism is based on the X chromosome alone may not represent the full picture.

genes and autism The first gene specifically linked to autism risk was identified in March 2004, but scientists suspect there may be from two to 100 genes involved in the development of autism. The way different symptoms of the AUTISM SPECTRUM DISORDERS (ASDs) affect family members and the wide variety of symptoms in ASD tell researchers there must be more than one gene. Although autism is a complex disorder, the identification of one gene linked to autism should theoretically simplify the search for others. Identifying these genes should lead to better diagnostic tests and treatments.

Some genes may place a person at greater risk for autism; these are called "susceptibility genes." Other genes may cause specific symptoms or determine how severe those symptoms are. Still other mutated genes might add to the symptoms of autism because the genes or their products are not working properly.

The link between genes and ASD is strengthened by results from twin studies, family member studies, and observations of disorders linked to autism.

Studies of Twins with Autism

Scientists have studied autism in both identical twins (who are genetically the same) and fraternal twins (who are genetically similar, but not identical). If one identical twin has autism, 60 percent of the time the other twin also will have autism. When one fraternal twin has autism, the chance that the other twin also has autism is much lower—about 5 percent. If genes were *not* involved in autism, the rate of autism would be the same for both types of twins.

Family Studies of Autism

Studies of family histories show that a sibling's chance of having autism is between 2 percent and 8 percent, which is much higher than the chance of someone in the general population. Also, some of the autism-like symptoms, such as delays in language development, occur more often in parents and brothers and sisters of people with autism than in families who have no members or relatives with ASDs. Because members of the same family are more likely to share genes, something about these genes' sequences appears to be related to autism.

Diagnosable Disorders and Autism

About 5 percent of the time, a person with autism also has a coexisting single-gene disorder, chromosome disorder, or other developmental disorder. This type of co-occurrence helps researchers who are trying to pinpoint the genes involved in autism. Similar disorders with similar symptoms may have similar genetic beginnings. When one disorder commonly occurs along with another, it could be that one is actually a risk factor for the other. This kind of information can provide clues to what actually happens in autism.

For example, many people with ASDs also have EPILEPSY, a condition marked by seizures. If scientists can understand what happens in epilepsy, they may also find clues to what happens in autism.

Searching for the Autism Gene

A "genome" includes all the genetic material in a person's cells—including DNA, genes, and chromosomes. Usually, researchers screen the genome of a family or a set of families that has more than one member with an ASD to look for common features and differences. Using genome-wide screens, scientists have identified a number of genes that might be involved in autism. Although some analyses suggest that there may be from two to 100 genes involved in ASDs, the strongest evidence points to areas on chromosomes 2, 7, 13, 15, 16, 17, and X.

Chromosome 2   Scientists know that areas of chromosome 2 are the neighborhoods for "homeobox" (HOX) genes, the group of genes that control growth and development very early in life. An individual has 38 different HOX genes in a chromosomal neighborhood, and each one directs the action of other genes in building the body and body systems. Expression of these HOX genes is critical to building the brain stem and the cerebellum, two areas of the brain where functions are disrupted in ASDs.

Chromosome 7   Researchers have found a strong link between this chromosome—especially a region called AUTS1—and autism. Most of the genome studies completed so far have found that AUTS1 plays some role in autism. In addition, evidence suggests that a region of chromosome 7 is also related to speech and language disorders. The fact that ASDs affect these functions suggests autism may involve this chromosome.

Chromosome 13   In one study, 35 percent of families with autism showed a link to chromosome 13. Researchers are now trying to replicate these findings with other populations of families affected by autism.

Chromosome 15   Genome-wide screens and other studies show that a part of this chromosome may play a role in autism. Genetic errors on this chromosome cause ANGELMAN SYNDROME and PRADER-WILLI SYNDROME, both of which share some behavioral symptoms with autism. Errors on chromosome 15 occur in up to 4 percent of patients with autism.

Chromosome 16   Genes found on this chromosome control a wide variety of functions that, if disrupted, cause problems that are similar or related to symptoms of autism. For example, a genetic error on this chromosome causes TUBEROUS SCLEROSIS COMPLEX, a disorder that shares many symptoms with autism. Like individuals with autism, those with tuberous sclerosis are at higher risk for seizures. Therefore, regions on this chromosome may be responsible for certain similar behavioral aspects of the two disorders.

Chromosome 17   A recent study found the strongest evidence of linkage on this chromosome among a set of more than 500 families whose male members were diagnosed with autism. Missing or disrupted genes on this chromosome can cause problems such as galactosemia, a metabolic disorder that, if left untreated, can result in mental retardation. Galactosemia causes some of the same symptoms as autism, as does OCD. For example, APRAXIA of speech has been reported in both galactosemia and autism, and OBSESSIVE COMPULSIVE DISORDER, which is marked by recurrent, unwanted thoughts (obsessions) and/or repetitive behaviors (compulsions), is often a problem seen in autistic individuals.

Chromosome 17 also contains the gene for the serotonin transporter, which allows nerve cells to collect SEROTONIN. Serotonin is involved in emotions and helps nerve cells communicate.

The X chromosome   Two disorders that share symptoms with autism (FRAGILE X SYNDROME and RETT DISORDER) are typically caused by genes on the X chromosome, which suggests that genes on this chromosome may also play a role in ASDs.

People usually have 46 chromosomes in most of their cells (23 from their mother and 23 from their father); after fertilization, the two individual sets form 23 pairs of chromosomes. The chromosomes in the 23rd pair are called the "sex chromosomes"—X and Y—whose combination determines a person's sex. Males usually have one X and one Y chromosome, and females usually have two X chromosomes.

The fact that more males than females have autism supports the idea that the disorder involves genes on the X chromosome. Females may be able to use their other X chromosome to function normally, while males, without such a spare, show symptoms of the condition.

Potential Genes

HOXA1 gene   Researchers have found evidence that autism may involve the HOXA1 gene, a homeobox gene that plays a critical role in the development of important brain structures, cranial nerves, the ear, and the skeleton of the head and neck. Researchers know that the HOXA1 gene is active very early in life (between the 20th and 24th days after conception) and that any problem with the gene's function causes problems with the development of these structures, including autism.

This gene is involved in DUANE SYNDROME, a rare disorder that causes eye movement problems and sometimes occurs with autism.

In one study of persons with autism, nearly 94 percent of participants had mutations in the same regions of HOXA1, which could mean that the region contributes to ASDs. In another study, nearly 40 percent of those with autism carried a specific mutation in the HOXA1 gene sequence—nearly twice as many as those who had the same change but who did not have autism and were not related to anyone with autism. In addition, 33 percent of those who did not have autism but were related to someone with autism also had the mutation in their HOXA1 gene.

These findings suggest that autism is not caused simply by an errant gene, but that some other factors must also be involved. If researchers can confirm an association between this mutation and ASDs, they may be able to use detection of the mutation as an early test for autism, allowing important interventions to start as early in life as possible.

Another study found that increased head size in ASD patients was associated with a different mutation in the HOXA1 gene. About 20 percent of persons with autism have large head size—it is one of the most consistently reported physical features of people with autism.

The reelin (RELN) gene   Located on chromosome 7, this gene plays a crucial role in the development of connections between cells of the nervous system. Researchers think that abnormal brain connections may play a role in autism. In addition, people with autism and their parents and siblings have lower levels of certain types of the reelin protein, which may mean that the gene is not functioning normally.

Gamma-aminobutyric acid (GABA) pathway genes   GABA compounds are neurotransmitters, which means they help different areas of the nervous system communicate with each other. GABA receptor genes are involved in early development of parts of the nervous system and help with communication between these parts throughout life.

A problem in the GABA pathway can cause some of the symptoms of ASDs. For instance, epilepsy may in part be caused by low levels of GABA compounds. Many people with autism also have epilepsy and low levels of GABA.

In studies of mice, disrupting the GABA pathway causes seizures, extreme reactions to touch and sound, and stereotyped actions—symptoms also common in autism. Research now focuses on whether medications used to treat these problems can also reduce some of the symptoms of autism.

Serotonin transporter gene   Located on chromosome 17, the serotonin transporter allows nerve cells to collect serotonin so that they can communicate with each other. Abnormal levels of serotonin appear to be involved in depression, alcoholism, obsessive-compulsive disorder, and many other problems.

Research shows that people with autism have levels of serotonin between 25 percent and 50 percent higher than persons without autism. High serotonin levels may explain why people with autism have problems showing emotion and handling sensory information, such as sounds, touch, and smells. This higher serotonin level may be caused by errors in the serotonin transporter gene.

Researchers are now studying whether medications that regulate serotonin levels may improve behavior in people with autism, and whether there are any abnormal patterns in the genes that make and regulate serotonin and its pathway components.

Isolating the genetic causes of autism should allow clinicians to develop better tests to identify at-risk children before they show symptoms of the disorder. Experts hope that the major genetic components of the disorder will be identified by 2009.

See also GENETIC MARKER.

genetic marker   A specific gene or section of DNA with an identifiable physical location on a chromosome that produces a recognizable trait. Scientists have been searching for genetic markers linked to AUTISM SPECTRUM DISORDERS (ASD) or autism, which would provide an easier way to diagnose these conditions.

Initial results suggest there may be a link between ASD and tiny sections of several chromosomes. Scientists are fairly certain there is more than one gene that influences the development of autism. In fact, they believe that many genes interact to result in autistic behavior.

By studying families with at least two autistic children, scientists have been able to narrow their search to a few small pieces of chromosomes (the carriers of genetic information).

They have found that in some autistic children, a small region of chromosome 15—an area that is highly unstable and prone to genetic rearrangement—is duplicated or deleted. The region also includes genes for PRADER-WILLI SYNDROME and ANGELMAN SYNDROME, two other disorders that can trigger autistic-like behavior. Further, it contains genes that recognize a powerful neurotransmitter in the brain called GABA (gamma-aminobutyric acid). Scientists have found evidence that at least one form of autism is associated with a genetic marker near a GABA receptor gene.

Researchers concluded that children with a particular genetic profile may have a specific subtype of autism that can be distinguished from other forms of autism. These children all have two copies of the same small region of chromosome 15, while nonautistic children have only one copy per chromosome.

Scientists hope that finding genes related to autism will help provide a better way to diagnose the condition. For example, autistic children share a pattern of behaviors—including speech delay, lack of social skills, and "stereotyped" or repetitive behaviors—that seem to cluster together with a specific genetic defect. But some of these children have seizures and low muscle tone, characteristics not necessarily associated with autism. These children all have a duplication of part of chromosome 15.

Studies show that the genetic errors that lead to autism are introduced when a piece of a chromosome breaks apart and recombines during the formation of sperm and eggs. As a result, in some children with autism there is an extra copy of a piece of chromosome 15, while in others the piece is missing. Scientists suspect that the gene or genes responsible for the behavioral changes we see in some children with autism are located in this area of chromosome 15. The scientists are not sure which of the genes in the region lead to autistic behaviors, but they have identified a few strong candidates.

Scientists have also found that the region of chromosome 7 is particularly susceptible to breaking apart and recombining with its chromosome pair. Apparently, in some cases this recombination is abnormal, and parts of the chromosome are not duplicated correctly. The result: a piece of chromosome 7 is turned upside down.

Researchers are narrowing down the potential candidate genes on a variety of other chromosomes by studying additional families and by using their existing genetic maps and genetic markers to test each potential gene candidate.

See also GENES AND AUTISM.

Gilliam Autism Rating Scale A test designed for use by teachers, parents, and professionals that helps to identify and diagnose autism in individuals ages three through 22 years and to estimate the severity of the problem. Items on the GARS are grouped into four subtests, assessing stereotyped behaviors, communication, social interaction, and developmental disturbances. The GARS also includes a summary score. The test can be completed in five to ten minutes by those who know about the child's behavior.

gluten-free (GF), casein-free (CF), and gluten-free casein-free (GFCF) diets These are three different types of diets that some families believe help improve some symptoms of autism. Gluten is a substance found mainly in wheat, oats, rye, and barley; casein is a protein found in milk products. There is some suggestion that a diet free from these two types of substances found in many foods may help improve concentration and prevent digestive problems in people with autism, although research has not substantiated this hypothesis. GFCF diets have been developed for those individuals who have allergic responses to gluten and casein.

Grandin, Temple An associate professor of animal science at Colorado State University and a well-known person with autism who has written books about her experiences with the condition. Grandin is the author of *Emergence: Labeled Autistic* and *Thinking in Pictures* and is a designer of livestock-handling facilities. Half of the cattle in North America are handled in facilities she has designed.

A popular speaker at colleges and autism conferences, she obtained her B.A. at Frankin Pierce College, her M.S. in animal science at Arizona State University, and her Ph.D. in animal science from the University of Illinois in 1989. Today she teaches courses on livestock behavior and facility design at Colorado State University and consults with the livestock industry on facility design, livestock handling, and animal welfare.

She has appeared on television shows such as *20/20, 48 Hours,* and *CNN Larry King Live* and has been featured in *People* magazine, the *New York Times, Forbes, U.S. News and World Report,* and *Time.* She has written more than 300 articles in both scientific journals and livestock periodicals on animal handling, welfare, and facility design. Grandin believes that her autistic condition has helped her understand the way that animals think. "Autism made school and social life hard," she writes in her book, *Animals in Translation.* "But it made animals easy."

guardianship A legal appointment by the court in which an individual or institution manages the estate of a person with autism judged incapable (not necessarily incompetent) of caring for his or her own affairs. Guardians (also called conservators) are also responsible for the care of people who are unable to care for themselves. A conservator/guardian also can be chosen to serve in the future when the parent is no longer able to serve.

In some states, guardians assist people while conservators manage estates. Many parents who have children with autism do not realize that when their children reach 18, they may no longer have legal authority over their care.

Haldol   See HALOPERIDOL.

haloperidol (Haldol)   An antipsychotic neuroleptic medication that was at one time the primary medical treatment of autism. However, the risk of serious side effects is significant in children, and although haloperidol was reported to improve some symptoms of autism, including motor stereotypies, withdrawal and hyperactivity, its side effects have limited its usefulness. Muscle spasms of the neck and back, twisting movements of the body, trembling of fingers and hands, and an inability to move the eyes are among the more common side effects.

Others include speaking or swallowing problems, loss of balance control, masklike face, severe restlessness or need to keep moving, and shuffling walk, stiffness of arms and legs, and weakness of arms and legs. Less often there may be decreased thirst; difficulty in urination; dizziness, light-headedness, or fainting; hallucinations; lip smacking or puckering; puffing of cheeks; rapid or wormlike movements of the tongue; skin rash; uncontrolled chewing movements; or uncontrolled movements of arms and legs.

Rarely, haloperidol may cause convulsions, difficult or fast breathing, fast or irregular pulse, high fever, high or low blood pressure, increased sweating, loss of bladder control, severe muscle stiffness, unusually pale skin, or unusual tiredness or weakness.

hand flapping   One type of repetitive movements that are typical of people with autism.

handicap   A term that refers to a disadvantage or impairment based on a disabling condition. Federal legislation—such as Public Law 94-142: the EDUCATION FOR ALL HANDICAPPED CHILDREN ACT OF 1975—uses "handicap" to identify the disadvantaged status of an individual with specific impairments as compared to others without such impairments.

However, the term "handicapped" is no longer considered an appropriate term to mean disability or disorder, because it places a perjorative emphasis on social status or defines an individual rather than suggesting a particular difference. In the same manner that many individuals challenge the use of the word "disability" because it by definition focuses on a negative condition, they may believe that "handicap" is best used in a legal context rather than in a social one.

head size   Small head circumference at birth followed by a rapid growth in head size in the first year of life may be the first physical warning sign of autism, according to a study published in 2003. Researchers' findings could lead to earlier identification of autistic children, who are now typically diagnosed at about age three. Experts say earlier intervention is more beneficial, and the study may help alert doctors to a possible, though not certain, diagnosis of autism in the first months of life. Experts hoped that head size might give doctors a physiological marker for identifying a child with autism. Currently, all doctors can do is watch for certain behaviors, most of which do not emerge until a child is older.

Heller's disease   Another name for CHILDHOOD DISINTEGRATIVE DISORDER.

hereditary factors   See GENES AND AUTISM; GENETIC MARKERS.

92

Higashi USA See Boston Higashi School.

higher cognitive functions A term that usually refers to complex thinking skills such as judgment, abstraction, problem-solving, and planning.

See also higher-order thinking.

higher-order thinking Advanced intellectual abilities that go beyond basic information processing. Higher-order thinking involves such abilities as concept formation, understanding rules, problem-solving skills, and the ability to look at information from multiple perspectives.

Students exercise their higher-order thinking abilities when they analyze, synthesize, and evaluate materials to which they have been exposed. The construction or creation of new material also requires higher-order thinking.

In general, abilities in the area of higher-order thinking are closely linked to intellectual capacity.

high-functioning autistic disorder Children who are autistic by definition yet are able to communicate, do not have overly severe social impairments, and have only minor deficits. Their IQ ratings are near normal, normal, or even high.

history of autism Most experts believe that before the discovery of the pattern of symptoms now known as autism, most people with the syndrome were considered either to be mentally retarded or insane. There have not been many historical descriptions that suggest autism. Of the few that exist, one of the best is of the Wild Boy of Aveyron, a youngster found in the 19th century and named Victor, who had grown up without human contact in the forest.

Thereafter, medical history was largely silent on the symptoms of what is now known as autism until the 20th century. In 1944 child psychiatrist Leo Kanner, M.D., studied 11 children who had apparently had a lack of interest in other people yet who were extremely interested in unusual aspects of inanimate objects. Kanner observed that these children often demonstrated qualities showing that they were not merely slow learners or emotionally disturbed. As a result, he invented a new category, which he called early infantile autism (sometimes called Kanner's syndrome).

Hans Asperger made the same discoveries at the same time, independently of Kanner, but the patients he identified all were able to speak; this is why the term Asperger's syndrome is often used to label autistic people who can speak (and whose early language development was intact).

Long before Kanner incorporated the term "autism" into his label, the word (coined in 1912 by Eugen Bleuler, who had already invented the term "schizophrenia") already had a meaning: "escape from reality." Kanner used the term because he believed the children gave the impression they were trying to escape from reality.

For several decades after the initial description of autism, research on it was impeded by a lack of consensus on its definition as well as by assumptions of continuity between autism and severe forms of mental illness in adults, particularly schizophrenia. The idea that autism was the earliest form of schizophrenia reflected three factors: an awareness of the severity of both conditions, an extremely broad view of schizophrenia among the scientists of the time, and Kanner's use of the word "autism," which had previously been used to describe the self-centered quality of thinking in schizophrenia rather than a lack of ability to relate socially.

It took many years before researchers and clinicians could be sure that autism and schizophrenia were indeed different conditions. Some early clinicians thought that perhaps autism could be caused by negative experience. Doctors had noticed that parents treated their autistic children without the warmth and affection normally observed between parent and child. At the time, doctors influenced by psychiatrist Sigmund Freud believed that if certain basic psychological bonds between parent and child fail to form, the child will fail to progress—and therefore, the idea of the cold "refrigeration mother" as the cause of autism was born. This Freudian theory of autism remained popular through the 1950s and into the 1960s. What Freudians failed to notice, however, is that the parents' stilted interaction with the child was actually the *result* of the child's autistic behavior. They also failed to note that autism is an extreme instance of a genetically inherited personality trait present to a milder extent in these parents.

Unfortunately, based upon these flawed theories of the basis of autism, some children were removed from their parents' home and placed in foster care to see if they would recover.

The syndrome identified by Kanner has been broadened somewhat since he first published his paper. Kanner reported a rate of occurrence of one in 10,000; more modern estimates suggest the rate is closer to 15 in 10,000. Kanner first identified people who were clearly not mentally retarded (since this was the unexplained group of people at the time). Since then, doctors have realized that some mentally retarded people have autistic symptoms whereas others do not; experts now believe the conditions overlap. This explains some of the difference in the reported rates of occurrence.

See also AUTISM, EARLY ONSET.

Hoffman, Dustin Gifted actor who portrayed an autistic man in the film *Rain Man* (1988). Although his performance was widely praised, the character illustrates just one point on a wide continuum of autistic personalities and skill levels. Some, but not all, individuals with autism excel in an area of interest (such as music) the way Hoffman's character did with math. Mark Rimland, son of autism expert Bernard Rimland, was one of the autistic individuals with whom Hoffman worked when preparing for the part.

holding therapy A treatment for AUTISTIC DISORDER in which the parent tries to make contact with the child by forced holding, a method devised by Columbia University psychiatrist Marth Welch. This method received widespread attention during the late 1970s when Dr. Welch first developed her theory. The method has some proponents who claim positive results but experts disagree with its intrusive nature and lack of evidence for its effectiveness.

During holding therapy, the parent tries to establish eye contact and share feelings verbally with the child, who is sitting or lying face to face with the parent. The parent should remain calm and offer comfort until the child stops resisting. This holding period may last just a few minutes up to hours at a time. A few very unfortunate outcomes have occurred when holding therapy was carried out in an extreme form. Some children have been injured and even smothered when they resisted the confinement of holding therapy.

hyperactivity Constant and excessive movement and activity. A child with hyperactivity may show restless movements. He or she may not be able to stop an action when directed to or to sit still for any period of time. Hyperactivity often occurs with inattentiveness and impulsivity. An affected child might have trouble sitting still, fidgets excessively, and moves about excessively even during sleep. Onset occurs before the age of seven years. Behaviors are chronic (present throughout the child's life), present throughout the child's day in many different settings, and are not due to other factors such as anxiety or depression.

In older children, symptoms of hyperactivity may be more subtle, displaying themselves in more subdued restlessness or fidgeting. Accompanying impulsivity may appear as a tendency to interrupt in class, problems waiting for one's turn, and other behaviors that often result in conflict with peers and family members.

hyperlexia A complex condition that includes an ability to read words at a far earlier developmental stage than is typical or earlier than one's abilities in other areas, such as talking. It is usually accompanied by an intense fascination with symbols such as letters and numbers. It also usually involves a significant difficulty in understanding verbal language and may present with problems with social skills, including difficulty interacting appropriately with peers and family members.

In addition, some children with hyperlexia may also develop expressive language skills in unusual ways, echoing what they hear without understanding the meaning, and failing to develop the ability to initiate conversations. They often exhibit a powerful need to maintain routines and ritualistic patterns of behavior, and have trouble with transitions and handling external sensory stimuli.

Children with hyperlexia often display very strong auditory and visual memory, but may have trouble understanding and reasoning in abstract rather than concrete and literal terms. Often, their approach to listening to others may be highly selective, and they can appear to be deaf.

Hyperlexia may share similar characteristics with autism, behavior disorders, language disorders, emotional disorders, ATTENTION DEFICIT DISORDER, hearing impairment, giftedness or, paradoxically, MENTAL RETARDATION.

Symptoms and Diagnostic Path

To develop effective teaching strategies, it is important to differentiate hyperlexia from other disorders. A thorough assessment by a speech and language pathologist who is familiar with hyperlexia is the first step. Psychological tests that emphasize visual processes rather than verbal skills can also help identify hyperlexia. Hearing, neurological, psychiatric, blood chemistry, and genetic evaluations can be performed to rule out other disorders but are not needed to identify hyperlexia.

Treatment Options and Outlook

The future of a hyperlexic child depends on developing language expression and comprehension skills. Intensive speech and language therapy and early intervention programs can help. The child's reading skills should be used as a primary means of developing language.

It is also important to teach the child appropriate social skills by providing opportunities for the child to interact with others whose behavior is more socially appropriate. Parents, teachers, and other professionals should work together to develop programs for each child.

idiot-savant   See AUTISTIC SAVANT.

imipramine (Tofranil)   A tricyclic antidepressant that has been used to treat people with autism, but which subsequently was found not to be especially helpful.

Side Effects

Side effects include dry mouth, blurred vision, constipation, fatigue, electrocardiogram changes, and weight gain.

immunization   A method of producing immunity to disease via vaccination. When a naturally occurring disease-causing germ infects the body, the immune system produces special proteins called antibodies to destroy the invader. If the same germ is encountered a second time, the immune system recognizes it and produces antibodies much more quickly, killing the germ before the disease can develop. That is why a person who had a disease such as measles as a child is immune from the disease if ever exposed again.

Vaccines work by the same principle. Vaccines are made from tiny amounts of bacteria or viruses (antigens) that are weakened or killed so that they are harmless to the body. But when introduced into the body, the immune system still makes antibodies against the vaccine's altered germs—so when the body later encounters the actual invading germ, it can fight off the disease. This is why a child who received a measles vaccine also would be immune to the disease if exposed later in life. A few vaccines produce immunity from a disease with just one dose, but most require two or more doses. For some vaccines (such as tetanus), peri-

odic booster shots for life are required to maintain immunity.

Immunization is not straightforward, however. As infectious diseases continue to decline, some people have become less interested in the consequences of preventable illnesses such as diphtheria and tetanus. Instead, they have become increasingly concerned about the risks associated with the vaccines themselves. Some vaccines are perceived by the public as carrying a risk, especially the pertussis part of the DPT (diphtheria-pertussis-tetanus) vaccine, which had been linked to seizures and other serious side effects. In response to these concerns, a safer acellular version of the pertussis vaccine is now in use.

Other concerns focused on the preservative thimerosal, a mercury compound, which used to be included in many vaccinations and which some parents believe has been linked to autism. A review by the Food and Drug Administration found no evidence of harm caused by doses of thimerosal in vaccines, except for minor local reactions. Nevertheless, in July 1999 the Public Health Service agencies, the American Academy of Pediatrics, and vaccine manufacturers agreed that thimerosal levels in vaccines should be reduced or eliminated as a precautionary measure. Today almost all vaccines for children are thimerosal free.

Medical experts argue that a vaccine is not licensed unless it is considered safe and its benefits far outweigh perceived risks. For a vaccine to be included on the annual Recommended Childhood Immunization Schedule for the United States, it must first be approved by the Advisory Committee on Immunization Practices from the Centers for Disease Control and Prevention, the American Academy of Pediatrics and the American Academy of Family Physicians. Scientists and physicians in these organizations carefully weigh the risks and benefits of newly developed vaccines, monitor the safety and effectiveness of existing vaccines, and track cases of vaccine-preventable diseases.

The topic of vaccine safety became prominent during the mid 1970s as lawsuits were filed on behalf of those presumably injured by the DPT vaccine. In order to reduce liability and respond to public health concerns, Congress passed the National Childhood Vaccine Injury Act (NCVIA) in 1986. Designed for citizens injured or killed by vaccines, this system provided a no-fault compensation alternative to suing vaccine manufacturers and providers. The act also created safety provisions to help educate the public about vaccine benefits and risks and required doctors to report adverse events after vaccination as well as keep records on vaccines administered and health problems that occurred following vaccination. The act also created incentives for the production of safer vaccines.

independent education evaluation (IEE) An evaluation of a student conducted by a qualified examiner who does not work for the school district. According to Public Law 94-142 (amended to the INDIVIDUALS WITH DISABILITIES EDUCATION ACT), parents have the right to have their child independently tested either to seek a more comprehensive assessment than is sometimes provided in a school setting or because they fear a school-based evaluation is biased or inaccurate.

An IEE would include the same elements as a school-mandated evaluation, focusing on measures of aptitude and achievement. Parents may obtain an evaluation at school district expense if they disagree with the evaluation arranged for by the school district.

If the parent wants the school district to pay for the tests, the district may ask (but not require) the parents to explain the reason why they object to the district's evaluation. The school district also may ask for an impartial hearing to show that its evaluation is appropriate. If the impartial hearing officer finds that the district evaluation is appropriate, parents still have the right to obtain an IEE—but the district does not have to pay for it. The school district may not unreasonably delay either providing the test or

calling an impartial hearing to defend the district's own evaluation.

independent living skills The ability to independently take care of personal needs and daily life tasks, such as dressing, preparing meals, eating, homemaking, maintaining personal hygiene (such as dressing, bathing, and toileting), communication, travel, and safety in the home.

Individualized Education Program (IEP) A written educational prescription developed for each child who qualifies for SPECIAL EDUCATION, describing what special education the child needs and what the school district will do to address those needs. School districts are required by law to develop these programs (sometimes called an Individualized Education Plan) in cooperation with parents. An IEP must be created for each exceptional child, according to the INDIVIDUALS WITH DISABILITIES EDUCATION ACT (IDEA).

An IEP is prepared at a team meeting attended by the parents, the child, the child's teacher, a school administrator, educational specialists, other professionals who are providing services to the child (such as a speech therapist or an occupational therapist), and a representative of the public agency that oversees special education. Any support the child needs, such as a trained one-on-one aide or assistive technology, needs to be discussed and written into the IEP.

An IEP must contain

- the child's present levels of educational performance
- annual and short-term educational goals
- the specific special education program and related services that will be provided
- the extent to which the child will participate in regular education programs with non-handicapped children
- a statement of when services will begin and how long they will last
- provisions for evaluating the effectiveness of the program and the student's performance

- statement of transition services for students 14 years of age or older

The team meets at least once a year, sometimes arranged to fall in the child's birthday month, to review the child's educational progress and needs, and to develop goals and objectives for the coming year. If parents decide their child needs a change in the program, they have the right to ask the school to call an IEP meeting at any time.

Individualized Education Program Committee   A group of people who meet to create an INDIVIDUAL-IZED EDUCATION PROGRAM (IEP) for a child who has been identified as learning disabled by a multidisciplinary team.

The committee should include a representative of the public school, the student's teacher, one or both parents, the student (when appropriate), and any other individuals deemed relevant by the school or parents such as an educational PSYCHOLO-GIST, speech teacher, legal expert, or advisor.

Individualized Family Service Program (IFSP)   A written plan developed with teachers and parents to outline special services to be provided to children of preschool age (often prior to or up to age three).

As stated in Public Law 99-457, Part H, families play a crucial part in a child's development from birth to age two; therefore, the individualized family services program is written to address the special needs of the child and the family.

According to the INDIVIDUALS WITH DISABILITIES EDUCATION ACT (IDEA), an IFSP must include

- present levels of the child's development (cognitive, physical, language/speech, psychosocial, and self-help)
- family resources and concerns regarding the child's development
- expected outcomes for the family and child including criteria, timelines, and assessment procedures
- specific intervention services necessary to meet the needs of the family and child

- projected start and end dates of services
- name of case manager
- steps needed for smooth transition from early intervention program to preschool program

See also EARLY INTERVENTION PROGRAM.

Individualized Habilitation Program (IHP)   A written statement that defines the goals for a developmentally disabled person (such as a person with AUTISTIC DISORDER) along with a description of how to attain those goals. The program must be approved by the developmentally disabled person or a guardian. The IHP is very much like an INDIVIDUALIZED EDUCATION PROGRAM (IEP), individual program plan (IPP), and individual work plan (IWP).

Individuals with Disabilities Education Act (IDEA), The   A federally mandated program that provides children with disabilities (including autism) access to a free appropriate public education and aims to improve the educational experience of such children.

Typically, children are placed in public schools and the school district pays for all necessary services. These will include, as needed, services by a SPEECH-LANGUAGE PATHOLOGIST, OCCUPATIONAL THERAPIST, school PSYCHOLOGIST, SOCIAL WORKER, school nurse, or aide.

However, each state has its own guidelines regarding how IDEA is applied, which means there may be substantial differences in services from state to state, and often from school district to school district. Although many school districts are knowledgeable about autism, recognizing that different strategies work for different children and providing effective support for both mainstream teachers and special education classrooms, some are not.

Sometimes, school administrators and parents disagree about what is an appropriate education for a particular child. School districts must furnish information about the parents' rights and responsibilities under the law.

IDEA was first enacted as the EDUCATION FOR ALL HANDICAPPED CHILDREN ACT OF 1975 (Public

Law 94-142), renamed in 1990 (Public Law 101-476), and amended (Public Law 102-119) in 1991. Under the IDEA, money is given to local school systems to educate children up to age 22; local schools are required to comply with the act as a condition of receiving funds.

Prior to IDEA's implementation in 1975, approximately one million children with disabilities were shut out of schools and hundreds of thousands more were denied appropriate services. Since IDEA was enacted, many of these children are learning and achieving at levels previously thought impossible—graduating from high school, going to college, and entering the workforce as productive citizens in unprecedented numbers.

Previously, 90 percent of children with developmental disabilities were housed in state institutions; today three times as many young people with disabilities are enrolled in colleges or universities, and twice as many of today's 20-year-olds with disabilities are working.

The IDEA provides that children covered by the act have access to a free and appropriate public education. By law, the public schools must prepare and carry out a set of instruction goals, or specific skills, for every child in a special education program. The list of skills is known as the child's INDIVIDUALIZED EDUCATION PROGRAM (IEP). The IEP is an agreement between the school and the family on the child's goals. When a child's IEP is developed, the parents are asked to attend the meeting. In general, students receiving services under the IDEA will take part in regular educational programs to some degree, and also receive special education services as described in their IEP. Parents have the right to receive a copy of the evaluation report and to receive a copy of the paperwork about the child's eligibility for special education.

There will be several people at this meeting, including a special education teacher, a representative of the public schools who is knowledgeable about the program, other individuals invited by the school or by the parents (who may want to bring a relative, a child care provider, an advocate or lawyer, or a supportive close friend who knows the child well). Parents play an important part in creating the program, as they know the child and his or her needs best.

Once a child's IEP is developed, a meeting is scheduled once a year to review the child's progress and to make any alterations to reflect changing needs. If a child is under three years of age and has special needs, he or she should be eligible for an early intervention program; this program is available in every state. Each state decides which agency will be the lead agency in the early intervention program. The early intervention services are provided by workers qualified to care for toddlers with disabilities and are usually in the child's home or a place familiar to the child. The services provided are written into an INDIVIDUALIZED FAMILY SERVICE PLAN (IFSP) that is reviewed at least once every six months. The plan will describe services that will be provided to the child but will also describe services for parents to help them in daily activities with their child and for siblings to help them adjust to having a brother or sister with disabilities.

Most students who fall under the IDEA are served within their own public school system, although in some cases students may attend a private educational institution with the school district assuming the cost.

Parents who are having a serious disagreement with school district officials may need the advice of an advocate or an attorney knowledgeable in special education. Some organizations and some law firms offer free legal advice in this area. If parents cannot reach an agreement with the school district, they may file for due process (an impartial hearing provided to parents who disagree with their child's placement). If, through due process or mediation parents reach an agreement but find the school district is still not fulfilling its end, parents may file a compliance complaint with their state's department of education.

infantile autism, residual state   A category in the *Diagnostic and Statistical Manual* that describes individuals who once met the criteria for autism but no longer do so, but who may retain some residual traits.

inflammation   Brain inflammation may play an important role in the development of autism, according to a study by researchers at Johns Hopkins University. Inflammation occurs when the immune system kicks into gear, triggering a rush of cells into the area, producing swelling.

In the study, researchers who analyzed frozen brain tissue from 11 deceased autism patients aged five to 44 discovered that inflammation is clearly a feature of the disease in certain brain areas. The autistic brains experienced active inflammation in various regions, but especially in the cerebellum. There also was ongoing inflammation in the fluid surrounding the brain and spinal cord, along with cytokines—powerful chemical messengers secreted by the immune system that lead to inflammation.

Scientists hope their findings will open up new possibilities for understanding the dynamic changes that occur, leading to new treatments and specific diagnostic tests that screen for inflammation in the spinal fluid of autistic patients. There is currently no blood or lab test to check for the disease.

inhibition   The ability to defer responses to unimportant distractions. The ability to control inappropriate impulsive responses or strategies while developing more effective or appropriate ones is essential to success in both academic and social settings.

insomnia and Asperger's syndrome   Children with ASPERGER'S SYNDROME (AS) have difficulty falling and staying asleep. Research suggests that neuropsychiatric problems inherent with AS predispose children both to insomnia and to anxiety and mood disorders. Therefore, a careful assessment of sleep quality should be an integral part of the treatment plan in these individuals.

insurance and autism   Although federal law deals with the issues of insurance coverage for people with autism and other PERVASIVE DEVELOPMENTAL DISORDERS (PDD), these laws may be vague and open to interpretation by the insurance industry. One of the major problems with these laws is that according to the guidelines of the *DSM-IV-TR,* autism is classified as a mental condition, which allows insurance

companies to place restrictions on coverage. If a state does not specifically mention autism as one of the conditions covered by insurance, companies may deny coverage for treatment. About 90 to 95 percent of insurance companies refuse outright to cover treatment for pervasive developmental disorders, although most will cover the cost of the initial diagnosis. Because there is no recognized cure for autism and the other AUTISM SPECTRUM DISORDERS, treatment may not be covered, although medications or treatments prescribed to ease symptoms might be covered. Sometimes insurance plans will not even cover any kind of psychological testing to rule in or rule out an autistic spectrum disorder, because they reason that this kind of screening is usually available through the school system.

Moreover, neurobiological disorders such as ASDs are often difficult to cover, because they are medically based illnesses with psychiatric symptoms. The insurer and health care providers may argue with each other about what kind of care is needed, who should deliver it, and who will pay for it.

Insurance companies that do cover these conditions may do so in a substandard way. For example, they may cover only short-term therapy programs or refuse to pay for necessary behavioral therapy, speech therapy, occupational therapy, or physical therapy. They may have no qualified practitioners in the plan but refuse to make outside referrals, or, as already mentioned, they may call PDD-NOS or atypical PDD a mental health issue rather than a medical problem and limit coverage.

In the United States, however, both case law and state legislation may support parents who say that treatment for autism and related disorders should be covered by their health insurance. For example, in 1988 *Kunin v. Benefit Trust Life Insurance Co.* (eventually affirmed by the U.S. Court of Appeals for the Ninth Circuit) established that because autism has organic causes, it is not a mental illness and so cannot be used as a basis for denying or limiting insurance benefits. Cases in some states have affirmed this conclusion in relation to other neurological disorders.

One piece of information parents should research is how the insurance company treats acquired nervous-system disorders, such as stroke, brain tumors, or traumatic brain injuries. If the insurance covers long-term care for these conditions, most states mandate equal benefits for patients with biologically based brain disorders.

Twelve states—Arkansas, Colorado, Connecticut, Indiana, Maine, Maryland, Minnesota, New Hampshire, North Carolina, Rhode Island, Texas, and Vermont—passed their own, more restrictive mental health parity laws, which supersede the federal regulations. Eleven other states have parity laws that are equal to the federal act, and others have less restrictive parity laws. Of the 12 with tighter restrictions, all of the laws are written in ways that should require coverage for PDDs. Colorado, Connecticut, Maine, New Hampshire, Rhode Island, and Texas specifically require coverage for autistic spectrum disorders and other "biologically based" mental illnesses. For parents and patients living in these states, this is a step in the right direction, although it remains to be seen how these laws will be enforced and what steps some insurers may take to evade responsibility.

intelligence The level of intellectual functioning and capacity of an individual; the ability to learn or understand. Some experts have suggested that intelligence is not a single phenomenon, but that there exist "multiple intelligences," a number of discrete "intelligences," and that an individual will possess a unique pattern of strengths and abilities across this range of intellectual functions.

Intelligence is measured by intelligence tests, which provide an "INTELLIGENCE QUOTIENT" (IQ), a measure of intellectual development that is the ratio of a child's mental age to his or her chronological age, multiplied by 100.

intelligence quotient (IQ) A measurement of intelligence based on performance on intelligence tests. Use of intelligence testing remains somewhat controversial because of the limitations of testing for specific abilities and knowledge and because of possible cultural bias in the design of tests. Nonetheless, IQ tests are used in educational and psychological settings in combination with other types of tests to evaluate an individual's mental capac-

ity and to recommend appropriate remediation or treatment.

For individuals with autism, however, standard IQ tests such as the Stanford-Binet and Wechsler are unreliable. These tests are designed to measure the intelligence of a person with typical language and forms of experience. While children with autism may have great perception strengths in some areas the tests will not measure, they most likely have deficits in other areas the tests do cover. This type of uneven development is quite typical of children with autism, with some superior skills and others that reveal significant delay.

IQ scores generally have a mean of 100, and range in classification from mentally retarded at the low end to very superior at the high end.

The concept of intelligence has existed for centuries, but it was not until this century that scientists began testing it—and debating whether or not they could do so accurately. Intelligence testing was developed in the late 19th century as France's Alfred Binet began work on tests of individual differences, which led him to study "subnormal" children in Paris schools. Several years later, Binet and Paris physician Theodore Simon recommended that an accurate diagnosis of intelligence be established for schoolchildren. The result was the Simon-Binet test of intelligence, which first appeared in 1905 and was revised in 1908.

Binet thought of the test as a tool for selecting students who needed special remedial teaching, not as a measure of absolute innate ability. The test was translated into English for the American audience in 1908 by Henry H. Goddard and revised several times, but it was not until 1916 that the test was standardized with the revision by Lewis M. Terman in the form we still know as the Stanford-Binet test.

In 1911, William Stern developed the idea of relating mental age to chronological age with his formulation of Intelligence Quotient. This simple formulation of $IQ = MA/CA \times 100$, where MA stands for mental age and CA stands for chronological age, gave a number to stand for the performance of the child. This allowed the IQ to be manipulated within statistical tests and to be used for prediction of later performance.

During World War I, the first massive use of psychological tests of intelligence was begun with the testing of military recruits. Hundreds of psychologists and graduate students in psychology were recruited to administer the tests. After the war, critics were outraged to find that the Army test suggested that southern and eastern Europeans were inferior to northern Europeans, and that blacks were inferior to whites. Some believe it was these test results that prompted restrictive immigration policies in America in 1924 and fanned the flames of racial prejudice against blacks and other minorities.

David Wechsler developed his tests in response to many of the criticisms of the Binet tests. In 1939, he introduced his Wechsler Adult Intelligence Scale (WAIS), the first of a series of tests still much in use.

Since that time there have been many intelligence tests produced, some specifically aimed at reducing cultural and background effects on pencil-and-paper tests. In 1969, the debate about the inherent versus the environmental bases of intelligence exploded with an article by psychologist Arthur Jensen in which he argued that these are inherent racial differences in intelligence. The debate continued into the last decade of the 20th century in response to further controversial work on intelligence and class structure in American life. In recent years, influential books by psychologist Howard Gardner and others have supported multiple intelligences over a single global factor in intelligence.

When a child with autism is tested in different skill areas, typically each score reflects a completely different IQ, but none of these scores can accurately predict an autistic person's potential. IQ tests cannot reveal what a child with autism can do, but they may highlight areas of strength or weakness.

interim alternative educational setting (IAES)

Most students with disabilities are disciplined as any other student would be, but in certain extraordinary circumstances, a suspension longer than 10 days would require education in an IAES, as students with disabilities must not be suspended for longer than 10 days. School officials may place students with disabilities in an alternative educational setting with or without parent consent. The interim alternative educational setting is determined by the INDIVIDUALIZED EDUCATION PROGRAM (IEP) commit-

tee and allows the student to continue to participate in general educational programs and receive special services as outlined on the IEP. If suspension is necessary for a longer period, an IAES may be put into place for up to 45 days.

intermediate care facility for the mentally retarded (ICR/MR)

A facility designed to nurture residents with mental retardation and other developmental disabilities, including autism, and to encourage them to be as independent as possible so that they can lead busy, active, and full lives. These facilities must provide 24-hour services, including a wide range of programs geared toward enhancing residents' maximum independent living capabilities and their ultimate return to a less restrictive living arrangement. Each facility has a unique atmosphere for residents requiring different levels of care.

ICFs are an optional Medicaid benefit and are licensed and certified to operate under federal Title XIX regulations of the Social Security Act. The Social Security Act created this benefit to fund "institutions" of four or more beds for people with mental retardation and specifies that these institutions must provide active treatment. Currently, all 50 states have at least one ICF/MR facility. The program serves about 129,000 people with mental retardation and other related conditions, all of whom must qualify for Medicaid assistance financially.

irlen lenses

A highly controversial treatment for autism not supported by research involving a special type of colored prism lens that supposedly treats autism, originally developed to treat dyslexia and other learning disabilities.

Many autistic individuals have difficulty paying attention to their visual environment or perceiving themselves in relation to their surroundings. These problems have been associated with a short attention span, easy distractibility, excessive eye movements, difficulty scanning or tracking movements, inability to catch a ball, extra cautiousness when walking up or down stairs, bumping into furniture, and even TOE WALKING.

Kanner, Leo (1894–1981)   Austrian child psychiatrist who was the first person to describe the condition now known as autism. Born in Klekotow, Austria, Kanner received his M.D. from the University of Berlin in 1921. He emigrated to the United States in 1924 to become assistant physician at a state hospital in South Dakota. Six years later, he was selected to develop the first child psychiatry service in a pediatric hospital, at Johns Hopkins Hospital in Baltimore, where he became associate professor of psychiatry in 1939.

Kanner was the first physician in the United States to be identified as a child psychiatrist, and his first textbook, *Child Psychiatry* (1935), was the first English language textbook that focused on the psychiatric problems of children.

In 1938, Kanner studied 11 children who apparently had a lack of interest in other people—yet they were extremely interested in unusual aspects of inanimate objects. His groundbreaking 1943 paper *Autistic Disturbances of Affective Contact,* together with the work of Hans ASPERGER, forms the basis of the modern study of autism. In this paper, Kanner focused on three defining characteristics of autism that are still used today: social isolation, language impairments, and insistence on sameness.

Before Kanner noticed and recorded a pattern of symptoms, such children would have been classified as emotionally disturbed or mentally retarded. Kanner observed that these children often demonstrated capabilities that showed that they were not merely slow learners, yet they did not fit the patterns of emotionally disturbed children. As a result, he invented a new category, which he called early infantile autism (then, also called Kanner's syndrome).

These 11 children resembled those with childhood schizophrenia, but several of their characteristics prompted Kanner to describe autism as a separate disorder: early onset, lack of hallucinations, and family histories. Almost all of the children showed signs of the disorder before the age of three; children with schizophrenia, on the other hand, did not have as many problems at an early age. In fact, most symptoms of childhood schizophrenia do not appear until age 10. In addition, these children had neither hallucinations nor delusions, which are classic signs of schizophrenia. They did exhibit bizarre behaviors and unusual perceptions. The families of these children showed much less evidence of psychosis than did families of children with schizophrenia.

Social isolation was the most important characteristic of the children whom Kanner studied. Unlike children with childhood schizophrenia, who withdrew from preexisting relationships, children with autism never formed these relationships in the first place. Kanner wrote in 1943 that "there is from the start an extreme autistic aloneness that, whenever possible, disregards, ignores, shuts out, anything that comes to the child from the outside."

Kanner also described the language problems in these autistic children, including ECHOLALIA (parrot-like repetition of a word or sentence just spoken by another person often without comprehension), extreme literalness, and switching pronouns. He believed these unusual speech patterns separated autistic children from those with schizophrenia.

His final defining characteristic of autism was insistence on sameness. The 11 children he studied were compulsive about following routines; environmental change—no matter how minor—caused them great distress. Their preference for consistency prompted the children to do whatever they could to avoid anything different or new.

Misconceptions

Although Kanner's description of autism was accurate, several of his ideas have since been proven incorrect. His biggest mistake was the idea that autism was an emotional disorder caused by inadequate parenting, especially from the mother. Kanner observed a range of similarities among the families of the patients he studied, including perfectionism, obsessiveness, and lack of humor. Although his sample was small, he suggested that the highly organized professional parents of his subjects might be emotionally aloof and that this aloofness could cause autism. Further biological research on the topic has concretely proved this theory to be false.

Kanner also believed that children with autism are of average or above average intelligence and have the potential for normal language development. He reached this conclusion because his small sample of autistic children indeed functioned at a much higher intellectual level than the average autistic child, with an IQ well over 70; all but one child had EXPRESSIVE LANGUAGE. Subsequent researchers since have found that the average autistic child has an IQ of about 50 and that at least 40 percent do not develop any expressive language at all. More recent research suggests that the average IQ is actually higher and a greater percent are capable of developing expressive language, perhaps as a result of better intervention. Kanner also failed to note that his subject pool included only families with extremely high intelligence and educational levels. Recent studies have determined the prevalence of autism is proportionally distributed throughout educational levels, social classes, races, and religious groups.

Kanner also believed that autism is more likely to occur in firstborn or only children. Although this idea was firmly entrenched for years, recent studies do not suggest there are more firstborn or only children with autism.

Although Kanner believed that autism was different from schizophrenia, he also described autism as the earliest form of schizophrenia. Hans Asperger made the same discoveries at the same time, independently of Kanner, but the patients he identified all were able to speak; this is why the term ASPERGER'S SYNDROME is often used to label autistic people who can speak and whose early language development was intact.

Long before Kanner incorporated the term "autism" into his label, the word already had a meaning: "escape from reality" (coined by Eugen Bleuler in 1912, who had already invented the term "schizophrenia"). Kanner used the term because he believed the children gave the impression that they were trying, or were actually trying, to escape from reality.

He became director of child psychiatry at Johns Hopkins in 1957, and retired two years later. He remained active until his death at age 87.

kinesthetic   One of the body's senses that refers to the acquisition of information from body movements. Like other forms of learning, kinesthetic learning involves the input of stimuli to specific channels in the brain, in this case through the motion of joints and muscles. Kinesthetic learning is best understood as the process of making movements automatic through practice and repetition, such as throwing a baseball or driving a car.

For individuals with strengths in kinesthetic areas, learning in basic skills might be supplemented with a kinesthetic approach. Walking or dancing movements, for example, might be used to represent concepts or steps in a sequence to aid recall.

kinesthetic method   Any situation in which learning takes place through the sense of movement.

Klonopin   See CLONAZEPAM.

Landau-Kleffner syndrome (LKS) A rare childhood neurological disorder (also known as acquired epileptiform aphasia) characterized by normal development followed by the appearance of autistic-like behaviors and the sudden or gradual development of the inability to understand or express language (APHASIA). This syndrome affects the parts of the brain that control comprehension and speech, usually appearing between the ages of five and seven years. LKS was first described in 1957 by Dr. W. M. Landau and Dr. F. R. Kleffner.

While in some cases LKS is believed to result from a lack of full development of various networks within the brain, other cases seem to be triggered by a viral infection. There have been no reports of children with a family history of this syndrome. Boys are more than twice as likely to be affected as girls.

Symptoms and Diagnostic Path

After the normal development of language for the first few years in childhood, affected individuals suddenly begin to have trouble understanding language—even recognizing their own names. They may have trouble understanding environmental sounds, such as a doorbell ringing or a baby crying, and they begin to have trouble speaking; some become unable to speak at all.

In addition to the aphasia, these children have a number of autistic-like behaviors, such as social withdrawal, insensitivity to pain, avoidance of touch, and bizarre repetitive or inappropriate play. There also may be a range of behavioral problems, such as temper tantrums, aggressiveness, HYPERACTIVITY, and ATTENTION problems. They may have trouble recognizing friends and family or even common objects, and they may lose control of bladder and bowels.

The disorder is difficult to diagnose and may be confused with autism, PERVASIVE DEVELOPMENTAL DISORDER, hearing loss, learning disability, auditory/verbal processing disorder, attention deficit hyperactivity disorder, MENTAL RETARDATION, childhood schizophrenia, or emotional/behavioral problems. Between 70 and 80 percent of children with this syndrome have SEIZURES, but the presence of seizures is not a requirement for diagnosis.

The sudden appearance of speech problems is the first indication of LKS. The diagnosis can be confirmed by an EEG, which will show signs of brain malfunction involving both cerebral hemispheres, although activity will be more prominent in the dominant cerebral hemisphere dealing with language function.

Treatment Options and Outlook

Treatment usually consists of anticonvulsants to control the epileptic seizures common in this condition. Early SPEECH THERAPY (including sign language) can be very effective in easing the language problems. Corticosteroids also have been shown to improve language abilities in some children. Eventually, these children will most likely need educational support in a SPECIAL EDUCATION classroom because of the significant language and speech problems.

A more controversial treatment involves a surgical technique called multiple subpial transection, in which the pathways of abnormal electrical brain activity are severed.

The prognosis is varied; some children may have a permanent severe language disorder, but most others may regain much of their language ability over months or years, usually by adolescence. In still others, symptoms may wax and wane. Typically, the later the condition develops, the better the prognosis. Seizures generally disappear by adulthood.

language   An organized communication system of symbols (verbal, gestured, or pictoral) that represents objects, actions, feelings, processes, and relationships. Every language has rules that govern how it is used.

language delay   A lag in the development of communication skills, in which these skills progress more slowly than would be expected based on age, environment, or specific deprivation or disease. Children with autism often have language delays, which typically means that language is developing in the right sequence, but at a slower-than-normal rate. They also may experience qualitative language impairments.

language disabilities   A range of deficits in linguistics, whether related to written or oral expressive language, or to auditory processing (the processing of sounds and meaning).

leaky gut syndrome   An increase in intestinal permeability that allows improperly digested peptides to enter the bloodstream and cross the blood-brain barrier, where they may mimic neurotransmitters and scramble sensory input. Some experts also believe that autism is related to leaky gut syndrome. In one study, altered intestinal permeability was found in 43 percent of autistic patients, but not found in any of the controls.

A healthy gastrointestinal tract, with its tightly packed cells lining the intestinal wall, is designed to absorb only small molecules needed by the body to function, such as amino acids, simple sugars, fatty acids, vitamins, and minerals. The intestines also contain special "carrier proteins" that bind to certain nutrients and transport them through the intestinal wall and into the bloodstream.

However, in leaky gut syndrome, the spaces between the cells of the intestinal wall become enlarged, which lessens the ability of the intestinal wall to keep out large undesirable molecules, so that they leak across the intestinal wall and into the body. When incompletely broken down foods enter the body, the immune system mounts an attack against the "foreigner," resulting in food allergies and sensitivities. The release of antibodies triggers inflammatory reactions when the foods are eaten again. The chronic inflammation lowers IgA levels. Sufficient levels of IgA are needed to protect the intestinal tract from clostridia and yeast. The decreasing IgA levels allow for even further microbe proliferation in the intestinal tract. Vitamin and mineral deficiencies are also found due to the leaky gut problem. Research implicates altered permeability of the intestinal wall in a large number of illnesses.

Many factors can increase the permeability of the intestinal wall, including alcohol and caffeine; antibiotic use; medications such as NSAIDs (nonsteroidal anti-inflammatory drugs), antacids, or aspirin; a high-carbohydrate diet; environmental contaminants; food additives; lack of digestive enzymes; foods and beverages contaminated by parasites such as *Giardia lamblia,* cryptosporidium, *Blastocystis hominis,* and others, or by bacteria such as *Helicobacter pylori,* klebsiella, citrobacter, and pseudomonas; and chronic stress.

Symptoms and Diagnostic Path
The most obvious problems resulting from a leaky gut are probably digestive symptoms such as bloating, flatulence, and abdominal discomfort; other problems include nutritional deficiencies and increased absorption of toxins.

Treatment Options and Outlook
Corticosteroids and prescription antibiotics may help acute episodes of pain, bleeding, or severe inflammation. For a more permanent treatment, it is important to reverse the leaky gut syndrome by completely changing the diet to a hypoallergenic plan. Sugar, white flour products, all gluten-containing grains (especially wheat, barley, oats, and rye), milk and dairy products, high fat foods, caffeine products, alcohol, and hidden food allergies determined by testing must all be eliminated for several years. Chewing food more thoroughly, eating frequent small meals, and eating more slowly can also help.

least restrictive environment (LRE)   The setting in which a child with autism (or other disability) can be educated with no more segregation than is absolutely necessary. Students with autism should have the opportunity to participate as fully as possible in school and school activities with classmates who are not disabled.

The concept of "least restrictive environment" is one of the most confusing and controversial in education for children with disabilities. As originally formulated in Public Law 94-142, children with disabilities were to be guaranteed a "free appropriate public education" in the "least restrictive environment," but it was not clear what that meant. The concept was more fully described in the INDIVIDUALS WITH DISABILITIES EDUCATION ACT (IDEA), which required that learning-disabled students be placed, when appropriate, in settings with nonspecial education students to provide maximum opportunities to learn in the least restrictive environment. Generally, a child with autism should be served in the regular classroom with as much interaction with nonhandicapped classmates as possible. A child with autism may be removed from the regular classroom only when the nature or severity of the disability is such that the education in regular classes cannot be achieved even with the use of supplementary aids and services.

However, for specific areas of intensive training, it is appropriate to remove a child from the regular classroom. The child's placement and services depend on the child's individual needs, not on administrative convenience.

Before a student's least restrictive environment is determined, the student's educational needs must be identified. After the school determines the student's educational strengths and needs, annual program goals and objectives are developed, which are part of the INDIVIDUALIZED EDUCATION PROGRAM (IEP). Only after the IEP is developed does the team consider the placement options. The school must make these decisions of placement when writing the child's IEP. Settings in regular education programs are considered less restrictive than special programs or schools.

There must be compelling educational reasons, based on the individual student's educational needs, for removing the student from the regular classroom. Those reasons must be listed on the IEP.

legal rights/protection   See INDIVIDUALS WITH DISABILITIES EDUCATION ACT; REHABILITATION ACT OF 1973.

Lemke, Leslie (1952–)   Blind musical savant with cerebral palsy who was featured on *60 Minutes* in the 1980s with several other savants.

Born prematurely in Milwaukee in 1952, Leslie Lemke developed brain damage, retinal problems and glaucoma, requiring the removal of his eyes in the first months of life. Given up for adoption by his mother, Lemke was taken in by foster mother May Lemke, 52, a nurse-governess who had raised five children of her own.

In a modest cottage on Lake Pewaukee where she lived with her husband, Joe, May taught the infant how to swallow so he could eat, and how to make sounds so he could communicate. When he was older, May strapped his body to hers to teach him how to walk. She placed his hands over hers as she played simple tunes on a piano. He responded to music and rhythm. He also had a remarkable memory and would often repeat a whole day's conversation, word for word. At first, Lemke played and sang the simple tunes his mother sang or the popular songs he heard on the radio.

But one evening when Leslie was about age 14, he listened to a TV program featuring Tchaikovsky's Piano Concerto No. 1. Later that night, Lemke sat down at the piano and flawlessly played the piece from beginning to end after hearing it just once.

As a way of sharing what she called God's gift of Leslie's music, May Lemke began having him play at concerts at the county fair, in churches, and at schools. In June 1980 Leslie gave a concert in Fond du Lac, Wisconsin. Wire services picked up his story, which prompted Walter Cronkite to feature Lemke on his CBS Evening News program in December 1980. Other programs, including *Donahue, That's Incredible,* and *Oprah* hosted the Lemkes, followed by *60 Minutes* in October 1983.

Lemke has given concerts throughout the United States and Japan, and in 1984 gave a command performance for the Crown Prince and Princess in Norway. Today he continues to give concerts, and also plays for free at schools, nursing homes, prisons, and churches.

In the 1980s, May Lemke was diagnosed with Alzheimer's disease; her youngest daughter Mary took both May and Leslie into her home in 1984, as May's Alzheimer's progressed. May died at Mary's home on November 6, 1993.

Leslie Lemke still lives with May's daughter, Mary Parker, in Arpin, Wisconsin. Although some savants stop playing when a parent dies, Leslie continues to play and occasionally performs. He can not only repeat a song accurately after hearing it only once, but he can improvise and compose new songs with his own words and effects. Yet he has never had a music lesson in his life. Today his concerts are infrequent, not because of Lemke's lack of energy or ability, but because of the effort involved in travel and Mary Parker's health limitations.

lifestyle planning   A record of what the family would like to happen to ensure the future of someone with a disability such as autism. This information is recorded in a "letter of intent" that, while not a legal document, is as important as a will and a SPECIAL NEEDS TRUST.

In lifestyle planning, parents need to make decisions about where their child will live, what education will be pursued, employment, social activities, religious affiliation, medical care, behavior management, advocacy, guardianship, trustees, and final arrangements.

In addition, detailed instructions need to be included for helping the person with the typical ACTIVITIES OF DAILY LIVING, such as bathing, dressing, feeding, and toileting. Rather than write a huge document describing how to do these things, experts recommend the family videotape how these activities are performed in different social settings. The ultimate goal is to make the transition from parental care to independent living, residency in a group home, or moving in with other family members as easy as possible.

living arrangements   Autism is a condition along a continuum, so it is possible to have only very mild effects or to be almost completely incapacitated by this disorder. Some adults with one of the AUTISM SPECTRUM DISORDERS (ASDs) are able to live entirely on their own, while others live in their own homes if they have help with major issues, such as personal finances or dealing with the government agencies. This assistance can be provided by family, a professional agency, or another type of provider.

Living with parents   Parents who choose to live with their autistic adult child may obtain government funds to help offset costs, including SUPPLEMENTAL SECURITY INCOME, Social Security Disability Insurance, and Medicaid waivers. Information about these programs is available from the Social Security Administration (SSA). An appointment with a local SSA office is a good first step to take in understanding the programs for which the young adult is eligible.

Foster homes   Some families share their homes with unrelated adults with disabilities. If the home owners teach self-care and housekeeping skills and arrange leisure activities, it is called a "skill-development" home.

Supervised group living   People with autism often live in group homes or apartments staffed by professionals who help the residents with basic needs, such as meal preparation, housekeeping, and personal care. Higher-functioning adults may be able to live in a home or apartment where support staff visit only a few times a week. These residents with autism usually prepare their own meals, go to work, and conduct other daily activities on their own.

Institutions   Although the trend in the past 30 years has been to avoid placing people with disabilities into long-term care institutions, this alternative is still available for individuals with autism who need intensive, constant supervision. Modern facilities are much more pleasant places to live than their predecessors, and staff members, treat residents as individuals with human needs, offering opportunities for recreation and simple but meaningful work.

low-functioning autistic disorder (LFAD)   A condition on the autistic spectrum that includes most of the people with autism (between 70 and 90 percent of all people with autism). LFAD is also three to four times more likely to occur in boys than girls.

Symptoms and Diagnostic Path

People with HIGH-FUNCTIONING AUTISTIC DISORDER (HFAD) and LFAD share many of the same symptoms, but those with LFAD tend to have a lower IQ, more symptoms, and more severe symptoms.

People with LFAD as a group have an average verbal and nonverbal IQ of about 55; an IQ of less than 70 is classified as mentally retarded. On the other hand, people with HFAD have a nonverbal IQ average like that of the general population (100), while verbal IQ is significantly less (85).

Most people with low-functioning autism are never capable of speech. Stereotyped and repetitive mannerisms and sensory abnormalities are common, and in some cases, such behaviors can lead to self-injury or aggressive responses directed outward when disruptions of ritualistic mannerisms or activities occur. Those with LFAD also have a higher rate of medical problems (especially EPILEPSY, which occurs in about 28 percent of those with low-functioning autism).

Most people with LFAD communicate by movements that are protests or requests. Self-injury and aggressive acts are used to communicate as well. However, in many cases of severe autism, the person is able to communicate through sign language, although this communication is still typically limited to a protest or a request, with a lack of focus on grammatical structure. Experts suspect that sign language is used more often than speech because autistic people capable of speech have problems with vocal volume, intonation, and stress patterns. Because understanding intonation is an important part of understanding stress within sentences and words, a problem in picking up intonation means the person will have trouble understanding words, sentences, and meaning in language. In addition, many autistic people take speech and interpretation quite literally; however, sign language does not require a person to infer meaning from words.

Treatment Options and Outlook

If a child with LFAD does not speak by the age of six, he or she will probably never be able to speak.

mainstreaming Placement of a disabled child with nondisabled peers in a regular classroom. Mainstreaming was introduced in the 1970s as a result of PUBLIC LAW 94-142, which mandated that special needs children be placed in the LEAST RESTRICTIVE ENVIRONMENT. Until the approval of P.L. 94-142 in 1975, most special needs children (from mildly to severely disabled), were educated in self-contained settings.

The philosophy of mainstreaming disabled children into the regular classroom comes from the idea that since most individuals will be "mainstreamed" into society, the integration of regular and special needs students should begin at an early age. It was also believed that school resources could be used more efficiently if special needs students were placed in the regular classroom. Mainstreaming also required regular educators to share the responsibility for disabled students with special educators. Conversely, mainstreaming benefits regular education students by increasing their understanding and tolerance of students with differences.

Longitudinal studies of mainstreaming over the past two decades indicate that mainstreaming is defined differently depending on the school and school district. In most school systems, mainstreaming involves placing a special needs student in the regular classroom setting for one subject area or a portion of the day, depending on what is best for the student. According to research, mainstreaming can be a valid alternative to self-contained classrooms, but it is not an appropriate practice for all special needs students. The student's need, teacher training, attitudes toward mainstreaming, and cost factors must all be carefully balanced.

Most students with learning disabilities are educated in the regular classroom while receiving support services. Although parents sometimes worry that their children's needs will not be met in a regular classroom setting, mainstreaming does not mean that special-education students are "dumped" into classes indiscriminately. Rather, students are placed in a regular classroom with support services so they can perform adequately. The concept of mainstreaming is a response to the fact that students can benefit from regular classroom placement if they get additional assistance at the same time. Forms of assistance might be the use of an aide, modification of instruction, more instruction time, and communication with the regular classroom teacher.

Parents of nondisabled children often complain that the disabled child might disrupt the class or take up too much of the teacher's time. Both are legitimate concerns, and if any child is so disruptive it interferes with the functioning of the class, then intervention is necessary.

Considerable time, energy, and planning go into every successful mainstreaming experience. Parents must be advocates for their children and provide input about the type and amount of mainstreaming that takes place, and they need to forge positive relationships with school personnel. This should be done during the development and implementation of the INDIVIDUALIZED EDUCATION PROGRAM (IEP).

Mainstreaming works when

- parents and teachers work together
- specific mainstreaming experiences are recorded in the child's IEP
- special education teachers meet with regular classroom teachers in the mainstreamed setting
- mainstream teachers get information on the special education student's strengths and needs as well as techniques considered helpful for the student's particular learning disability

- mainstream teachers have time to consult with special education teachers to discuss student progress
- regular students are given information to better understand students with special needs

medications for autism Medication to control behavioral symptoms is one of the most common treatments for autism today, but no single drug can control all autism symptoms completely. Medications used to treat autism fall into several categories, including antipsychotics, antiepileptics, blood pressure medications, antidepressants, stimulants, and other types of drugs.

Antipsychotics

One of the most common types of medications and the most widely studied for autism are the ANTIPSYCHOTICS, which help to control aggressive behaviors. Originally developed for treating schizophrenia, these drugs have been found to decrease hyperactivity, irritability, repetitive behaviors, withdrawal, and aggression in individuals with autism. (However, autism and psychosis are not in any way related.) Four that have been approved for the treatment of autism are clozapine (Clozaril), RISPERIDONE (RISPERDAL), olanzapine (Zyprexa) and quetiapine (Seroquel), but only risperidone has been investigated in a controlled study of adults with autism. Like the antidepressants, these drugs all have potential side effects, including sedation.

Risperdal is probably the most commonly used antipsychotic, which can help lessen aggression, agitation, and explosive behaviors. It has been studied extensively in treatment of autism and works well. As with any medication, there can be side effects, which may include a sedative effect, weight gain, dizziness, and muscular stiffness.

Two other antipsychotics, Zyprexa and Seroquel, have the same effects as Risperdal and the same side effects. However, Zyprexa does not cause muscular stiffness, and Seroquel causes less of a problem with weight gain.

Clozapine (Clozaril) has not yet been studied extensively, but so far it appears to have the same benefits as Risperdal. However, because Clozaril can cause serious bone marrow suppression, biweekly blood tests are required to ensure that the side effects are not becoming problematic.

Antiepileptic Drugs

ANTIEPILEPTIC MEDICATION also controls the aggressive behaviors in people with autism by helping to stabilize brain activity. However, these drugs require regular blood testing in order to ensure that liver or bone marrow damage does not occur.

Valproate (Depakote) is a common antiepileptic that can lessen explosive behaviors and aggression. Since many children with autism also have seizure disorders, Depakote has the added benefit of treating both behavior problems and seizures. Most of the side effects (such as a sedative effect and an upset stomach) are not severe. However, in rare cases, Depakote can cause liver damage, so frequent blood tests are required to monitor the level of this drug in the blood.

Carbamazapine (Tegretol) is another antiepileptic medication that has the same benefits as Depakote. This drug may cause a rash or bone marrow problems.

Blood Pressure Medications

Certain medications used to treat high blood pressure have shown promise in alleviating the aggressive behaviors common in autism. Although experts are not sure why these drugs work, for some children they do stem aggressiveness and emotional outbursts. Of these, propranolol (Inderal) and pindolol (Visken) both seem to lessen aggression and explosions.

Side effects include a sedative effect, aggravation of asthmatic symptoms, and light-headedness or fainting due to lowered blood pressure.

Antidepressants and Antianxiety Medications

Although there are no psychiatric medications that can directly target autism itself, many ANTIDEPRESSANTS and antianxiety medications can be used to treat specific symptoms often found in autism, such as aggression, self-injury, anxiety, depression, OBSESSIVE-COMPULSIVE DISORDER, and attention deficit hyperactivity disorder (ADHD).

In particular, selective serotonin reuptake inhibitors (SSRIs) have been effective in treating depression, obsessive-compulsive behaviors, and anxiety that are sometimes present in autism. Because researchers have consistently found abnormally high levels of the neurotransmitter SEROTONIN in the blood of a third of individuals with autism, experts suggest that the SSRI drugs (that lower serotonin levels) could potentially reverse some of the symptoms in autism. Three drugs that have been studied as a possible autism treatment are the SSRIs fluvoxAMINE (LUVOX) and FLUOXETINE (PROZAC) and the tricyclic antidepressant CLOMIPRAMINE (ANAFRANIL). Studies have shown that they may reduce the frequency and intensity of repetitive behaviors, and may decrease irritability, tantrums, and aggressive behavior. Some children have shown improvements in EYE CONTACT and responsiveness.

Other antidepressant and antianxiety drugs, such as Elavil, Wellbutrin, Valium, Ativan, and Xanax, have not been studied as much in regard to autism but may have a role in treating behavioral symptoms. However, all these drugs have potential side effects, which should be discussed before treatment is started.

For some classes of drugs, the doses that can reduce symptoms such as aggression or anxiety are much lower for people with autism than for other patients. For example, the best dose for SSRI drugs such as Prozac and Zoloft may be only one-third of the typical starting dose for depressed patients. Too high a dose in patients with autism may trigger agitation or insomnia.

There is no medical test to determine which antidepressant medication will work best; a "trial and error" approach works best, as dosages need to be adjusted differently for each person, and one medication may be ineffective or have negative effects while others are helpful.

Although psychiatric medications are widely used to treat the symptoms of autism and they can be helpful to many older children and adults, some experts are concerned about their use in younger children. There is relatively little research on their use for children with autism, and almost no studies on the long-term developmental effects, especially for the newer medications.

Stimulants

Stimulants such as Ritalin, Adderall, and Dexedine, used to treat hyperactivity in children, have also been prescribed for children with autism. Although few studies have been done, these drugs may increase focus and decrease impulsivity and hyperactivity in autism, particularly in higher-functioning children. Dosages need to be carefully monitored, however, because behavioral side effects are often dose-related.

Other Medications

Lithium—a medication more typically used to treat bipolar disorder—is also effective in calming explosive outbursts and agitation. However, its negative effects on the thyroid have led many physicians to avoid this drug for autistic patients. Lithium also can cause weight gain, stomach upset, and frequent urination, and requires regular blood tests and cardiac testing.

Gabapentin (Neurontin) and lamotrigine (Lamictal) are other medications that may have potential benefit in the treatment of autism but that have not been studied sufficiently to be recommended for use with children. These medications seem to provide the same benefits as Depakote, as well as the same side effects, but insufficient data exists on their overall effect.

mental retardation Below-average intellectual functioning abilities as determined by IQ tests, and low adaptive functioning such as self-care and independence skills. (An IQ of 100 is considered "average.") Between 75 and 80 percent of people with AUTISM SPECTRUM DISORDERS are also mentally retarded. Of these, 15 to 20 percent are considered severely retarded, with IQs below 35. However, not everyone with autism has a low IQ; in fact, more than 10 percent of people with autism have an average or above-average IQ. A few show exceptional intelligence. Most people who are mentally retarded develop skills at about the same level in different areas, but individuals with autism typically have deficits in certain skill areas (most often in social skills and communication) with distinct abilities in other areas.

Traditionally, an individual is considered to have mental retardation if IQ is below 70; there are significant limitations in two or more adaptive skill areas; and if the condition has been present from childhood. Intelligence testing alone is only part of the assessment of mental retardation. A person with impaired intellectual functioning who does not have impairments in adaptive skill areas may not be diagnosed as having mental retardation. "Adaptive skill areas" include those daily living skills needed to live, work, and play in the community, such as communication, self care, home living, social skills, leisure, health and safety, self direction, functional academics, community involvement, and work. Adaptive skills are assessed in the person's typical environment across all aspects of life. Psychologists and educators assess adaptive behavior by interviews with people who know the person as well as by tests completed by people who know the person.

Interpreting an IQ score for a person with autism is uniquely difficult, however, because most intelligence tests are not designed for people with autism, who tend to perceive or relate to their environment in atypical ways. When tested, some areas of ability are normal or even above average, and some areas may be especially weak. For example, a child with autism may do extremely well on the parts of the test that measure visual skills, but earn low scores on the language subtests. Although it has been estimated that up to 75 percent of people with autism are also mentally retarded, research studies have often used inappropriate IQ tests (such as verbal tests with nonverbal children) to estimate intelligence level.

The effects of mental retardation vary considerably among people, just as the range of ability varies considerably among people who do not have mental retardation. About 87 percent are mildly affected, and will be only a little slower than average in learning new information and skills. As children, their mental retardation is not easy to see, and may not be identified until school age. As adults, many individuals with mental retardation will be able to lead independent lives in the community.

The remaining 13 percent of people with mental retardation (those with IQs under 50) will have serious limits in function. However, with early intervention, a good education, and appropriate supports as an adult, all can lead satisfying lives in the community.

People with mental retardation may have trouble communicating, interacting with others, and being independent. There also may be concerns with regard to understanding health and safety issues. Not all skills are necessarily impaired, and individuals with mental retardation may learn to function independently in many areas. However, education programs, providing skilled assistance and ongoing support, are necessary for determining appropriate living and work environments.

While the term "mental retardation" still exists as a clinical diagnosis, contemporary usage is moving toward terms such as "developmental disabilities," which some believe do not carry the same negative connotations or misuse. In the past, those who were retarded were traditionally divided by IQ scores into "educable," "trainable" and "custodial." Today, the more commonly used terms include "mild," "moderate," "severe," or "profound" categories, based on the level of functioning and IQ. Individuals with mental retardation are not a homogenous group, but have widely differing levels of function.

"Mild retardation" is used to specify an individual whose IQ test scores lie between 55 and 69, and correspond to an educators' label of "educable retarded." The individual is capable of learning basic academic subjects. Many people with mild retardation are able to live and work independently.

"Moderate retardation" is a classification used to specify an individual whose IQ test scores are between 40 and 55; it corresponds to the earlier label of "trainable." These individuals can usually learn functional academics and vocational skills. They often achieve coached employment goals and live with limited assistance.

"Severe" and "profound" mental retardation applies to individuals with IQ scores below 25. These are the most seriously impaired, often characterized by physical and sensory impairment as well as mental retardation. They can sometimes achieve supported employment goals; more typically they can function at the level of sheltered employment. They generally require significant assistance with daily living skills.

If a child with autism is going to have an IQ test, parents should request nonverbal intelligence tests that do not require language skills, such as the Test for Nonverbal Intelligence (TONI). Furthermore, regardless of the result, autistic children will develop more skills as they grow older, and appropriate therapies and education can help them reach their true potential.

mirror neurons   Cells, in a part of the brain called the premotor cortex, that fire when a person performs an action or when the person sees someone else perform the action. Mirror neurons were first identified in macaque monkeys in the early 1990s, when they were called "monkey-see, monkey-do cells." Scientists noticed that these cells fired both when a monkey performed an action itself and when it observed another living creature perform that same action.

Although it has been impossible to directly study these neurons in people (since human subjects cannot be implanted with electrodes), several indirect brain-imaging measures, including electroencephalograph (EEG), have confirmed the presence of a mirror neuron system in humans. When these cells are working normally, seeing is doing. Scientists believe that the human mirror neuron system is involved not only in making and observing movement, but also in more complex mental processes such as language, for instance, or being able to imitate and learn from others' actions or decode their intentions and empathize with their pain. These are all areas with which autistic people have problems. Because the hallmark of autism is a problem in these sorts of social interaction and communication skills, research has suggested that a dysfunctional mirror neuron system may explain the symptoms of autism.

In autistic individuals, the brain circuits that enable people to perceive and understand the actions of others do not behave in the usual way, according to researchers from the University of California, San Diego. According to their research, EEG recordings of 10 individuals with autism showed a dysfunctional mirror neuron system—their mirror neurons respond only to what they do and not to what others do.

The San Diego team collected EEG data in 10 males with AUTISM SPECTRUM DISORDERS who were considered "high-functioning" (defined as having age-appropriate verbal comprehension and production and IQs above 80) and 10 age- and gender-matched control subjects. The EEG data was analyzed suppressing a type of brain wave (called "mu") that is blocked when the brain is engaged in doing, seeing, or imagining action, and correlates with the activity of the mirror neuron system. In most people, this mu wave is suppressed both in response to their own movement and to observing the movement of others. Subjects were tested while they moved their own hands and while they watched videos of visual white noise, of bouncing balls, and of a moving hand.

As expected, the mu wave was suppressed in the control subjects both when they moved and when they watched another human move. In other words, their mirror neuron systems acted normally. The mirror neurons of the subjects with autism spectrum disorders, however, responded only to their own movement.

The findings provide evidence that individuals with autism have a dysfunctional mirror neuron system, which may contribute to many of their symptoms—especially those that involve understanding and responding appropriately to others' behavior.

Although EEGs are not designed to measure the mu brain rhythms of low-functioning children with autism because their repetitive movements confound EEG signals, it could be used as a tool for earlier diagnosis of high-functioning autistics, whose disorder today is typically not recognized until age four or later.

Earlier diagnosis in turn could lead to earlier interventions. One treatment possibility suggested by the study's findings is biofeedback. In fact, the mu wave rhythm involved is one that patients most readily learn to control. By imagining action, subjects are able to move a paddle in a computer game of Pong after just four to six hours of practice. Because this mu rhythm is one that everyone has access to at will, it could be used in therapy.

Alternatively, ordinary mirrors could be used in treatment to fool the brain. Researchers have treated amputees who experience pain in their missing limbs by using a mirror reflection of the healthy limb to fool the brain into believing that the missing limb has been restored to pain-free motion. Since autistics' mirror neurons respond to their own motion, researchers hope that their brains might be tricked into believing their own reflected movements are the movements of another human being.

For the first time, researchers have been able to relate symptoms unique to autism (loss of empathy and the abilitiy to imitate) to the function of a brain circuit (the mirror neuron system). Researchers are now studying whether another problem of autism—the ability to understand metaphors—might be related to mirror neurons as well.

Modified Checklist for Autism in Toddlers (M-CHAT) A simple, self-administered parental questionnaire for use during regular pediatric visits, designed to screen for AUTISTIC DISORDER in children. The M-CHAT is an expanded American version of the original CHECKLIST FOR AUTISM IN TODDLERS (CHAT) formulated in the United Kingdom, which was a simple screening tool for identification of autistic children at 18 months of age. The M-CHAT tests for AUTISM SPECTRUM DISORDERS against normally developing children. A child fails the checklist when two or more critical items are failed, or when any three items are failed.

M-CHAT was redesigned to improve the sensitivity of the CHAT and position it better for an American audience; M-CHAT had a better sensitivity than the original CHAT because children up to 24 months of age were screened, with the aim of identifying those who might regress between 18 and 24 months.

The M-CHAT consists of 23 questions—nine questions from the original CHAT and an additional 14 questions addressing core symptoms in young autistic children. The original observational part of the test (that is, section B) was omitted. In the M-CHAT, the more questions children fail, the higher their risk of having autism.

multisystem developmental disorder A term developed by Dr. Stanley Greenspan, a child psychiatrist and expert on autism, for an autistic-like set of symptoms.

muscle tone Research has suggested that about 30 percent of children with autism have a moderate-to-severe loss of muscle tone that can limit their gross and fine motor skills. These children also tend to have low potassium levels, which is significant because potassium aids in good muscle tone.

musical savant An individual who can identify exact musical pitches and play back a complex piece of music after hearing it once. This type of unusual ability typically appears in a person with AUTISTIC DISORDER. The most common savant skill among autistic people is related to music.

This musical superiority may be a result of an abnormally high sensitivity to fine pitch differences in sounds, according to some researchers. This enhanced sensitivity to different pitches may account for the observation that some autistic individuals excel at musical perception tasks and for the ability of musical savants to determine absolute pitch.

The difference between a normal musician and a musical savant is that the normal musician usually plays from written scores, whereas musical savants always play initially by ear. The immediate recall of musical fragments by savants is usually not a literal reproduction of the material heard. Instead, the savant preserves essential musical structural regularities present in the original music.

See also AUTISTIC SAVANT; SAVANT SYNDROME.

National Institutes of Health Autism Coordinating Committee (NIH/ACC)   A government committee designed to enhance the quality, pace, and coordination of efforts at the National Institutes of Health to find a cure for autism. Founded in 1997 at the request of Congress, the NIH/ACC has been instrumental in the research into, understanding of, and advances in treatment of autism.

NIH Institutes that are members of the NIH/ACC include: National Institute of Child Health and Human Development (NICHD), National Institute on Deafness and Other Communication Disorders, National Institute of Mental Health (NIMH), National Institute of Neurological Disorders and Stroke, and National Institute of Environmental Health Sciences. In addition, other NIH Institutes, centers, and offices, as well as other federal agencies and parents' groups, participate in NIH/ACC meetings focusing on specific topics. The directors of the NIMH and NICHD co-chair the NIH/ACC.

The NIH/ACC is also involved in the broader federal Interagency Autism Coordinating Committee (IACC) that is composed of representatives from various component agencies of the U.S. Department of Health and Human Services, including the NICHD, as well as other governmental organizations. The IACC is chaired by the director of NIMH.

natural language paradigm   The older name for PIVOTAL RESPONSE TRAINING.

neuroleptic   A class of antipsychotic drug that has been used for several decades to treat individuals with autism. However, the need for long-term use and the danger of unwanted side effects have limited their effectiveness. Examples of neuroleptics used to treat autism include HALOPERIDAL (Haldol) and pimozide.

More recently, newer versions of neuroleptics, called "atypical neuroleptics," have been developed to treat autism patients' symptoms without causing some of the unpleasant side effects of more traditional neuroleptics. Some of these unpleasant side effects include tardive dyskinesia (jerky, uncontrollable movements), slowed thinking, parkinsonism, or dystonia (postural spasms). Atypical neuroleptics include clozapine and RISPERIDONE (RISPERDAL).

The results of a number of preliminary studies suggest that risperidone and other atypical neuroleptics may help reduce repetitive behaviors, aggression, and impulsivity and improve social relatedness in children, adolescents, and adults with autism. Relatively low doses of risperidone appear to be effective. Although the exact reason why atypical neuroleptics work is unclear, scientists suspect that the drug's effects on neurotransmitters (SEROTONIN and dopamine) may explain the beneficial effects on social behavior.

neurologically typical   A term used to refer to people who do not have autism.

neurologist   A physician specializing in brain function. Neurologists can assess and treat with medication a variety of neurological conditions and disorders, and can perform detailed examinations of all the neurological structures in the body, including the nerves of the head and neck, muscular strength and movement, sensation, balance, and reflex testing. In some cases, detailed questions about memory, speech and language, and other cognitive functions are part of the examination.

Neurologists also use other common tests, including CAT (computerized axial tomography) and MRI (magnetic resonance imaging) scans to provide detailed pictures of the brain, spinal structures, and blood vessels. A neurologist can also perform a lumbar puncture (spinal tap) to obtain a patient's cerebrospinal fluid for analysis. Some neurologists interpret EEG (electroencephalography) used in the evaluation of seizure disorders. In addition, neurologists use many types of drugs to treat problems involving the nervous system. A neurologist may send a patient for a surgical evaluation, but does not perform surgery.

A neurologist must complete a four-year premedical university degree and four years of medical school followed by at least three years of specialty training in an accredited neurology residency program. After residency training, neurologists may choose to enroll in a one- or two-year fellowship program, which offers the opportunity to focus on a subspecialty of neurology such as stroke, dementia, or movement disorders. After completing the educational requirements, neurologists may seek certification from the American Board of Psychiatry and Neurology (ABPN). To be eligible for certification, an applicant must be a licensed physician with the required years of residency who has passed both a written and an oral exam administered by the ABPN.

neuropsychologist   A psychologist who focuses on the relationship between behavior and neurological functions. A pediatrician, medical specialist such as a neurologist, or school specialist might suggest a referral to a neuropsychologist for an evaluation. This is especially likely if a child's abilities are complicated or difficult to assess, if there are thinking problems or behavior patterns that might be closely linked to disrupted brain function, or if the child might have some kind of actual brain damage. Neuropsychologists are trained to think about the link between brain function and behavior.

The more a problem has to do with a child's capacity to learn or master skills or appears to be linked to a problem with brain function, the more the child would need a neuropsychologist.

Clinical neuropsychologists have a Ph.D., Psy.D., or Ed.D. from a university or professional school, usually with the same kind of experience that a clinical psychologist needs but sometimes in different areas of psychology such as "school" or "counseling." They also have specialized education in neuropsychology and neuroscience, including at least two years of postdoctoral training in a clinical setting, and often have passed a national board certification exam. Those holding an ABCN/ABPP Diploma in Clinical Neuropsychology have the clearest evidence of competence as clinical neuropsychologists.

See also NEUROPSYCHOLOGY.

neuropsychology   The study of the relationship between brain function and behavior. This field includes NEUROPSYCHOLOGISTS who work in experimental and clinical settings; experimental neuropsychologists, who work with both human and animal models; and clinical neuropsychologists, who look for procedures that will help people with neurologically based disorders by studying brain and behavior relationships.

neurotransmitter   A chemical messenger in the brain that is released from the ends of a brain cell and carries information across the gap between cells, where it arrives at specific sites on a receiving cell.

Examples of neurotransmitters include acetylcholine, dopamine, epinephrine, SEROTONIN and various neuropeptides. Treatment for attention disorders involving medications focuses primarily on regulating the action of neurotransmitters.

nonfluent aphasia   A language disorder, characterized by little speech and poor articulation, in which a person uses primarily nouns and verbs; automatic responses such as "yes" and "no" prevail. This condition is also called Broca's APHASIA.

Nonspeech Test for Receptive/Expressive Language   A test designed to provide a systematic way for observing, recording, and summarizing the variety of ways an individual may communicate. This tool determines a person's skills as a communicator, whether speech or nonverbal means are used for communication.

obsessive-compulsive disorder (OCD) An anxiety disorder, characterized by severe obsessions and/or compulsions, that is sometimes present in people with AUTISTIC DISORDER. OCD affects men and women about equally, occurring in about one in 50 people (or about 3.3 million adult Americans). It can occur at any time but usually first appears in the teens or early adulthood. A third of adults with OCD experienced their first symptoms as children. Evidence suggests that OCD might run in families. Left untreated, obsessions and the need to perform rituals can take over a person's life. OCD is often a chronic, relapsing illness.

There is growing evidence that OCD is caused by a physical problem in the brain, not because of family problems or because of attitudes learned in childhood, such as an emphasis on cleanliness, or a belief that certain thoughts are dangerous or unacceptable.

Brain scans using positron emission tomography (PET) have found that those with OCD have different patterns of brain activity from people with other mental illnesses or people with no mental illness at all. In addition, PET scans show that in patients with OCD, both behavioral therapy and medication produce changes in a part of the brain called the caudate nucleus.

Symptoms and Diagnostic Path

People with OCD suffer intensely from recurrent, unwanted thoughts (obsessions) or rituals (compulsions), which they feel they cannot control. Rituals such as handwashing, counting, checking, or cleaning are often performed as a way of preventing obsessive thoughts or making them go away. Performing these rituals, however, provides only temporary relief, and not performing them markedly increases anxiety. The symptoms may come and go, may get better over time, or they can grow progressively worse.

Often, people with OCD may avoid situations in which they might have to confront their obsessions, or they may try unsuccessfully to use alcohol or drugs to calm themselves. Severe OCD can keep someone from working or from carrying out normal responsibilities at home, but more often it does not develop to those extremes.

Many healthy people have some of the symptoms of OCD, such as checking the stove several times before leaving the house. But the disorder is diagnosed only when such activities consume at least an hour a day, are very distressing, and interfere with daily life. Most adults with this condition know that what they are doing is senseless, but they cannot stop. However, children with OCD may not realize that their behavior is unusual.

In addition to autism, OCD is often linked with other anxiety disorders, major depression, TOURETTE SYNDROME, and attention deficit hyperactivity disorder.

Treatment Options and Outlook

A combination of medication and psychotherapy is often helpful for most patients; some individuals respond best to one therapy, some to another. Medications that are effective are the antidepressants FLUVOXAMINE, paroxetine, sertraline, CLOMIPRAMINE, and FLUOXETINE. Others are showing promise and may soon be available. Behavioral therapy (specifically "exposure and response prevention") is also helpful in treating OCD. This type of therapy involves exposing the person to whatever triggers the problem and then helping the person avoid the usual ritual. This might involve having the patient touch something dirty and then not wash his hands. This therapy is often successful in patients who complete a behavioral therapy program, although results have been less favorable in some people who have both OCD and depression.

occupational therapists   Professionals who work directly with individuals with impaired physical or motor functions caused by disease, injury, or surgical or other medical interventions. Occupational therapists work with individuals who have conditions that are mentally, physically, developmentally, or emotionally disabling, such as autism, and help them to develop, recover, or maintain daily living and work skills. They not only help clients improve basic motor functions and reasoning abilities, but also compensate for permanent loss of function. Their goal is to help clients have independent, productive, and satisfying lives.

Occupational therapists may work exclusively with individuals in a particular age group or with particular disabilities. In schools, for example, they evaluate children's abilities, recommend and provide therapy, modify classroom equipment, and in general, help children participate as fully as possible in school programs and activities.

Occupational therapists help clients perform activities of all types, such as using a computer. Physical exercises may be used to increase strength and dexterity, while paper and pencil exercises may be chosen to improve visual acuity and the ability to discern patterns. An autistic client with coordination problems might be assigned exercises to improve hand-eye coordination. Occupational therapists also use computer programs to help clients improve decision making, abstract reasoning, problem solving, and perceptual skills, as well as memory, sequencing, and coordination—all of which are important for independent living.

In mental health settings, they may treat individuals who are low-functioning autistics, choosing activities that help them learn to cope with daily life, such as time management skills, budgeting, shopping, homemaking, and use of public transportation.

Occupational therapists must have at least a bachelor's degree in occupational therapy, and the profession is regulated in all states. To obtain a license, applicants must graduate from an accredited educational program and pass a national certification examination. Those who pass the test are called "registered occupational therapist." Occupational therapy course work includes physical, biological, and behavioral sciences and the application of occupational therapy theory and skills. Completion of six months of supervised fieldwork is also required.

occupational therapy (OT)   A type of treatment that can help improve the sensory needs of children with autism, who often have lessened or heightened sensitivity to sound, sight, smell, touch, and taste. The ultimate goal of traditional OT is to help the child participate in daily life tasks and activities as independently as possible, such as playing, enjoying school, eating, dressing, and sleeping—activities that are often a problem for children with autism. OT should be a major component of a treatment plan for autistic children.

OT often focuses on improving fine motor skills, such as brushing teeth, feeding, and writing; or boosting sensory motor skills, including balance (vestibular system), awareness of body position (proprioceptive system), and touch (tactile system).

After the occupational therapist identifies a specific problem, each child is provided with an individualized treatment plan that directly involves parents. Occupational therapy usually takes place in a large, sensory-enriched gym with lots of swinging, spinning, tactile, visual, auditory, and taste opportunities. Typically, therapy may include sensory integration activities such as massage, firm touch, swinging, and bouncing.

oppositional defiant disorder (ODD)   A pattern of negativism characterized by angry, hostile, and impulsive behavior in opposition to authority figures. It often appears together with AUTISTIC DISORDER; occasionally, a child who is autistic alone may be misdiagnosed as having ODD. In fact, it is extremely rare for a physician to see a child with only ODD.

ODD is an antisocial disorder of early to middle childhood that may evolve into a conduct disorder, usually diagnosed before the age of 12; children with oppositional defiant disorder defy adult rules, are angry, and often lose their tempers. These individuals may often be out of control, overstimulated, or understimulated, showing behavioral patterns that are difficult to explain and that often disrupt an entire household.

ODD is considered less severe than conduct disorder, and may involve behaviors that include overt resistance to rules and instructions, lying, and violations of other social norms.

This is the most common psychiatric problem in children, which affects more than 5 percent of them; in younger children it is more common in boys than girls, but as they grow older, the rate is the same in both. Usually, the child has another psychiatric disorder, or may have autistic disorder. Children with ODD develop signs of mood disorders or anxiety as they get older; by the time these children reach the end of elementary school, about 25 percent will have disabling mood or anxiety problems.

Symptoms and Diagnostic Path

The criteria for ODD include a pattern of negative, hostile, defiant behavior lasting at least six months. Any child could be oppositional upon occasion, especially during times of fatigue or stress. The difference between ODD and occasional arguments, backtalk, or disobedience is that with ODD, the child's hostile, uncooperative behavior is so continuous that it is blatantly unusual compared to other children of the same age. Often, children with ODD annoy others or challenge authority on purpose, making their symptoms much more difficult to live with. The disturbance in behavior causes significant problems with social, school, or job functioning.

At least four of the following symptoms must be present for a diagnosis. The individual often

- gets angry and argues
- actively defies or refuses to comply with the requests or rules of an authority figure
- deliberately annoys people
- blames others for mistakes or misbehavior
- is touchy or easily annoyed by others
- feels resentful
- is spiteful and vindictive

All of the criteria above include the word "often," which may mean different things to different people.

After all, these behaviors occur to a varying degree in all normal children. Researches have found that "often" is best solved by the following criteria:

- At least four times a week the person is angry and resentful and deliberately annoys people.
- At least twice a week the person is touchy or easily annoyed by others, loses his temper, argues, and actively defies or refuses to comply with requests or rules of authority figures.
- In the last three months, the person is spiteful and vindictive and blames others for his or her mistakes or misbehavior.

The problems usually begin in childhood, between ages one to three, and appear to run in families. If a parent is alcoholic and has been in trouble with the law, the children are almost three times as likely to have ODD. Biological, genetic, and environmental factors may play an interweaving role. Some experts believe ODD may be linked to how a child was disciplined. Family interaction patterns often need to be examined to fully understand and work on changing the opposition.

Treatment Options and Outlook

Unfortunately, many studies suggest that children with ODD do not always respond well to treatment. Although there have not been major research breakthroughs in finding good ways to handle this condition, there have been some small improvements, especially with interventions based on improved parenting.

Children with these problems typically benefit from some form of structured behavior management program at home and school which should include clear and specific commands and reinforcing positive behaviors. In addition, the child should be exposed to consistent negative consequences given calmly in response to inappropriate behaviors. Parents and caregivers also should try to provide more positive incentives than reprimands. These strategies should be used both calmly and consistently enough to keep behavior problems from worsening to the meltdown point. Training the parent in these techniques and working with the child in therapy tends to be effective.

patterning A series of exercises designed to improve the "neurologic organization" of a child's neurologic impairments. These exercises are performed over many hours during the day by several persons who manipulate a child's head and extremities in patterns purporting to simulate prenatal and postnatal movements of nonimpaired children. Patterning has been advocated for more than 40 years for treating children with brain damage and other disorders, such as autism, learning disabilities, Down syndrome, and cerebral palsy but is no longer accepted as helpful by a number of organizations, including the American Academy of Pediatrics (AAP), which condemns patterning as "based on an outmoded and oversimplified theory of brain development." Current information does not support the claims of proponents that this treatment is useful, the academy states, and considers its use "unwarranted."

Patterning is based on the neurologic organization theory of brain function, which many experts today believe is an oversimplified concept of hemispheric dominance and the relationship of sequential development, and which notes that failure to complete any stage of neurologic organization harms all subsequent stages. According to this theory, the best way to treat a damaged nervous system is to regress to more primitive modes of function and to practice them; most cases of autism, MENTAL RETARDATION, learning problems, and behavior disorders are caused by brain damage or improper neurologic organization, and these problems lie on a single continuum of brain damage, for which the most effective treatment is patterning.

However, the AAP and other experts disagree, noting that the lack of dominance or sideness probably is not an important factor in the cause or treatment of autism. "Several careful reviews of

the theory have concluded that it is unsupported, contradicted, or without merit based on scientific study," according to the AAP statement.

In most cases, any improvement in patients undergoing patterning can be accounted for based on growth and development, the intensive practice of certain isolated skills, or the nonspecific effects of intensive stimulation.

Mainstream experts have been concerned about patterning because promotional methods had made it difficult for parents to refuse treatment for their children without having their motivation and adequacy as parents questioned. Moreover, dire health consequences for children are implied if parents do not make arrangements to have their child begin patterning.

Several treatment options are offered, ranging from a home program to an intensive treatment program, which states that each succeeding option "offers greater chance of success." Participation in the intensive treatment program requires completion of three of five preceding programs, is by invitation only for the "most capable families," and potentially could deplete substantially a family's financial resources. In fact, the AAP warns, the patterning regimens can be so demanding, time-consuming, and inflexible that they may place considerable stress on parents and lead them to neglect other family members.

Patterning programs use a developmental profile designed by the Institute for the Achievement of Human Potential both to assess a child's neurologic functioning and to document change over time. However, the validity of using this profile for these areas has not been demonstrated nor has it been compared with currently accepted methods of measuring a child's development. In addition to making claims that a number of conditions may be improved or cured by patterning, proponents of the program assert that patterning can make healthy children superior in physical and cognitive skills. According to providers of patterning therapy, most children with autism who are treated are claimed to achieve at least one of the goals of normal physical, intellectual, or social growth.

"The lack of supporting evidence for the use of this therapy," the AAP warns, "brings into question once again its effectiveness in neurologically impaired children."

Peabody Picture Vocabulary Test–III   This test measures an individual's receptive vocabulary for standard American English. Measuring one facet of general intelligence (vocabulary), it takes a relatively short period of time to administer and may be used as an initial screening device.

PECS   An acronym for Picture Exchange Communication System, a type of treatment in which a child attaches meanings to words through pictures, useful in both verbal and nonverbal children, as a way of producing spontaneous communication. Difficulty with communication is one of the main problems endured by people with AUTISM SPECTRUM DISORDERS. While some children develop verbal language, others never speak. An augmented communication program such as PECS can help get language started, as well as provide a way of communicating for those children who do not talk.

Developed at the Delaware Autistic Program, PECS has been recognized around the world for focusing on the initiation component of communication. Moreover, it does not require expensive materials or equipment, and can be used in a variety of settings. Instead, it used APPLIED BEHAVIORAL ANALYSIS methods to teach children to exchange a picture for something they want (an item or activity).

First a student is taught to exchange a picture of a desired item with a teacher, who honors the request right away. Verbal prompts are not used. The teacher then teaches how to discriminate symbols, and then how to put them together in sentences. At the same time, children are taught to comment and answer direct questions. It is helpful

to have two trainers available in the initial part of the program, when it is most intensive.

PECS advantages are that it is clear, intentional, and initiated by the child. The child hands the teacher or parent a picture, and the child's request is immediately understood. This method also makes it easy for the child with autism to communicate with anyone.

pediatric autoimmune neuropsychiatric disorders associated with strep infection (PANDAS)   A recently described subgroup of childhood disorders, such as TOURETTE SYNDROME (TS) and OBSESSIVE-COMPULSIVE DISORDER (OCD), that may be related to a preceding streptococcal infection. Over the last few years, in addition to OCD and TS, AUTISTIC DISORDER has also been considered, although not yet accepted, to fit under the PANDAS umbrella. This new theory is controversial, and the link has not yet been proven.

The evidence for autism as part of the PANDAS spectrum remains circumstantial. A study of 18 children with autism demonstrated a higher frequency of a marker linked to PANDAS (D8/17 positive B cells) than did a control group. The D8/17 positive children had more severe repetitive behaviors and significantly higher compulsion scores, suggesting that autism may have an autoimmune basis in a subset of patients, which in itself remains controversial.

Peek, Kim   (1951–   )   A "megasavant" who was the inspiration for the character of Raymond Babbit in the Oscar-winning movie *Rain Man* starring Dustin Hoffman as an autistic savant. However, Peek is not autistic.

Peek was born on November 11, 1951, with an enlarged head (an encephalocele). Subsequent brain scans revealed significant brain damage: a missing corpus callosum (the connecting tissue between the left and right hemispheres), no anterior commissure, and damage to the CEREBELLUM. By age 16 months, Peek was able to memorize every book that was read to him. At age three he was reading by himself and looking up terms in a dictionary, but he did not walk until age four. At that time he was also obsessed with numbers and arithmetic, reading telephone directories and adding columns of telephone numbers. He enjoyed totaling the numbers on automobile license plates as well.

Peek is the only person ever to be diagnosed as a "megasavant"; his brain appears to be unique. While his motor skills are underdeveloped, he has the capability of total recall and remembers almost everything he has read since age three. But after years of having his son tested, Fran Peek decided it was not important to understand why his son's brain worked the way it did. What was most important was that he become as self-reliant as possible.

Peek's expertise includes at least 14 subject areas, including history, politics, geography (especially the roads and highways in the United States and Canada), professional sports (including baseball, basketball, football, Kentucky Derby winners, and so on), the space program, movies, actors, the Bible, Mormon Church doctrine and history, calendar calculations, literature, authors, telephone area codes, major zip codes, and all TV stations and their markets. He can identify most classical music compositions and tell the date the music was written and the composer's birth date and place of birth and death. He has read—and can recall—more than 7,600 books. He also has the unique ability to read two pages simultaneously, one with each eye, with 98 percent retention.

Peek met screenwriter Barry Morrow in Texas and astonished him with his mental abilities. Morrow decided to write a script inspired by Peek's abilities; that script eventually evolved into *Rain Man*. The original script underwent a number of modifications; although Peek was the initial inspiration for the story, Raymond Babbitt is a composite savant with abilities drawn from a number of living individuals.

In preparation for playing the part of Raymond Babbitt, actor Dustin Hoffman met Peek and his father in February 1987. That day, according to Peek's father Fran, Kim shared with Hoffman facts about British monarchs, the Bible, baseball, horse racing, dates, times, places, composers, melodies, movies, geography, the space program, authors, and literature. When Hoffman accepted his Oscar in March 1989, he thanked Kim Peek for "making *Rain Man* a reality," although Hoffman also spent time with several other savants and their families as well.

Since 1969, Kim has worked at a day workshop for adults with disabilities, preparing payroll checks from work sheet hours without the aid of calculators or adding machines.

After the movie, due to numerous requests for appearances, Peek became far more self-confident and able to talk to people and travels all over the country with his father to discuss his message: recognize and respect differences in others and treat them as you want them to treat you.

He has appeared on many TV programs, including *20/20* and *Good Morning America*. Peek and his father continue to travel throughout the United States and Canada to share Peek's message of inspiration. His father, Fran Peek, wrote a book about his son: *The Real Rain Man* (Harkness Publishing Consultants, 1996).

perseveration   Persistent repetition of a behavior or activity regardless of the result, or having trouble switching from one activity to another. In addition, one can show perseveration in ideas or interest by consistently focusing on a narrow topic area, such as the geography of western Europe. Extreme examples of perseveration may be seen in individuals with autism, for whom repetitive hand motions, rocking, or other movements are common characteristics. More typical examples in childhood might involve singing a song from a video again and again.

In a school setting, perseveration can be used to describe the fixation on a specific element in a broader task, such as spending all of the time of an exam on a single essay question. This type of behavior may be caused by inflexible strategies and problems in shifting from one task to another.

pervasive developmental disorder–not otherwise specified (PDD-NOS)   A type of AUTISM SPECTRUM DISORDER characterized by significantly impaired social interactions or stereotyped behaviors without all of the features of autism or ASPERGER'S SYDROME. Children with Asperger's syndrome or PDD-NOS tend to function at a higher level than children with autism, and may be able to function independently.

If a diagnosis of PDD-NOS is made, rather than autism, the diagnosticians should clearly specify the behaviors present. Evaluation reports are more useful if they are specific and become more helpful for parents and professionals in later years when reevaluations are conducted.

pervasive developmental disorders (PDD) A term used in the *DSM-IV-TR* for a group of disorders that encompasses AUTISTIC DISORDER and similar conditions, characterized by varying degrees of difficulty with communication skills, social interactions, and restricted, repetitive and stereotyped patterns of behavior. The term is gradually being replaced with AUTISM SPECTRUM DISORDERS. The PDDs range from a mild form (ASPERGER'S SYNDROME) to a severe form (AUTISTIC DISORDER). If a child has symptoms of either of these disorders, but does not meet the specific criteria for either, the diagnosis is called PERVASIVE DEVELOPMENTAL DISORDER–NOT OTHERWISE SPECIFIED (PDD-NOS). The other two rare, very severe disorders that are included in the autism spectrum disorders are RETT DISORDER and CHILDHOOD DISINTEGRATIVE DISORDER. (More recently, many experts tend to exclude Rett disorder from the autism spectrum disorders.)

Each of these disorders has specific diagnostic criteria as outlined by the *Diagnostic and Statistical Manual of Mental Disorders (DSM-IV-TR)*. Autism (or autistic disorder) is the most common of the five PDDs, affecting an estimated one in 250 births, according to the U.S. Centers for Disease Control and Prevention. Rett's is the least common of the five.

The term "pervasive developmental disorders" was first used in the 1980s to describe a group of disorders that shared symptoms or characteristics. Unfortunately, the term occasionally causes confusion, because one of the disorders included under PDD has a very similar name—PDD-NOS (pervasive developmental disorder–not otherwise specified). As a result, PDD and PDD-NOS are sometimes used interchangeably. PDD has since been replaced by the more common term autism spectrum disorders.

Since no medical tests can be performed to indicate the presence of autism or any other of the spectrum disorders, the diagnosis is based upon the presence or absence of specific behaviors. For example, a child may be diagnosed as having PDD-NOS if he or she has some behaviors that are seen in autism, but does not meet the full criteria for having autism.

Pervasive Developmental Disorders Screening Test-II (PDDST-II) An easily administered assessment tool designed to screen for several AUTISM SPECTRUM DISORDERS, including AUTISTIC DISORDER, pervasive developmental delay, and ASPERGER'S SYNDROME, in children as young as 18 months. Designed to be a parent-report screening measure, the test helps to identify children with these problems in early childhood so that intervention can begin as soon as possible. As such, it does not include a full description of early signs of autism but does reflect those early signs that can be reported by parents and later correlated with a correct diagnosis.

phenolsulphertransferase (PST) deficiency The theory that some children with autism have low levels of sulphate, or an enzyme that uses sulphate called phenol-sulphotransferase-P. This means that these children will be unable to get rid of amines and phenolic compounds once the body no longer has any use for them. These compounds then remain in their bodies and may cause adverse effects, including effects in the brain.

Treatment Options and Outlook

Treatment for this condition involves dietary changes and EPSOM SALTS BATHS.

physical therapy A series of treatments, including exercise and massage, that are designed to improve function of the body's larger muscles through physical activities, thus improving strength, coordination, and movement. Children with autism often have limited gross and fine motor skills, so physical therapy can help improve function in these areas. Specifically, physical therapists work on improving a child's gross motor skills, such as running, reaching, and lifting. Physical therapists also may work in conjunction with occupational therapists to improve a child's SENSORY INTEGRATION.

See also OCCUPATIONAL THERAPY.

pica The urge to eat nonfood items, such as dirt, sand, paint, plaster, or paper. About 30 percent of children with AUTISTIC DISORDER have moderate to severe pica. Pica can expose the child to heavy metal poisoning, especially if there is lead in the paint or in the soil.

picture exchange communication system See PECS.

Pillault, Christophe (1982–) French AUTISTIC SAVANT in art who creates mystical paintings with his hands, although unable to use his fingers or talk, walk, or feed himself.

Born in Iran to a French father and an Iranian mother and now living in France, he discovered painting in 1993, encouraged by his SPECIAL EDUCATION teacher and his mother, Jacqueline. Although he cannot speak, he expresses himself using acrylic on paper, canvas, and cardboard. His fingerprints on the backs of his paintings are his signature.

His haunting, mystical paintings of ethereal beings were introduced to the United States in 1998 at the Mills Pond House Gallery in Smithtown, Long Island; he also has exhibited and won prizes throughout France, Italy, and Japan. One of his paintings was featured on the cover of the 2003 DAN! (Defeat Autism Now!) conference program; his art is also included in Art of the Mind, the permanent art collection of the M.I.N.D. Institute in California.

pivotal response training (PRT) A behavioral treatment based on the principles of APPLIED BEHAVIOR ANALYSIS (ABA) that uses natural learning opportunities to alter certain behaviors in children with autism, improving communication, behavior, and social skills. Researchers have identified two "pivotal behaviors" that affect a wide range of behavior in children with autism: motivation and responsivity to multiple cues. Rather than teaching thousands of behaviors one at a time, PRT concentrates on these pivotal behaviors. Experts believe that PRT is able to increase the generation of new skills while increasing the motivation of children to perform these behaviors they are learning.

PRT works on boosting motivation by giving children choices, emphasizing taking turns, reinforcing attempts, and interspersing maintenance tasks.

The product of 20 years of research from Robert and Lynn Koegel, cofounders of the Autism Research Center at the University of California/Santa Barbara, this approach helps improve a child's communication and language skills, even in extremely challenging cases, and fosters social interactions and friendships with typically developing peers. PRT also reduces disruptive behaviors by combining functional assessment with self-management strategies and is an aid to early identification and intervention for autism. PRT also reduces ritualistic behaviors, broadens a child's interests, and improves performance in school activities and on homework.

Because PRT works with each child's natural motivations and stresses functional communication over rote learning, this comprehensive model helps children develop skills they can really use. However, research suggests that this treatment works better with some children than others; studies are ongoing to try to pinpoint which children can best be helped by PRT.

positive behavior support (PBS) A broad approach for resolving problem behaviors displayed by people with autism spectrum disorders, including SELF-INJURIOUS BEHAVIOR, aggression, tantrums, and repetitive behaviors. It is based on and derived from the theory of APPLIED BEHAVIOR ANALYSIS and many of the intervention procedures are derived from this discipline.

PBS requires that procedures be positive and respect the dignity of the person, featuring individualized interventions based on an understanding of the person and his or her environment. PBS interventions usually consist of more than one strategy and involve collaboration among more than one caregiver and support provider. PBS goals should include improvements in social relationships and other lifestyle enhancements, as well as reductions in problem behavior.

The process begins with the formation of a support team, which consists of the most relevant individuals in the person's life, such as family members, teachers, and friends. The team members are usually responsible for implementing the positive behavior support plan.

The next step is to establish an agreement on the broad goals that a support plan should seek to achieve. Once the support team defines their common vision, then a functional behavior assessment is conducted, gathering information about the problem behavior. Armed with the support plan and the functional behavior assessment, the team writes a positive behavior support plan that includes a number of components:

- strategies for teaching and increasing skills that are intended to replace the problem behaviors
- strategies for preventing the problems before they occur
- strategies for dealing with the problems if or when they do occur
- strategies for monitoring progress

As time goes on, the support team often meets to evaluate progress and make adjustments to the plan, as necessary.

Prader-Willi syndrome (PWS) A genetic disorder sometimes associated with (but not a subtype of) AUTISTIC DISORDER because both conditions share some behaviors. These include language and motor development delays; learning disabilities; feeding problems in infancy; sleep problems; obsessive-compulsive behaviors such as repetitive thoughts and verbalizations, collecting and hoarding of possessions, and skin picking; a strong need for routine and predictability; and a high pain threshold. Frustration or schedule changes can easily trigger loss of emotional control in someone with PWS, ranging from tears to temper tantrums to physical aggression.

Prader-Willi syndrome affects about one out of 10,000 to 15,000 people—both males and females, and all races.

Most individuals suffering from this disorder are missing a small portion of the critical genes on chromosome 15, which appears to come from the paternal side of the family. A few individuals with Prader-Willi are missing the entire chromosome from the father, inheriting instead two chromosome 15s from the mother. When a small portion of chromosome 15 is missing and comes from the maternal side, the person may suffer from ANGELMAN SYNDROME, another condition with some similarities to autism.

Occasionally (less than 2 percent of the time), a genetic mutation that does not affect the parent is passed on to the child, and in these families more than one child may be affected. A similar disorder can be acquired after birth if the hypothalamus is damaged through injury or surgery.

Symptoms and Diagnostic Path

Despite the similarities with autism as listed above, the classical features of this disorder are quite distinctive, and include an obsession with food often associated with impulsive eating, compact body build, underdeveloped sexual characteristics, and poor muscle tone. Signs of Prader-Willi may be seen at birth, with very small size and floppy muscles. Infant boys may have undescended testicles. Because of their obsession with food, many people afflicted with Prader-Willi syndrome are overweight. Most individuals afflicted with this condition also have mild MENTAL RETARDATION, and IQ seldom exceeds 80. However, children with Prader-Willi generally are very pleasant, happy, and smile frequently.

Treatment Options and Outlook

Recent studies have shown that growth hormone treatment can improve growth and decrease the percent of body fat, as well as improve physical strength and agility. A micropenis (very small penis) in the male infant may be corrected with a short course of testosterone. Hormone replacement can correct hypogonadism at puberty.

The most effective form of treatment for minimizing difficult behaviors in people suffering from Prader-Willi syndrome is behavior modification, with careful environmental structuring and consistent use of positive behavior management and supports. In general, medications do not appear to be very effective for these individuals, although psychotropic medications can help some patients.

With treatment, people with PWS can expect to graduate, get a job, and even move away from their family home. However, they do need a significant amount of support from their families and from school, work, and residential service providers to achieve these goals while avoiding obesity. Even individuals with normal IQ need lifelong diet supervision and protection from food availability.

In the past, many people with PWS died in adolescence or young adulthood, but today preventing obesity can enable those with the syndrome to live a normal life span. Ongoing research may provide discoveries that will enable patients to live more independent lives.

pregnancy factors   Pregnancy factors and preterm delivery may be associated with the risk of autism, according to a study supported in part by the Centers for Disease Control and Prevention (CDC). Breech presentation at birth, delivery before 35 weeks, and low birth weight at delivery are specific risk factors.

The research, which involved national study of all 698 Danish children with autism born after 1972 and diagnosed before 2000, focused on perinatal risk factors such as delivery and newborn characteristics, pregnancy characteristics, and parental characteristics, among other things.

At present, the study only identifies possible associations. Additional research is needed to determine if the factors identified actually play a role in causing autism.

prognosis   A prediction of the probable course and outcome of a disease or ailment. How well a person with autism is able to function can vary dramatically, ranging from individuals who require nearly complete custodial care to those who can function independently. Adult independence can be linked directly to both the severity of the disorder in the individual and the quality, quantity, and onset of the treatment.

Most adults with autism are either living at home with their parents or living in a group home. Some

higher-functioning people live in a supported-living situation with modest assistance, and a very few are able to live independently. Some are able to work, either in volunteer work, sheltered workshops, or private employment, but many do not. Although each person with autism is different, in general people with autism function best at highly structured jobs featuring lots of repetition. These may include computer operators, office workers, assembly line workers, or employees at sheltered workshops.

Adults with PERVASIVE DEVELOPMENTAL DISORDER–NOT OTHERWISE SPECIFIED (PDD-NOS) and ASPERGER'S SYNDROME generally are more likely to live independently, and they are more likely to work, although they often have trouble finding and maintaining a job. The major reason for chronic unemployment is not a lack of job skills, but rather limited social skills. This is why it is important to encourage appropriate social skills early in the life of children with autism, so they will one day be able to live and work as independently as possible.

Some of the most successful people on the autism spectrum who have good jobs have developed expertise in a specialized skill that others value. If a person makes himself or herself very good at something, this can help make up for some difficulties with social skills. Good fields for higher functioning people on the spectrum are architectural drafting, computer programming, language translation, special education, library science, the sciences, and sometimes music. In fact, many experts believe that some brilliant scientists and musicians have a mild form of Asperger's syndrome. Individuals with autism who are most successful often have good mentors either in high school, college, or on the job who can help channel interests into careers.

Untreated sensory oversensitivity can severely limit a person's ability to tolerate a workplace environment. Eliminating fluorescent lights will often help, but untreated sound sensitivity has caused some individuals on the autism spectrum to quit good jobs because ringing telephones hurt their ears. Some experts believe that sensory sensitivity may be reduced by AUDITORY INTEGRATION TRAINING, diets, IRLEN LENSES, conventional psychiatric medications, or vitamin supplementation.

Today, the educational and treatment options are much better than in the past and should continue to improve in the future. However, it is often up to parents to find those services, determine which are the most appropriate for their child, and ensure that they are properly implemented. Parents are a child's most powerful advocates and teachers. With the right mix of interventions, most children with autism will be able to improve and lead a happy, fulfilled life.

See also GRANDIN, TEMPLE.

prosopagnosia   A rare type of neurological condition in which patients have special problems recognizing human faces. Prosopagnosia is a form of agnosia—a condition in which patients fail to recognize objects even though they show no signs of sensory problems. Prosopagnosia has nothing to do with a person's ability to see faces—someone with perfect vision can suffer from prosopagnosia. It is also unrelated to the person's IQ.

Experts believe that prosopagnosia occurs when that special brain center dedicated to face recognition becomes damaged or is otherwise unable to perform its function. Anecdotal evidence suggests that prosopagnosia is especially common in people with autism and ASPERGER'S SYNDROME, but few scientific studies have examined this aspect. Evidence suggests that individuals with prosopagnosia identify other people by observing their clothing, hairstyles, beards, gait, and voice.

Prosopagnosia was first observed and documented several hundred years before Christ, but it was not named until 1947.

See also FACE RECOGNITION.

psychological evaluation   A type of test that is sometimes used as part of a general assessment of an individual's learning difficulties, especially when there are other significant behavioral, social, or emotional elements involved. In cases where symptoms or behavior might indicate the presence of a significant psychological problem, a psychological evaluation may be necessary to determine whether psychological or emotional factors may be involved in an individual's performance or behavior or to rule out such possible conditions as depression, OBSESSIVE-COMPULSIVE DISORDER, or a personality disorder.

psychologist   A mental health expert who specializes in the diagnosis and treatment of mental or emotional problems. A psychologist studies and understands brain and behavior processes from a scientific viewpoint and applies this knowledge to help people understand, explain and change behavior. Clinical psychologists often use a range of assessment tools, including intelligence testing, to assess, diagnose, and treat patients. Psychologists can treat learning disabilities by helping the person explore upsetting thoughts and feelings and helping find more positive ways to channel emotions. They also develop standardized assessment tools to measure behavior and therapeutic interventions to help people improve their ability to function as individuals and in groups.

A psychologist usually holds a doctoral degree (Ph.D., Psy.D., or Ed.D.) from a university or professional school. Generally, a psychologist in clinical practice will have a degree in clinical psychology (although it might be in counseling psychology). With the exception of the Psy.D. (a purely clinical degree), all psychologists have had extensive training in research, having completed a doctoral dissertation as a major part of the training. In fact, the psychologist's training in research is what most distinguishes a psychologist from other providers of mental health treatment. In addition to research training, the psychologist will have completed one or more clinical internships.

psychologist, educational   A Ph.D.-level mental health expert who specializes in assessment and consultation relating to educational issues, including the assessment of learning disabilities. Educational psychologists use a range of assessment tools, including intelligence and academic achievement testing.

Special educational needs, learning difficulties, dyslexia, behavior problems, and the guidance of gifted children all fall within the scope of the educational psychologist's expertise. The educational psychologist is qualified to give advice based upon expert assessment and observation of the child's strengths and weaknesses, drawing upon a knowledge of child psychology, child development, and education.

Psychologists use a range of techniques to put together a picture of the child's strengths and difficulties and identify important factors affecting the child's learning and behavior. Individual tests of intelligence will give a profile of the child's verbal and nonverbal thinking skills and may identify specific areas of strength and weakness that need to be taken into account. Information is also gathered through structured classroom observation as well as interviews with teachers and parents. Getting an objective picture helps understanding and provides a framework for discussing solutions to problems.

psychologist, school A professionally trained PSYCHOLOGIST who specializes in working with preschool and school-age children, adolescents, and their teachers and families to help make education for students a positive and rewarding experience.

School psychologists address many issues such as crisis intervention, social skills training, behavioral management techniques, self-esteem, attention deficit disorders, post-traumatic stress disorders, and special education regulations. A school psychologist is also trained in counseling and crisis intervention and is often involved in one-on-one counseling and in group counseling with elementary and high school students.

In addition, school psychologists administer and interpret intelligence tests and achievement tests and complete social-emotional assessments (such as tests of personality, affect, or behavior problems). They are primarily responsible in helping schools make an educational diagnosis of learning disabilities such as attention deficit disorder. One of the main roles of the school psychologist is to administer a variety of psychoeducational tests to students who are experiencing academic or behavioral problems in the classroom. Based on these test results and information collected from the student's teachers and parents, the school psychologist helps the schools determine if a student is eligibile for special education services.

School psychologists work with students who have vastly different educational problems and needs, including learning disabilities, traumatic brain injuries, emotional and behavioral disorders, autism, intellectual disabilities, and developmental delays.

School psychologists earn a bachelor's degree followed by an advanced degree—usually a mas-

ter's degree plus 30 graduate credits. Many school psychology programs across the country offer a specialist degree as well, which is a master's degree plus 30 credits. The specialist's degree is an intermediary degree between a masters and a Ph.D. In fact, most states require a specialist's degree (or its equivalent) in order to become certified as a school psychologist. Training focuses on mental health, child development, learning, and motivation.

There are several differences between a school psychologist and a school counselor. Unlike school psychologists, school counselors are not required to have a master's degree or a specialist's degree. In addition, counselors are not trained or qualified to administer and interpret psychological and social-emotional assessments, nor are they able to make educational diagnoses of handicapping conditions as required by federal law. Many counselors spend their school day doing guidance in the classrooms.

School psychologists usually must be certified in the state in which services are to be provided. This can also be done at the national level through the National School Psychology Certification Board (NSPCB) or the National Association of School Psychologists (NASP). Each state has different requirements, and not all states accept NSPCB, but all states accept the NASP certification. They do not necessarily have to be licensed by the state as clinical psychologists (required to formally diagnose autism and other developmental disabilities and mental disorders).

Public Law 94-142 (Education for All Handicapped Children Act of 1975) A federal law that provides funds to states that maintain certain standards in their education of handicapped children, such as providing a free and appropriate education in a least restrictive environment. It was renamed the INDIVIDUALS WITH DISABILITIES EDUCATION ACT (IDEA) in 1990.

Purkinje cells A type of brain cell that, when in short supply, may be related to autism. This link was uncovered during autopsies on autistic people, but the reason behind any such link is presently unknown.

The Real Life Rating Scale (RLRS) A test used to assess the effects of treatment on 47 behaviors of people with autism, including motor, social, affective, language, and sensory skills. The RLRS can be used in everyday settings by nonprofessional raters.

receptive language The forms of language that are received as input: listening and reading. Listening and reading are receptive skills that involve feeding information into the brain, as opposed to speaking and writing, which are the expressive forms of language. Most individuals maintain similar capacity for receptive and expressive, oral and written language function, but those with learning problems may have specific deficits in one or more of these areas.

refrigerator mother Slang term used in a pejorative way to describe mothers of autistic children. The phrase was used in descriptions of the Freudian psychological theory of the cause of (infantile) autism, implying that emotionally distant, cold mothers were the cause of autism in their children. This theory is no longer accepted as a cause of autism.

Rehabilitation Act of 1973 (RA), Section 504 A major piece of legislation requiring that schools not discriminate against children with disabilities (including AUTISTIC DISORDER) and that they provide children with reasonable accommodations. Under some circumstances, these "reasonable accommodations" may include the provision of services.

While the INDIVIDUALS WITH DISABILITIES EDUCATION ACT (IDEA) focuses on "free appropriate pub-

lic education" for children with disabilities, Section 504 of the Rehabilitation Act is intended to prohibit discrimination against individuals with handicaps in programs receiving federal financial assistance. The RA is more general in scope, and its definition of handicapped is somewhat broader than that of the IDEA.

Unlike the IDEA, which applies primarily to public elementary and secondary education for children with disabilities, the Rehabilitation Act also applies to post-secondary institutions that receive federal funds in any form. To fall under the protection of the RA, an individual must meet the definition of "handicapped" as defined in the act, be "otherwise qualified," and be denied employment or education "solely by reason" of the handicapping condition. In addition, the act requires that an employer or educational institution must make "reasonable accommodations" for the handicapping condition.

Eligibility

Eligibility for Section 504 is based on the existence of an identified physical or mental condition that substantially limits a major life activity. As learning is considered a major life activity, children diagnosed with autistic disorder are entitled to the protections of Section 504 if the disability is substantially limiting their ability to learn. Children who are not eligible for special education may still be guaranteed access to related services if they meet the Section 504 eligibility criteria.

Evaluation

Although Section 504 requires nondiscriminatory testing, there are far fewer regulations placed on the testing procedure than are required for IDEA. In addition, unlike IDEA, Section 504 does not discuss the frequency of testing or the role outside evaluations may play nor require parental consent for testing. It does require that an evaluation be conducted before a child receives a remediation plan and before any changes are made to the plan.

Section 504 Plan

If the child is eligible for services under Section 504, the school district must develop a "Section 504 plan." However, the regulations do not dictate the frequency of review of the 504 plan, and do not specify the right of parents to participate in its development.

In general, Section 504 provides a faster, more flexible, and less stigmatizing procedure for obtaining some accommodations and services for children with disabilities than IDEA. By virtue of the looser eligibility criteria, some children may receive protection who are not eligible for services or protection under IDEA, and less information is needed to obtain eligibility. Thus, Section 504 can provide an efficient way to obtain limited assistance without the stigma and bureaucratic procedures attached to IDEA.

There are some benefits under IDEA, however:

- a wider range of service options
- far more extensive procedures for parent participation and procedural safeguards
- far more specific degree of regulation than that found in Section 504

If a child has behavioral problems that could lead to the possibility of excessive discipline, suspension, and expulsion, parents should be particularly aware of the less rigorous safeguards provided by Section 504.

relationship development intervention (RDI) A new method for teaching children how to develop relationships, first with their parents and later with their peers. The method focuses on teaching the development of social skills and friendships, which is a core problem for most people with AUTISTIC DISORDER.

repetitive behaviors Odd repetitive motions, such as repeatedly flapping the arms or toe walking, are a common symptom of autism and the AUTISM SPECTRUM DISORDERS. These behaviors might be obvious or subtle.

Repetitive behavior sometimes is expressed by having a persistent, intense preoccupation. For example, the child might be obsessed with learning all about vacuum cleaners, train schedules, or lighthouses. Often there is great interest in numbers, symbols, or science topics. Children with autism often spend hours lining up their cars and trains in a certain way instead of manipulating them in pretend play. If someone accidentally moves one of the toys out of alignment, the child typically loses control and gets extremely upset, because children with autism need and demand absolute consistency in their environment. A slight change in any routine, such as a later mealtime, a change in dress, or going to school at a different time or by a different route can be extremely disturbing. Experts suspect that such a need for order and sameness may lend some stability in a world of confusion.

residual state autism See INFANTILE AUTISM, RESIDUAL STATE.

Rett disorder (Rett syndrome) A rare, progressive disorder of developmental arrest that occurs almost exclusively in girls, producing autistic-like behavior, learning disabilities, poor muscle tone, aimless hand-wringing movements, difficulty expressing feelings, poor eye contact, seizures, slow brain and skull growth, shortened life expectancy, and walking abnormalities. This condition is considered to be one of the five disorders under the umbrella term AUTISM SPECTRUM DISORDERS (ASD) as listed in the *DSM-IV-TR.* It is included as an ASD because there is some potential confusion with autism, particularly in the preschool years. However, the course and onset of this condition are distinctive.

Although the gene mutation that causes Rett also occurs in some cases of autism, suggesting that they are related conditions, Rett occurs mostly in girls, whereas autism occurs much more often in boys. Both conditions feature a loss of speech and emotional contact, but Rett disorder also causes lagging head growth and loss of purposeful hand skills and mobility (APRAXIA), which are not part of autism. Girls with Rett enjoy affection and almost always prefer people to objects, whereas children with autism prefer objects to people. For these reasons, many experts now no longer consider Rett disorder to be a condition on the autism spectrum.

The syndrome, which is caused by a faulty X chromosome, appears in about one of every 10,000 to 15,000 live female births. Once considered a condition exclusively of girls, experts now believe that boys can have Rett disorder, but that in boys the condition is usually fatal before birth. The difference between boys and girls occurs because girls have two X chromosomes, only one of which is active in any particular cell. This means that only about half the cells in a girl's nervous system will actually have the defective Rett gene. Because boys have a single X chromosome, *all* of their cells must use the faulty version of the gene, which experts believe results in fatal defects.

The condition was first described in 1954, when Viennese physician Andreas Rett first noticed this syndrome in two girls as they sat in his waiting room, making the same repetitive hand-writhing motions. When he compared their medical histories, he discovered striking similarities. Upon further investigation, he located six other girls with similar symptoms among his patients. After filming these girls, he began traveling throughout Europe looking for other similar children.

At about the same time, Swedish physician Bengt Hagberg noticed his young female patients who shared similar symptoms. In 1966, Dr. Rett published his findings in several German medical journals, followed by a description of the disease in English in 1977. Finally, in 1983 an article on the disorder appeared in the *Annals of Neurology* written by Dr. Hagberg, who honored its pioneering researcher by naming the condition Rett disorder.

Rett is classified as a developmental disease because it does not cause the brain to degenerate. Instead, it interferes with the maturation of certain areas of the brain that control basic processes, including the frontal, motor, and temporal cortex; brainstem; basal forebrain; and basal ganglia. These areas are also critical to the normal development of the cortex in late infancy; Rett destroys the brain areas that control both movement and emotion. This probably occurs when subsets of brain cells and their synapses are disrupted during a very dynamic phase of brain development during the first few months of life, when synapses are normally being overproduced, only to be trimmed back later to the normal adult number.

The specific genetic problem was discovered in 1999: a mutation of the MECP2 gene on the X chromosome. This mutation is found in up to 75 percent of typical and atypical cases of Rett. Experts suspect that overproduction of these proteins triggers the nervous system deterioration characteristic of the disease. The role of the MECP2 gene is to silence other genes when they are no longer needed in development. (Most genes are active for only a specific period in development and then shut off forever.) The MECP2 mutation makes the turn-off mechanism fail, allowing other genes to stay active when they are no longer needed, and allowing proteins and enzymes to build up and become toxic to the central nervous system.

Mutations in MECP2 almost always occur spontaneously rather than through heredity, which means that parents rarely pass on the disease to their children. The chance of having more than one child with Rett disorder is less than 1 percent, which means that more than 99 percent of the time, the mutation is sporadic and is not repeated in a family.

Symptoms and Diagnostic Path

Although rarely fatal in girls, Rett disorder nevertheless causes permanent impairment. Individuals with Rett disorder often experience autistic-like behavior in the early stages. Other symptoms may include toe walking, sleep problems, wide-based gait, teeth grinding and difficulty chewing, slowed growth, seizures, cognitive disabilities, and breathing difficulties such as hyperventilation, breath holding, and air swallowing. It is difficult to determine the IQ of a child with Rett disorder because of the apraxia and lack of verbal communication skills, since most traditional testing methods require speech and the use of the hands.

Apraxia is a fundamental and severely handicapping aspect of the condition that can interfere with all types of movement, including eye gaze and speech. Some children start to use single words and word combinations before they lose this ability.

There are four stages of Rett disorder, which usually begins in early childhood and follows an irreversible course. Typically, the child develops normally for the first months of life.

Stage I (early onset) generally begins between six and 18 months of age and often is overlooked because symptoms may be somewhat vague, and parents and doctors may not notice the subtle slowing of development at first. The infant may begin to show less eye contact and lose interest in toys. There may be delays in gross motor skills such as sitting or crawling. Hand-wringing and decreasing head growth may occur, but not enough to draw attention. This stage usually lasts for a few months but can persist for more than a year.

Stage II (the rapid destructive stage) usually begins between ages one and four and may last for weeks or months. This stage may begin quickly or more slowly, as purposeful hand skills and spoken language are lost. The characteristic hand movements begin to emerge during this stage and often include wringing, washing, clapping, or tapping, as well as repeatedly moving the hands to the mouth. Hands are sometimes clasped behind the back or held at the sides, with random touching, grasping, and releasing. The movements persist while the child is awake but disappear during sleep. Breathing irregularities such as episodes of apnea and hyperventilation may occur, although breathing is usually normal during sleep. Some girls at this stage also display autistic-like symptoms such as loss of social interaction and communication. There may be general irritability and sleep irregularities, with unsteady gait and problems initiating motor movements. Slowing of head growth is usually noticed during this stage.

Stage III (the plateau or pseudo-stationary stage) usually begins between ages two and 10 and can last for years. Apraxia, walking problems, and seizures are prominent during this stage. However, there may be improvement in behavior, with less irritability, crying, and autistic-like behavior. An individual in Stage III may show more interest in her surroundings, and her alertness, attention span, and communication skills may improve. Many girls remain in this stage for most of their lives.

The last stage, **Stage IV**—called the late motor deterioration stage—can last for years or decades and is characterized by problems in walking. Muscle weakness, rigidity, spasticity, and scoliosis are other prominent features. Girls who were previously able to walk may stop walking. Generally, there is no decline in cognition, communication, or hand skills in Stage IV. Repetitive hand movements may decrease, and eye gaze usually improves.

A girl's problems may include seizures, which can be severe, although they tend to become less intense in later adolescence. Disorganized breathing patterns also may occur, but this too will improve with age. Mild to severe scoliosis is a prominent feature of girls with Rett disorder.

In the past, diagnosing the disorder before age four or five years old was difficult, and so the condition was often misdiagnosed as autism, cerebral palsy, or nonspecific developmental delay. But the discovery of the genetic mutation has led to a genetic blood test that can improve the accuracy of early diagnosis.

The first step in getting a diagnosis is to get the blood test for the malfunctioning gene. There are more than 100 mutations in the MECP2 gene that causes Rett, and mutations have been found in more than 80 percent of girls who match the diagnostic criteria for the disorder. For the remaining 20 percent who do not appear to have an MECP2 mutation yet do exhibit the symptoms, experts suspect that their mutations are located in a part of the very large MECP2 gene not yet screened. At present, it is possible to have Rett with a negative blood test. And because researchers now understand that the MECP2 mutation also causes other disorders, it is possible to have the MECP2 gene mutation and not have Rett disorder.

After the blood test has been taken, the doctor will assess the child's early growth and development, evaluate the medical history, and check the child's physical and neurological signs. To come up with a diagnosis, specialists use a Rett disorder diagnostic criteria worksheet that outlines one of three categories: classic Rett disorder, provisional Rett, and atypical Rett.

There are several different types of Rett disorder. Classical Rett disorder is diagnosed in those children who meet all the diagnostic criteria guidelines.

"Provisional" Rett is diagnosed in a child if there is *some* evidence of symptoms between ages one and three. "Atypical Rett syndrome" is diagnosed if symptoms begin earlier (soon after birth) or later (beyond 18 months of age, sometimes as late as age three or four), speech and hand skill abnormalities are milder, or it is found in a boy (very rare).

Other conditions mimic Rett disorder and must be ruled out, including Angelman syndrome, PRADER-WILLI SYNDROME, metabolic disorders, storage diseases, mitochondrial disorders, and Batten Disease.

Genetic testing is also available for sisters of girls with Rett disorder and an identified MECP2 mutation to determine if they are asymptomatic carriers of the disorder, which is an extremely rare possibility.

Treatment Options and Outlook

There is no cure for Rett disorder, but there are several treatment options, including behavioral training to teach communication and other functional skills, and medication for seizures that may occur. In addition, the child should be monitored for scoliosis and possible heart abnormalities. Occupational therapy can help children develop skills needed for self care, such as dressing and feeding; physiotherapy and hydrotherapy may prolong mobility.

Some children may need special equipment and aids such as braces to treat scoliosis, splints to modify hand movements, and nutritional programs to help them maintain adequate weight. Special academic, social, vocational, and support services may also be required in some cases.

Predicting the severity of Rett disorder in any child is not easy, but in spite of the severe problems this condition causes, most girls with Rett survive at least into their 40s. Most girls can learn to use the toilet and many can learn to feed themselves by hand or with utensils with some assistance. Some girls can learn to use assistive devices to communicate.

Girls and women with Rett can continue to learn and have fun with family and friends well into middle age and beyond, experiencing a full range of emotions as they participate in social, educational, and recreational activities.

risperidone (Risperdal) An antipsychotic drug found effective for the treatment of tantrums, aggression, or self-injurious behavior in children with AUTISTIC DISORDER. However, scientists caution that side effects and the lack of a clear benefit with regard to core symptoms of autism indicate that risperidone should be reserved for treatment of moderate-to-severe behavioral problems associated with the disorder.

This medication works by blocking brain receptors for dopamine and serotonin, two chemical messengers in the brain, and has been found to be effective in treating adults with schizophrenia. However, there are few large studies on the safety and efficacy of antipsychotics in children with autism.

safety issues Living with a person with autism means that difficult behaviors can make safety a lifelong problem. An individual with autism may engage in a wide variety of unsafe behaviors, including climbing, throwing or breaking items, jumping, sweeping items off surfaces, dumping drawers and bins, and climbing out of or breaking windows. In addition, people with autism may put items in appliances, flush things down the toilet, touch a stove burner, turn on hot faucets, insert items into electrical sockets, chew on wires, play with matches, or crawl in a washer or dryer.

Because children with autism do not understand the results of their actions, it becomes very important to make sure the home is as safe and protected as possible.

Arrange the Furniture

If a child often runs out of a room along the same route, the furniture should be arranged so the child is unable to escape. Furniture should be moved away from shelves or places where the child may climb, and surfaces should be kept clear. Items should be kept out of reach on shelves or locked away, and gates can prevent falls down steps.

Locks

Locks should be placed on exterior doors to protect individuals who run away or leave the home without supervision. Locks also should be placed on interior doors and on cabinets to which the individual should not have free access.

If parents need to prevent wandering at night, locks on the child's bedroom door must be able to open with a keyhole/key, a hook-and-eye lock, or a slide-bolt. It is imperative that parents have immediate access to the room where the door is locked in the event of fire, flood, or other emergency. Some parents place the lock key above the doorframe of the room to have quick access.

Poisonous items must also be locked away, including detergents, chemicals, cleaning supplies, pesticides, medications, and small items that a child may mouth or chew.

Safeguard Windows

Specialized window locks will prevent a child from climbing out the window. If a child breaks glass or pounds windows, the glass should be replaced with Plexiglas to prevent injury. Some parents place wooden boards over windows to prevent injury or escape.

Electrical Outlets and Applicances

Electrical outlets should be covered or removed and plastic knob covers used for doors, faucets, ovens, and stove burners. The door to the washer or dryer, appliances, or power tools should be locked. All wiring for appliances and electronics must be concealed; individuals with autism are curious about how things work and are unaware of dangerous situations.

Eating Utensils and Place Settings

If a child typically throws utensils, forks and spoons can be tied with nylon string and attached to the chair or leg of the table. If the child throws or sweeps plates, bowls, and cups, these items can be fastened to the table with Velcro. Plastic or rubber plates, bowls, and cups should be used to prevent shattering.

Social Safety Stories

Parents can develop SOCIAL STORIES with photographs, pictures, and words about the purpose of smoke detectors, fire drills, fire alarms, the importance of avoiding fire, and so on. (A social story is a short, personalized tale that explains the subtle cues in social situations and breaks down a situation or task into easy-to-follow steps.) Parents should read the stories to the child on a regular basis. Photos or pictures can help the child understand what they should or should not do.

savant syndrome   A condition in which a person with a developmental disability (such as AUTISTIC DISORDER) exhibits unusual areas of brilliant ability. Savant syndrome is rare, however; only one out of ten people with autistic disorder have any savant abilities at all. Still, although only 10 percent have some savant abilities, that percentage is much higher than for people with other developmental disabilities (one in 2,000).

Some people with autism have particular savant skills that are remarkable only in contrast to the handicap (called "talented savants"). A few others with a much rarer form of the condition exhibit a brilliant ability not just unusual in contrast to the handicap, but so outstanding it would be incredible even if the skill was exhibited by a nonautistic person (called "prodigious savant"). There are fewer than 100 reported cases of prodigious savants in the world. The character played by Dustin Hoffman in the movie *Rain Man* was a prodigious savant who displayed incredible memory feats. Real-life prodigious savants include Leslie Lemke (music), Kodi Lee (piano), Alonzo Clemens (sculpting), Richard Wawro (painting), Stephen Wiltshire (drawing), and Tony DeBlois (music). DeBlois, for example, can play 20 instruments and has committed an estimated 8,000 songs to memory.

The condition was first named "idiot savant" in 1887 by J. Langdon Down, M.D. (who also gave his name to a syndrome of MENTAL RETARDATION known as Down syndrome). In the 19th century, the word "idiot" was an accepted classification of mental retardation (IQ below 25), and the word "savant" was derived from the French word *savoir* ("to know"). Today the term "idiot savant" has been abandoned because of its negative connotations.

The condition can be congenital (often linked to premature birth) or acquired in an otherwise normal individual after brain injury or disease. It occurs in boys more often than girls in about a 6:1 ratio. Typically, savant skills appear in one of six areas: calendar calculating; lightning calculating and mathematical ability; art (drawing or sculpting); music (usually piano); mechanical abilities; and spatial skills. A few individuals exhibit unusual language abilities.

Other skills much less often reported include map memorizing, visual measurement, extrasensory perception, and enhanced sense of touch and smell. The most common savant skill is musical ability; a combination of musical genius, blindness, and autism is not unusual. In some cases, the individual has a single special skill, while others exhibit several skills—but whatever the skill, it is always linked with an incredible memory.

There are a variety of theories to explain savant syndrome, although no one has been able to trace the origin of the talent precisely. The unusual skill could be due to genetics or to a lack of ability to think abstractly. Newer imaging studies reveal left hemisphere damage in savants, which suggests that the most plausible explanation for savant syndrome might be left brain damage with right brain compensation. It is not surprising that many savants struggle with language and comprehension skills (primarily left brain functions), but often have amazing skills in music, mathematics, and calculation (primarily right brain skills). This right brain compensation could be coupled with corresponding damage to higher level cognitive memory, so that lower level, habit memory takes over.

Whatever the cause, once established, the skills are typically enhanced by intense concentration, practice, and reinforcement by family and teachers. However, not all autistic savants function at a high level; the disorder consists of a spectrum of disability ranging from profoundly impaired to high functioning. For many years experts were afraid that helping a savant achieve a higher level of functioning with treatment would trigger a loss of special skills. That has not turned out to be the case. Instead, training the talented savant increases socialization, language, and independence. In fact, the special skills of the savant can become a treatment tool. Some schools include children with savant syndrome in classes for the gifted and talented.

school programs for autism Early intervention programs are available for children younger than age three; children over age three are eligible for preschool and school programs. In some cases, a separate program for special needs children may be the best choice for an autistic child. For higher-functioning children with autism, integration into a regular school setting may be more appropriate, as long as there is enough support (such as an aide).

It is important that parents work with their child's teacher on an INDIVIDUALIZED EDUCATION PROGRAM (IEP), which outlines in great detail what specific steps will be taken to help educate the child. Additionally, meeting with the child's classmates and/or their parents can be helpful in encouraging other students to interact positively with the autistic child.

In some states, home therapy programs (such as APPLIED BEHAVIOR ANALYSIS or speech therapy) may be funded by the school district, rather than through the state. However, it may take considerable effort to convince the school district to provide those services.

scotopic sensitivity syndrome A visual-perceptual problem that occurs in some people with AUTISTIC DISORDER, characterized by a variety of perceptual distortions when reading or looking at their environment. Scotopic sensitivity is triggered by one or more components of light, such as the source (for example, fluorescent lighting or the sun), reflection or glare, brightness, color, or color contrast. As a result, an afflicted person may experience light sensitivity; inefficient reading; difficulty with high contrast; tunnel vision or difficulty reading groups of letters; and problems maintaining attention.

The IRLEN LENS system, developed by Helen Irlen, was designed to treat scotopic sensitivity, using two methods: the use of colored transparencies or overlays to improve reading, and tinted glasses to improve visual perception.

For some people, letters or words on a page may appear to move, vibrate, or jiggle. The white background may overtake and dominate the person's perceptual system, and the black print of the text may fade into the background. People may also have trouble reading for a long period of time, developing headaches or feeling dizzy. Some experts believe that some individuals' visual systems are excessively stimulated by a high contrast between black print on a white background, which thus interferes with the reading process. Transparencies or overlays are used to reduce these problems while reading. A colored overlay, such as a light blue transparency placed over the text, will reduce the contrast between black and white as well as reduce the dominance of the white background. The best color of the transparency depends on each person's unique visual-perceptual system.

In addition to reading problems, people with scotopic sensitivity may have trouble perceiving their surroundings. Some of these autistic individuals have reported improvements after wearing special tinted glasses prescribed by Helen Irlen at one of her 76 diagnostic clinics located around the world. These individuals report seeing better, feeling more relaxed, being less bothered by sunlight or indoor lighting, and/or having fewer perceptual distortions, which can affect small and gross motor coordination.

screening instruments for autism A group of tests developed to quickly gather information about a child's social and communicative development within medical settings that are used to help diagnose autism. These tests include the CHILDHOOD AUTISM RATING SCALE, the CHECKLIST FOR AUTISM IN TODDLERS, the modified Checklist for Autism in Toddlers, the Screening Tool for Autism in Two-Year-Olds, and the SOCIAL COMMUNICATION QUESTIONNAIRE (SCQ) (for children four years of age and older).

During the last few years, additional screening instruments have been designed specifically to check for ASPERGER'S SYNDROME (AS) and higher functioning autism. These tests include the autism spectrum screening questionnaire (ASSQ), the Australian scale for Asperger's syndrome, and the CHILDHOOD ASPERGER'S SYNDROME TEST. These tests concentrate on social and behavioral impairments in children without significant language problems. A "well-child" check-up should include one of these developmental screening tests. If a child's pediatrician does not routinely check the child with such a test, parents should ask that it be done. Autism can be difficult to detect in very young children, yet early identification is critical because those who receive early treatment have the best prognosis over the long term.

If a screening test suggests the possibility of one of the autistic spectrum disorders (ASDs), a second round of diagnostic tests are begun that are more comprehensive and can accurately rule in or rule out an ASD or other developmental problem. This evaluation may be done by a multidisciplinary team that includes a PSYCHOLOGIST, a NEUROLOGIST, a psychiatrist, a speech-language therapist, or other professionals who diagnose children with ASD. Because ASDs are complex disorders that may involve other neurological or genetic problems, a comprehensive evaluation should include neurologic and genetic assessment, along with in-depth cognitive and language testing. In addition, tests developed specifically for diagnosing autism are often used. These include the AUTISM DIAGNOSTIC INTERVIEW–REVISED (ADI-R) and the AUTISM DIAGNOSTIC OBSERVATION SCALE (ADOS-G).

Childhood Autism Rating Scale (CARS)

This assessment, which is based on observed behavior of children over age two, was developed in the early 1970s by Eric Schopler and the Treatment and Education of Autistic and Related Communication Handicapped Children (TEACCH) program staff in North Carolina to formalize observations of the child's behavior throughout the day. Using a 15-point scale, professionals evaluate a child's relationship to people, body movements, adaptation to change, listening response, and verbal communication. This test helps to identify children with autism and to distinguish them from developmentally disabled children who are not autistic.

Brief, convenient, and suitable for use with any child older than two, the CARS makes it much easier for clinicians and educators to recognize and classify autistic children. Developed over a 15-year period, CARS includes items drawn from five prominent systems for diagnosing autism. Each item covers a particular characteristic, ability, or behavior. After observing the child and examining relevant information from parent reports and other records, the examiner rates the child on each item. Using

a seven-point scale, the examiner indicates the degree to which the child's behavior deviates from that of a normal child of the same age. A total score is computed by summing the individual ratings on each of the 15 items. Children who score above a given point are categorized as autistic, and can be subcategorized as mild-to-moderate or severe.

The Checklist for Autism in Toddlers (CHAT)

A simple screening tool used by pediatricians to screen for autism at 18 months of age, CHAT was developed in the United Kingdom by Simon Baron-Cohen in the early 1990s. This test features a short questionnaire with two sections, one prepared by the parents and the other by the child's family doctor or pediatrician.

Section A of the CHAT is a self-administered questionnaire for parents, with nine "yes or no" questions addressing rough and tumble play, social interest, motor development, social play, pretend play, pointing to ask for something, functional play, and showing. Section B of the CHAT consists of five items recorded by the physician who observes the child. The five items address the child's eye contact, ability to follow a point given by another person, pretend play, ability to point to an object, and ability to make a tower of blocks. Children are considered likely to have autism if they fail the CHAT at 18 months and fail again at 19 months. It is estimated that consistent failure in three key areas (pointing, gaze monitoring, and pretend play) at 18 months indicates a greater than 80 percent risk of having autism.

Modified Checklist for Autism in Toddlers (M-CHAT)

Because of the poor sensitivity of the original CHAT a Modified Checklist for Autism in Toddlers (M-CHAT), consisting of 23 questions, with nine questions from the original CHAT and an additional 14 addressing core symptoms present among young autistic children, was designed in the United States. The original CHAT observational part (section B) was omitted.

The simpler M-CHAT, developed by Marianne Barton, Diana Robins, and Deborah Fein, asks parents to rate how their child usually behaves. The M-CHAT was designed as a simple, self-administered, parental questionnaire for use during regular pediatric visits. The more questions a child fails, the higher his or her risk of having autism.

Researchers found that M-CHAT was more sensitive in identifying children with autism than the original CHAT because children up to age 24 months were screened, with the aim of identifying those who might regress between 18 and 24 months. The original CHAT was administered during the 18 month checkup. The six most relevant questions of the M-CHAT address the following: interest in other children, imitation, protodeclarative pointing, gaze monitoring, bringing objects to show parents, and responses to calling. Joint attention was addressed in the original CHAT, whereas the other areas were addressed only in the M-CHAT.

Screening Tool for Autism in Two-Year-Olds (STAT)

This test, developed by Wendy Stone, uses direct observations to study behavioral features that seem to indicate autism in children under age two, focusing on three skills areas (play, motor imitation, and joint attention).

The STAT is a play-based screening tool in which the examiner presents 12 activities to the child. The activities assess the child's play, communication, and imitation skills, as these are common difficulties for young children with autism. There is a scoring cutoff that indicates whether a child is at risk or not at risk for an autism diagnosis. An "at risk" score indicates the need for further evaluation.

Social Communication Questionnaire (SCQ)

Previously known as the Autism Screening Questionnaire, this assessment features a 40-item screening scale that has been used with children aged four and older (with a mental age of at least two years) to help evaluate communication skills and social functioning. Designed by Michael Rutter, M.D., Anthony Bailey, M.D., and Catherine Lord, Ph.D., it is available in a "lifetime" and "current" form, each composed of 40 "yes or no" questions. Both forms can be given directly to the parent or physician, who can answer the questions without supervision.

The "lifetime" form focuses on the child's entire developmental history to come up with a total score that is interpreted in relation to specific cut-off points. The score identifies children who may have autism and should be referred for a more complete evaluation, using the Autism Diagnostic Interview–Revised or the Autism Diagnostic Observation Schedule.

The "current" form looks at the child's behavior over the most recent three months and produces results that can be helpful in treatment planning, educational intervention, and measurement of change over time.

In addition to its screening and educational applications, the SCQ can also be used to compare symptom levels of different groups, such as children with developmental language disorders or youngsters with medical conditions typically associated with ASDs.

Because this screening test is short, easily administered, and relatively inexpensive, it allows clinicians and educators to routinely screen children for ASD.

Autism Spectrum Screening Questionnaire (ASSQ)

This ASD screening questionnaire includes 27 statements replied to with "no," "somewhat," or "yes," and includes statements such as: "Is regarded as eccentric professor by other children" and "Expresses sounds involuntarily, clears throat, grunts, smacks, cries, or screams."

The ASSQ is a useful brief screening device for identifying autism spectrum disorders, by assessing symptoms characteristic of Asperger's syndrome and other high-functioning autism spectrum disorders in children and adolescents with normal intelligence or mild mental retardation. Data for parent and teacher ratings in a clinical sample are presented along with various measures of realibility and validity.

Australian Scale for Asperger's Syndrome

This screening tool includes 24 questions responded to on a six-point scale from "rarely" to "frequently"; five items are answered yes or no. Zero is the expected response; two to six indicates the posibility of AS. The questionnaire of 25 items is designed to identify behaviors and abilities indicative of Asperger's syndrome in children during their primary school years. This is the age at which the unusual pattern of behavior and abilities is most conspicuous.

Childhood Asperger's Syndrome Test (CAST)

Far too often, Asperger's syndrome is identified much too late; it should be possible to identify the condition in elementary school children ages five to 11. The Autism Research Centre developed CAST to screen for Asperger's syndrome and related social and communication conditions in children aged four to 11 years in a nonclinical setting. This 38-item yes/no screening measure is designed for parents to answer about their children, and is based on the core features of the autism spectrum disorder. If parents suspect an autism spectrum disorder, they can complete this test, and take it to their primary care provider. Authors are Fiona Scott, Simon Baron-Cohen, Patrick Bolton, and Carol Brayne.

secretin   A hormone produced by the small intestine that helps in digestion. Currently, the U.S. Food and Drug Administration (FDA) approves a single dose of secretin only for use in diagnosing digestive problems; there are no data on the safety of repeated doses over time.

In the 1990s, news reports described a few persons with autism whose behavior improved after receiving secretin during a diagnostic test, including improvements in sleep patterns, eye contact, language skills, and alertness.

However, a series of clinical trials found no difference in improvement between those taking secretin and those taking placebo, according to studies supported by the National Institute of Child Health and Human Development and the Network on the Neurobiology and Genetics of Autism: Collaborative Programs of Excellence in Autism (CPEAs). In fact, of the five case-controlled clinical trials published on secretin, none showed secretin performing any better than placebo, no matter what the dosage or frequency. For this reason, the FDA does not recommend secretin as a treatment for AUTISM SPECTRUM DISORDERS.

seizures   As many as one quarter of all individuals with autism experience seizures, some in early childhood and others as they go through puberty (changes in hormone levels may trigger seizures). Seizures, caused by abnormal electrical activity in the brain made worse by lack of sleep or high fever, can produce a temporary loss of consciousness (a "blackout"), unusual movements, staring spells, or convulsions.

Symptoms and Diagnostic Path

People with autism may experience seizures that can range from mild (gazing into space for a few seconds) to severe, grand mal seizures. Many autistic individuals have subclinical seizures that are not easily noticeable, but which can significantly affect mental function.

An electroencephalogram (EEG), which records the electric currents developed in the brain via electrodes applied to the scalp, can help confirm seizures. A short one- or two-hour EEG may not be able to detect any abnormal activity, so a 24-hour EEG may be necessary.

Treatment Options and Outlook

In most cases, anticonvulsant medications can help stabilize brain activity and control both the seizures and some of the behavioral problems typical of autism. However, these drugs require regular blood testing in order to ensure that liver or bone marrow damage does not occur.

Valproate (Depakote) is a common anticonvulsant drug that can lessen seizures; most of the side effects (such as a sedative effect and an upset stomach) are not severe. However, in rare cases, Depakote can cause liver damage, so frequent blood tests are required to monitor the level of this drug in the blood. Carbamazapine (Tegretol) is another antiepileptic medication that has the same benefits as Depakote. This drug may cause a rash or bone marrow problems. While medications can be used to reduce seizure activity, a child's health must be checked regularly because these drugs can be harmful.

There is also some evidence that certain nutritional supplements, such as vitamin B_6 and dimethylglycine (DMG), can provide an alternative to drugs.

See also EPILEPSY.

self-injurious behavior   Any behavior that damages the person's own tissues, such as that which causes bruises, redness, and open wounds. Individuals with AUTISTIC DISORDER sometimes engage in this type of extreme behavior, including head-banging, hand-biting, and excessive scratching or rubbing.

Some forms of self-injury may be caused by overarousal (such as frustration), so that the self-injury acts as a release, subsequently lowering the arousal. In other cases, self-injury may be a form of repetitive, ritualistic behavior that provides some form of sensory stimulation or arousal.

sensorimotor   This term pertains to brain activity other than cognition or automatic functions such as breathing, circulation, and sleep. Sensorimotor activity includes voluntary movement and senses like sight, touch, and hearing.

sensory integration   The process of taking in sensory information, organizing this information in the central nervous system, and using the information to respond appropriately in order to function smoothly in daily life. Sensory integration is a continual process as the central nervous system matures.

Individuals with autism frequently have unusual responses to various forms of sensory input. Autistic children may seek out unusual amounts of certain types of sensations (referred to as self-stimulation) but be extremely hypersensitive to others. Improving sensory processing may help some of these children develop more productive contacts with people and environments.

Sensory experiences include touch, movement, body awareness, sight, sound, and the pull of gravity. As the brain organizes and interprets this information, it provides a crucial foundation for later, more complex learning and behavior. For most people, effective sensory integration occurs automatically and unconsciously, without effort. For others, however, the process is inefficient, demanding effort and attention with no guarantee of accuracy.

Sensory integration normally develops in the course of ordinary childhood activities. But for some children with autism, some clinicians believe that sensory integration does not develop as efficiently as it should.

The concept of sensory integration comes from a body of work developed by OCCUPATIONAL THERA-PIST A. Jean Ayres, Ph.D., who was interested in the way in which sensory processing and motor planning disorders interfere with daily life function and learning. This theory has been developed and refined by the research of Dr. Ayres, as well as other occupational and PHYSICAL THERAPISTS.

Children with sensory integration problems may have trouble using a pencil, playing with toys, or taking care of personal tasks, such as getting dressed. Some children with this problem are so afraid of movement that ordinary swings, slides, or jungle gyms trigger fear and insecurity. On the other hand, some children whose problems lie at the opposite extreme are uninhibited and overly active, often falling and running headlong into dangerous situations. In each of these cases, some clinicians believe a sensory integrative problem may be an underlying factor. Its far-reaching effects can interfere with academic learning, social skills, even self esteem.

However, the concept of sensory integration is not well accepted in the medical community, and there is no peer-reviewed research supporting sensory integration therapy.

See also SENSORY INTEGRATION DYSFUNCTION.

sensory integration dysfunction   A controversial theory that hypothesizes inefficient brain processing of information received through the senses. Many individuals with autism appear to have trouble detecting, discriminating, or integrating sensations. This complex neurological problem is thought to lead to either sensory seeking or sensory avoiding patterns, or a motor planning problem called dyspraxia.

Sensory Seekers

These children are thought to have nervous systems that do not always process sensory input that is sent to the brain. As a result, they respond too strongly to sensations. Children who are underresponsive to sensation seek out more intense or longer duration sensory experiences. They may

• be hyperactive as they seek more and more movement input

• be unaware of touch or pain, or touch others too often or too hard (may seem aggressive)

- engage in unsafe behaviors, such as climbing too high
- enjoy sounds that are too loud, such as TV or radio volume

Sensory Avoiders

At the other end of the spectrum are those children who are thought to have nervous systems that feel sensation too easily or too much so that they are overly responsive to sensation. As a result, they may have "fight or flight" responses to sensation, a condition called "sensory defensiveness." They may

- respond to being touched with aggression or withdrawal
- be afraid of, or become sick with, movement and heights
- be very cautious and unwilling to take risks or try new things
- be uncomfortable in loud or busy environments such as sports events or malls
- be very picky eaters or overly sensitive to food smells

Treatment

SENSORY INTEGRATION dysfunction is postulated to be a neurological problem that affects behavior and learning. Medicine cannot cure the problem, but the field of OCCUPATIONAL THERAPY has developed a treatment (sensory integration therapy) that tries to address the child's underlying problems in processing sensations. However, there is no sound empirical research supporting sensory integration therapy.

Treatment may include guiding the child through activities that challenge the child's ability to respond appropriately to sensory input by making a successful, organized response. Training of specific skills is not usually the focus of this kind of therapy. Such services are important, but they are not the same as therapy using a sensory integrative approach. Instead, sensory integration therapy focuses on such activities that provide sensory input, such as brushing the child's skin, swinging him about, providing deep pressure to joints and other body parts, and other experiences.

The motivation of the child plays a crucial role in the selection of the activities in a sensory inte-grative approach. Most children tend to seek out activities that provide the best sensory experiences at that particular point in their development. It is this active involvement and exploration that enable the child to become a more mature, efficient organizer of sensory information.

sensory problems Many children with AUTISM SPECTRUM DISORDERS are extremely sensitive to sounds, textures, tastes, light, temperature, or smells. For some of these children, the feel of clothes touching their skin is almost unbearable. For others, some sounds (a vacuum cleaner, a ringing telephone, a sudden storm, even the sound of waves lapping the shoreline) are so painful that they cover their ears and scream. These problems can involve not only hypersensitivity but hyposensitivity to stimulation as well, so that a broken bone will not elicit a whimper, but a light touch can make the child scream with alarm. Others are hyposensitive and have a high tolerance to pain.

Normal perceptions allow children to learn from what they see, feel, or hear, but if that sensory information is faulty, their experiences of the world can be confusing or even frightening. When the ability to recognize sensory information breaks down, a number of problems in learning, development, or behavior may develop.

It appears that the brain of a child with an autism spectrum disorder is unable to balance the senses appropriately. The resulting sensory problems typical of autism can range from mild to severe.

See also SENSORY INTEGRATION; SENSORY INTEGRATION DYSFUNCTION.

Sequenced Inventory of Communication Development–Revised A diagnostic test that evaluates the communication abilities of children with and without retardation who are functioning between age four months and four years. It can be used in treating a young child with language disorders, MENTAL RETARDATION, and specific language problems. It has been used successfully with children with sensory impairments and with children with varying degrees of retardation.

sequencing skills The ability to order elements correctly. Sequencing skills may be motor (sequencing body movements smoothly) or linguistic (sequencing words appropriately into sentences) as well as keeping track of the correct order of stimuli.

serotonin A brain chemical that functions as a neurotransmitter, playing a part in communication within the nervous system. Thought to be involved in inducing sleep, sensory perception, temperature regulation, and control of mood, serotonin also has been implicated as a factor in some cases of autism since the 1961 finding of high levels of serotonin in the blood of patients with autism. Also elevated are the levels of the serotonin precursor tryptophan; the higher the tryptophan, the worse the symptoms, according to some studies.

On the other hand, however, the defect in serotonin metabolism may be a marker for a tendency to experience autism but not cause the disorder. Relatives of autistic children are found to have a variety of serotonin-metabolism disorders, but not the autism itself. Some individuals with autism who are treated with serotonin inhibitors experience less ritualistic behavior and aggression.

shaken baby syndrome Forceful shaking of an infant or young child by the arms, legs, chest, or shoulders that can cause brain damage leading to AUTISTIC DISORDER, MENTAL RETARDATION, speech and learning disabilities, paralysis, seizures, hearing loss, and death.

A baby's head and neck are especially vulnerable to injury because the head is so large and the neck muscles are still weak. In addition, the baby's brain and blood vessels are very fragile and are easily damaged by whiplash motions such as shaking, jerking, and jolting.

About 50,000 cases of shaken baby syndrome occur each year in the United States; one shaken baby in four dies as a result of this abuse. Head trauma is the most frequent cause of permanent damage or death among abused infants and children, and shaking accounts for a significant number of those cases. Some studies estimate that 15

percent of children's deaths are due to battering or shaking and an additional 15 percent are possible cases of shaking. The victims of shaken baby syndrome range in age from a few days to five years, with an average age of six to eight months.

While shaken baby abuse is not limited to any special group of people, 65 to 90 percent of shakers are men. In the United States, adult males in their early 20s who are the baby's father or the mother's boyfriend are typically the shakers. Females who injure babies by shaking them are more likely to be baby-sitters or childcare providers than mothers.

Severe shaking often begins in response to frustration over a baby's crying or toileting problems. The adult shaker also may be jealous of the attention that the child receives from a partner.

Shaken baby syndrome is also known as abusive head trauma, shaken brain trauma, pediatric traumatic brain injury, whiplash shaken infant syndrome, and shaken impact syndrome.

Symptoms and Diagnostic Path
A variety of symptoms may point to shaken baby syndrome, including

- altered consciousness: unconscious or semiconscious
- blood pooling in eyes or brain
- breathing problems
- head turned to one side, swollen head, or inability to lift or turn head
- lethargy
- pupil abnormality: pinpoint or dilated, unresponsive to light
- rib cage damage
- seizures or spasms
- skin paleness or blue color
- spinal cord damage
- vomiting

In addition, a baby who has been shaken may experience poor sucking or swallowing, decreased appetite, lack of smiling or vocalizing, rigidity, or be unable to focus his eyes or track movement.

Shaken baby syndrome is difficult to diagnose unless someone accurately describes what happens. Physicians often report that a child with possible shaken baby syndrome is brought for medical attention due to falls, difficulty breathing, seizures, vomiting, altered consciousness, or choking. The caregiver may report that the child was shaken to try to resuscitate it. Babies with severe or lethal shaken baby syndrome are typically brought to the hospital unconscious with a closed head injury.

To diagnose shaken baby syndrome, physicians look for bleeding in the retina of the eyes (this will be very rare in a normal fall), along with blood in the brain or increased head size indicating buildup of fluid in the tissues of the brain. Damage to the spinal cord and broken ribs from grasping the baby too hard are other signs of shaken baby syndrome. Computed tomography (CT) and magnetic resonance imaging (MRI) scans can reveal injuries in the brain, but are not regularly used because of their expense.

A milder form of this syndrome may be missed or misdiagnosed. Subtle symptoms that may be the result of shaken baby syndrome are often attributed to mild viral illnesses, feeding dysfunction, or infant colic. These include a history of poor feeding, vomiting or flu-like symptoms with no accompanying fever or diarrhea, lethargy, and irritability over a period of time. Without early medical intervention, the child may be at risk for further damage or even death, depending on the continued occurrences of shaking.

Treatment Options and Outlook

An infant who survives the initial shaking may require medical, behavioral, and educational assistance. In addition, children may need speech and language therapy, vision therapy, physical therapy, occupational therapy, and special education services. Some may need the assistance of feeding experts and behavioral consultants.

similar conditions A number of conditions share similar symptoms with autism, including CHILDHOOD DISINTEGRATIVE DISORDER, deafness, galactosemia, LANDAU-KLEFFNER SYNDROME, phenylketonuria, and RETT DISORDER.

Childhood Disintegrative Disorder (CDD)

Much rarer than autism, this is a serious condition in which a child older than age three suddenly stops developing normally and regresses to a much lower level of functioning, typically after a serious illness such as an infection of the brain and nervous system. The disorder is associated with seizures and is more common in boys. Patients with the condition usually require lifelong care. CDD was first described in 1908, many years before autism, but it has only recently been officially recognized. Although apparently rare, experts believe the condition probably has often been incorrectly diagnosed. Fewer than two children per 100,000 with an AUTISM SPECTRUM DISORDER could be classified as having CDD.

Deafness

Some children who have symptoms similar to autism have been discovered instead to be deaf. For this reason, a child should always have his hearing checked before being identified as autistic.

Galactosemia

This inborn error in carbohydrate metabolism refers to an inability to metabolize galactose, and its symptoms are sometimes confused with those of autism.

Landau-Kleffner Syndrome

This is a very rare disorder in which a child develops normally and begins to speak until between three and seven years. At this point, the child begins to lose receptive language while retaining some expressive language and experiences "telegraphic" speech with few verbs. The child seems to be frustrated and is puzzled by these changes, and begins to show autistic-like behaviors. These children have normal or above normal nonverbal IQ scores but abnormal electroencephalograms, with or without seizures. Some practitioners suspect that some cases of childhood disintegrative disorder or late onset autism may in fact be Landau-Kleffner syndrome.

Phenylketonuria (PKU)

This genetic disorder of metabolism will cause brain damage during the first years of life unless special dietary measures are taken. It is caused by lack of an enzyme that converts the amino acid phenylalanine into another amino acid (tyrosine). The extra phenylalanine builds up in body fluids and converts to several chemicals that damage the brain. Symptoms include MENTAL RETARDATION as well as some of the symptoms of autism. Fortunately, today PKU-related brain damage has been minimized because all children are screened for the disorder immediately after birth.

Rett Disorder

This rare neurological disorder occurs in girls, who show normal development before regressing. The initial symptoms include some that are associated with autism.

A child with Rett usually experiences an early period of apparently normal or near-normal development until ages six to 18 months, when a period of temporary stagnation or regression begins. At this point, the child loses the ability to communicate and to purposefully use the hands. Soon, stereotyped hand-writhing movements, gait disturbances, and slowing of the rate of head growth develop. Other problems may include seizures and disorganized breathing patterns. APRAXIA (the inability to program the body to perform motor movements) is the most profound and severely handicapping aspect of this condition, which can interfere with every body movement, including eye gaze and speech. Rett is most often misdiagnosed as autism, cerebral palsy, or nonspecific developmental delay.

sleep problems   As many as 65 percent of children with AUTISTIC DISORDER have abnormal sleep patterns. Adequate sleep is particularly important in these individuals because sleep disturbances may worsen other symptoms, exacerbating the disruptive daytime behavior typical of autistic children.

Treatment Options and Outlook

Melatonin has been very useful in helping many autistic individuals fall asleep. Other popular interventions include using 5-HTP and implementing a behavior modification program designed to induce sleep. Vigorous exercise will help a child sleep.

Other sleep aids include a weighted blanket or tight fitting mummy-type sleeping bag.

social cognition   A term used by social and developmental PSYCHOLOGISTS to refer to how people come to be concerned about the actions, thoughts, and feelings of others. This area of study examines how social perceptions develop, how individuals make social judgments, and how others affect an individual's self-concept.

Social Communication Questionnaire (SCQ)   This brief assessment (previously known as the Autism Screening Questionnaire [ASQ]) helps evaluate communication skills and social functioning in children who may have autism or AUTISM SPECTRUM DISORDERS (ASDs). Completed by a parent or other primary caregiver in less than 10 minutes, the SCQ is a cost-effective way to determine whether an individual should be referred for a complete diagnostic evaluation. The questionnaire can be used to evaluate anyone over age four, as long as the person's mental age is more than two years.

It is available in two forms ("lifetime" and "current") each composed of just 40 yes-or-no questions. Both forms can be given directly to the parent, who can answer the questions without supervision. The lifetime form focuses on the child's entire developmental history, providing a score that identifies individuals who may have autism and should be referred for a more complete evaluation with an assessment such as the AUTISM DIAGNOSTIC INTERVIEW–REVISED (ADI-R) or the AUTISM DIAGNOSTIC OBSERVATION SCALE (ADOS).

Moving from developmental history to the present, the current form looks at the child's behavior over the most recent three months, producing results that can be used to plan treatment and educational objectives.

Because the SCQ is inexpensive, easy, and quick to administer, clinicians and educators can routinely screen children for ASDs.

social problems   Most children with AUTISM SPECTRUM DISORDERS (ASDs) seem to have great problems learning how to deal with others in everyday human interactions. Normal infants are extremely social, very early beginning to look at others, turn toward voices, grasp a finger, and smile.

Infants with autism, however—often even in the first few months of life—do not interact at all, avoid eye contact, and sometimes arch their backs in an effort to distance themselves. At best, these babies seem indifferent to others—even their parents— and seem to prefer being alone. Some children with autism passively accept cuddling while others actively resist touching another person at all.

As these children get older, they rarely seek comfort from others or respond to parents' emotions in a typical way. Scientists suggest that children with autism are attached to their parents, but the way they express this attachment is unusual and difficult to understand. Parents typically feel as if their child does not care about them—or anyone—at all, and many are deeply saddened by this lack of the typical attachment behavior.

As children with autism get older, their social problems only worsen as they must deal with the complexity of human society. They seem to have trouble learning to interpret what others are thinking and feeling, and most totally miss more subtle social facial cues (such as a smile, a wink, or a grimace). To a child who misses or does not understand these cues, the request: "Come here!" always means the same thing, whether the speaker is smiling and extending her arms for a hug or frowning and shaking her finger. Unable to interpret gestures and facial expressions, these children find the social world a bewildering and sometimes frightening place.

People with autism also have trouble understanding that others have different feelings and goals than they have. This difficulty means people with autism are often unable to predict or understand other people's actions.

Children with autism tend to lose control when they are angry, frustrated, or in a new or overwhelming environment. At these times, they may hurl objects, break things, attack others, or hurt themselves by banging their heads, pulling their hair, or biting their arms. Often, people with ASD also have trouble regulating their emotions, so that they may cry, scream, or be disruptive in public in

ways that seem inappropriate to others. This makes it even harder to find friends.

Social Security assistance Families with limited incomes (under about $25,000 to $35,000 a year, depending on family size and assets) can apply to the U.S. Social Security agency to obtain money to help children with a disability. For more information, parents should contact their local Social Security office.

social skills Many children with AUTISTIC DISORDER or any of the AUTISM SPECTRUM DISORDERS (ASD) also exhibit problems with social skills; indeed, impaired social functioning is a central feature of ASD. Most children learn basic social skills quickly and easily, such as taking turns, starting a conversation, or inviting another child to play. For children with an ASD, the process is much more difficult. Many healthy children learn these basic skills simply by exposure to social situations, but children with ASD often need to be taught these skills explicitly. Typically, these children have trouble with reciprocity, initiating interactions, maintaining eye contact, sharing enjoyment, empathy, and inferring the interests of others.

The cause of these problems varies from an inherent problem in the brain, such as a dysfunctional limbic system, to the lack of opportunity to acquire skills because of social withdrawal.

Sadly, this lack of social skills makes it hard for the child to develop and maintain meaningful and fulfilling personal relationships. The popular idea that individuals with an autism spectrum disorder are not interested in social interactions is often inaccurate. In fact, many individuals with ASD do very much want to be involved socially, but they do not have the necessary skills to interact effectively. This lack can lead to feelings of social anxiety in some children, including a racing heart, sweaty palms, noticeable shaking, and concentration problems.

As a result, children with ASD often avoid social situations and subsequently they do not develop social skills. When a child always avoids social encounters, she never gets the chance to learn social interaction skills. In some individuals, these social skill deficits lead to negative peer interactions, peer rejection, isolation, axiety, depression, substance abuse, and even suicidal thoughts. Others simply learn how to amuse themselves with solitary activities and hobbies.

See also SOCIAL SKILLS TRAINING.

social skills training   A type of behavioral therapy in which a therapist describes and models appropriate behaviors (such as waiting for a turn, sharing toys, asking for help, or responding to teasing). Through role-playing, a child has an opportunity to practice these skills in a therapeutic setting.

See also SOCIAL SKILLS.

social stories   Scripts that are read out loud to individuals as a way to clarify social expectations, teach the "rules" of society, and encourage self-management in social situations. The scripts are individualized for each patient and reread until the behavior is learned. They often include pictures, photographs, or music. Although proponents believe that the behavior of autistic individuals improves with this repetition, there is no scientific evidence supporting this claim.

Developed in 1991 by therapist Carol Gray as a tool for teaching SOCIAL SKILLS to children with autism, social stories address the child's ability to understand or recognize feelings, points of view, or others' plans. Through a story developed about a particular situation or event, the child is given as much information as possible to help understand the appropriate response. The stories typically have three sentence types:

- descriptive sentences addressing where, who, what, and why
- perspective sentences that provide some understanding of the thoughts and emotions of others
- directive sentences that suggest a response

Before using social stories with an autistic child, it is important to identify the child's social skills and determine what situations are difficult. Situations that are frightening, produce tantrums or cry-

ing, or make a child withdraw or want to escape are all appropriate for social stories. However, it is important to address the child's misunderstanding of the situation. A child who cries when a teacher leaves the room may be doing so because of fears or frustration. Therefore, a story about crying will not address the reason for the behavior. Instead, a story about what scares the child and how to deal with those feelings will be more effective.

social worker   A social worker is a mental health professional who provides intervention and treatment to clients who are referred to an agency or through typical school channels. These professionals work as part of a team, providing consultation regarding further assessment or actions for individuals with medical and/or psychological issues, including parents and children. A social worker must have a degree in social work from a college or university program accredited by the Council on Social Work Education.

The undergraduate degree is the bachelor of social work (BSW); graduate degrees include the master of social work (MSW) and the doctorate in social work (DSW) or Ph.D. An MSW is required to provide therapy. Degree programs involve classroom study as well as practical field experience. The bachelor's degree prepares graduates for generalist entry-level work, whereas the master's degree is for more advanced clinical practice. A DSW or Ph.D. is useful for doing research or teaching at the university level.

Most states require practicing social workers to be licensed, certified, or registered, although standards vary.

Son-Rise   The title of a book by Barry Neil Kaufman about his autistic son. It is also the name of a program, started by Kaufman, for treating/educating autistic children.

See also SON-RISE PROGRAM.

Son-Rise Program   A comprehensive system of treatment and education designed for children with autism and other developmental disabilities to dramatically improve skills in all areas of learning, development, and communication. The program was developed in the 1980s by Neil and Samahria Lyte Kaufman in an effort to reach their autistic son Raun.

The Son-Rise Program offers techniques for designing, implementing, and maintaining a stimulating, high-energy, one-on-one, home-based, child-centered program. According to the program, children with autism have the potential for extraordinary healing and growth if parents and caregivers join children instead of opposing them. The program places parents as key teachers, therapists, and directors of their own programs and utilizes the home as the most nurturing environment in which to help their children.

The Son-Rise Program suggests that respect and deep caring are the most important factors that affect a child's motivation to learn, so love and acceptance are meaningful parts of every teaching process. Employing this attitude, program teachers seek to create bonding and a safe environment. The program insists that joining in a child's repetitive and ritualistic behaviors is the key to unlocking the mystery of these behaviors and promotes eye contact and social development. The program advocates teaching through interactive play and using energy, excitement, and enthusiasm to engage the child. In addition, a nonjudgmental and optimistic attitude boosts the child's enjoyment and attention.

As with most programs for autistic people, Son-Rise has both proponents—who praise the results—and critics, who complain that the program misleads some parents with an overly optimistic outlook on autism and potential treatments.

The program was developed by the Kaufmans after experts advised them to institutionalize their severely autistic son because of his condition. Instead, the Kaufmans designed an innovative home-based, child-centered program in an attempt to reach their child.

The Kaufmans point to Raun as evidence of the success of their program; he eventually graduated from an Ivy League university and currently teaches families and individuals at the Autism Treatment Center of America. However, there is currently no sound research showing that other children receiving Son-Rise therapy can obtain the level of positive outcome that the Kaufmans describe for Raun.

After the publication of their bestselling books *Son-Rise* and *Son-Rise: The Miracle Continues* and the award-winning NBC-TV movie *Son-Rise: A Miracle of Love,* the Kaufmans were flooded with requests for help. In response, the Kaufmans established The Option Institute and the Autism Treatment Center of America, where they have offered the Son-Rise Program since 1983. Today they have written 12 books that have been published in 22 languages. Individuals from more than 60 countries on six continents have attended programs at the Autism Treatment Center of America in Massachusetts and at various international outreach programs.

special education   Educational services and programs that may be appropriate for students with special learning needs, including autism. The history of special education can be traced at least as far back as Plato's recommendation that children with extraordinary intellectual ability should be provided special leadership training. In the 16th century special education was practiced when Pedro Ponce de Leon taught deaf Spanish children to speak, read, and write. In the 18th century Jean-Marc-Gaspard Itard (1775–1838) developed special education techniques with Victor, the so-called WILD BOY OF AVEYRON. During the late 18th and early 19th centuries, special education procedures for teaching some school skills to pupils with sensory handicaps were supported by Thomas Hopkins Gallaudet. For example, individuals with profound hearing loss were taught meanings for printed words by repeated simultaneous presentations of a printed word and a picture of what the word represented.

About the same time, attempts to educate individuals with MENTAL RETARDATION or with emotional or behavioral disorders increased in number and degree of success, as exemplified in the work of the American educator Samuel Gridley Howe (1801–76). Successful attempts to educate the deaf and blind led to scientific methods for teaching the disabled in Europe. For example, Maria Montessori, a pediatrician and innovative educator, used multi-sensory methods to teach mentally retarded and culturally deprived children in Rome in the late 19th century.

In the 20th century, the enactment and implementation of compulsory education laws led to an increasing need for special education services. In most developed countries, addressing the educational needs of the disabled has become a common goal. However, it was not until the mid-1970s, with the passage of the EDUCATION FOR ALL HANDICAPPED CHILDREN ACT OF 1975 (Public Law 94-142), that the education of autistic children carried the force of law in the United States. This revolutionary legislation, guaranteeing a free and appropriate education for all children, paved the way for a rapid expansion of the field of special education that continues to this day.

PL 94-142, renamed INDIVIDUALS WITH DISABILITIES EDUCATION ACT (IDEA) in 1990, requires students with disabilities to be placed in the LEAST RESTRICTIVE ENVIRONMENT (LRE) available in order to avoid segregating students with disabilities.

Schools that comply with the laws receive more money from the federal government to offset part of the costs of providing special education services. The federal government also requires that schools report the number of special education students they serve. During the 1989–90 school year, more than 4.5 million children received such services. About 85 percent of these children were between the ages of six and 17.

Special equipment is used extensively with students who have problems with vision or hearing. Such equipment might include computers to convert printed materials into synthetic speech, and special desks, chairs, writing devices, and school buses may help students with physical handicaps. Special ramps and wide doors, swimming pools, and schoolrooms specially equipped with hearing-aid transmitting equipment are all part of special education.

Special services for exceptional individuals include speech language training, physical and occupational therapies, counseling, and vocational training for students with mental retardation.

The most common elements of special education are the specialized instructional techniques, such as:

- AMERICAN SIGN LANGUAGE
- other augmentative communication methods

- programmed instruction procedures designed to present information in small steps
- behavior modification techniques (such as a TOKEN ECONOMY)

While most special education for children with autism takes place in regular public schools, some classes are provided in special public or private day or residential schools, public or private hospitals, and, in some cases, the homes of individuals whose disabilities prevent them from attending school. Most individuals with disabilities do not require an entire program of services apart from conventional instruction, but rather only a modification of features.

When children are considered able to benefit from participation with other children, they are usually taught in the normal school program. This process, known as mainstreaming, was believed to be consistent with the legal mandate for education in the least restrictive environment. More than two-thirds of students with disabilities receive most of their education in regular education classes.

If a child's handicap is not severe, a special education teacher works with the regular classroom teacher to develop skills. In other cases, an assistant teacher may be able to care for a student's specific needs. For individuals with more serious problems, special education may be provided in a separate classroom for part of the school day; students with severe learning and behavioral problems may remain in a separate special education room all day. The ratio of students to teachers is usually much lower in a special education classroom than in an ordinary classroom.

With the development of assistive technologies, the field of special education continues to evolve, although its goal remains the same as it was from the beginning—to educate and integrate individuals with disabilities into society.

special needs trusts A special irrevocable trust that can be established in most states for children with disabilities that holds title to property for the benefit of a child or adult who has a disability. A trust can hold cash, personal property, or real property, or can be the beneficiary of life insurance proceeds. In a special needs trust, a guardian decides how to spend money on a child. (Otherwise, children with assets over about $2,000 would be ineligible to receive state and federal services.)

To determine the supplemental needs of the person, a monthly budget is established based on today's needs while projecting for the future. Then, by using a reasonable rate of return on principal, the family identifies how much money is needed to fund the trust. In addition, the life expectancy of the person must be considered and then the need projected into the future using an inflation factor. Once this is done, the family must identify the resources to be used to fund the trust. These may include stocks, mutual funds, IRAs, 401(k)s, real estate, the family home, life insurance, and so on. Professional management for investing the assets may be done by the trustee, or the trustee may hire advisors.

These trusts are the best way for relatives to leave money to a child with autism, because this money does not affect the child's eligibility for government services. In addition to working out the financial details, it is very useful for parents to write suggestions about how they want the child cared for. An attorney who specializes in special needs trusts should set up the trust.

A disabled person who expects an inheritance may also establish a special needs trust, since receiving these funds might otherwise disqualify the person from public benefits. In many situations, a trust can also be established after the disabled person has received an extraordinary amount of money, although in this case a court order might be required.

See also ESTATE PLANNING; GUARDIANSHIP.

specific learning disabilities   A legal term that plays a central role in legislation governing learning disabilities. As described in Public Law 94-142 (amended by PL 101-76), specific learning disability means a disorder in one or more of the basic psychological processes involved in understanding or in using spoken or written language. This may manifest itself in an imperfect ability to listen, think, speak, read, write, spell, or to do mathematical calculations. The term includes such conditions

as perceptual handicaps, brain injury, minimal brain dysfunction, dyslexia, and developmental APHASIA. The term does not include children who have problems that are primarily caused by visual, hearing, or motor problems, MENTAL RETARDATION, or emotional disturbance or children of environmental, cultural, or economic disadvantage.

speech-language pathologist   An expert who specializes in the assessment and treatment of speech, language, and voice disorders. Also known as a speech pathologist or speech therapist, the speech-language pathologist evaluates and treats individuals with communication problems resulting from AUTISTIC DISORDER, hearing loss, brain injury, cleft palate, emotional problems, development delays, or stroke. He or she also provides clinical therapy to help those with speech and language disorders and their families understand the disorder and develop better communication skills.

Speech-language pathologists administer screening tests and recommend the type of speech language treatment that may be necessary, which might include a specific program of exercises to improve language ability or speech, together with support from the client's family and friends. They also conduct research to develop new and better ways to diagnose and treat speech/language problems, work with children who have language delays and speech problems, and provide treatment to people who stutter and to those with voice and articulation problems.

Educational requirements include a master's degree in speech-language pathology, more than 300 hours of supervised clinical experience, and successful completion of a certifying exam. Those who meet the strict requirements of the American Speech-Language and Hearing Association are awarded the certificate of clinical competence.

speech-language therapist   See SPEECH-LANGUAGE PATHOLOGIST.

speech therapy   A type of treatment that may be beneficial to many autistic children, but since often only one to two hours per week is available, it probably has only modest benefit unless integrated with other home and school programs. Sign language and the picture exchange communication system (PECS) may also be very helpful in developing speech. Speech therapists should work on helping the child to hear hard consonant sounds such as the "c" in "cup." It is often helpful if the therapist stretches out and enunciates the consonant sounds.

STAART network   An autism research network (Studies to Advance Autism Research and Treatment) including eight centers of excellence in autism research mandated by Congress as part of its Children's Health Act of 2000. STAART was begun by the five institutes of the National Institutes of Health Autism Coordinating Committee. Each of the eight centers will contribute to the autism research base in the areas of causes, diagnosis, early detection, prevention, and treatment.

Most of the eight STAART centers are currently evaluating and treating patients as well as enrolling them into clinical trials. The centers include Boston University, Kennedy Krieger Institute, Mt. Sinai Medical School, University of California/Los Angeles, University of North Carolina/Chapel Hill, University of Rochester, University of Washington, and Yale University.

Studies include

- early characteristics of autism: outpatient treatment study that will identify factors that distinguish children aged 18 to 24 months with autism from children with developmental delay and those with normal development as well as examine the efficacy of intensive behavioral therapy in children with autism
- diet and behavior in young children with autism: outpatient treatment study to determine whether a gluten- and casein-free diet has specific benefits for children with autism aged 30 to 54 months
- citalopram for children with autism and repetitive behavior: outpatient treatment study. This study will determine the efficacy and safety of citalopram compared to placebo in the treat-

ment of children aged five to 17 with autism in locations across the United States
- relationship training for children with autism and their peers: outpatient treatment study. This study will determine whether peer interaction training interventions are effective in enhancing the social relationships of children aged six to 11 years with autism in Los Angeles, California.

See also COLLABORATIVE PROGRAMS OF EXCELLENCE IN AUTISM (in Appendix V).

state services   Most states will provide some services for children with autism, primarily funded by the federal Medicaid program. However, many states have waiting lists for a limited number of slots, and the quality of services varies widely state to state.

Most states have one set of services for children under age three (early intervention), and a second set of services for older children and adults. Typical state services for people with autism include respite, habilitation, speech therapy, and OCCUPATIONAL THERAPY.

In order to qualify for services, children or adults must be specifically diagnosed with AUTISTIC DISORDER by a licensed psychiatrist or psychologist with training in childhood development. The applicant also must meet three of seven functional limitations: self-care, receptive and expressive language, learning, mobility, self-direction, capacity for independent living, and economic self-sufficiency.

statistics   Autism is one of the four major developmental disabilities, and its incidence *appears* to be increasing dramatically. Nationwide, at least 1.5 million Americans have some form of autism, and it now affects one in every 166 births—or 24,000 of the 4 million children born every year, according to the Centers for Disease Control and Prevention (CDC). The CDC also notes that the number of children diagnosed with autism, ASPERGER'S SYNDROME, and other PERVASIVE DEVELOPMENTAL DISORDERS increased sixfold from 1994 to 2003.

Although more cases of autism are being identified, it is not clear why—or if the number of autism cases has truly increased. Since there appears to be more than one cause of autism, there may be more than one reason for the increase. Some of the increase may result from better education about the symptoms of autism or from more accurate diagnoses of autism. The new definition of autism as a spectrum disorder means that even people with mild symptoms can be classified as having an AUTISM SPECTRUM DISORDER (ASD), which could also account for the increase in identified cases. As research moves forward using the current definition of ASDs, more definite numbers may be available to answer this question.

The most accurate statistics on the prevalence of autism come from California, which has a systematic centralized reporting system of all diagnoses of autism. The California data show that autism is rising rapidly, from one per 2,500 in 1970 to one per 285 in 1999. Similar results have been reported for other states by the U.S. Department of Education. Whereas autism once accounted for 3 percent of all developmental disabilities, in California it now accounts for 45 percent of all new developmental disabilities. Other countries report similar increases. In the United States overall, studies estimate that as many as 12 in every 10,000 children have autism or a related condition, according to the U.S. Department of Health and Human Services in 1999.

Some of the increase in autism cases in which speech is delayed may be the result of better diagnosis and awareness, but the report from California reveals that this only explains a small part of the increase. However, the increase in the milder variant of autism (Asperger's syndrome) may indeed be due to better, earlier diagnosis. In Asperger's syndrome, there is no significant speech delay and early childhood behavior is much more normal.

Most experts suspect the primary reason for the increase in autism cases is certainly due to environmental factors, not genetics, since there is no such thing as a "genetic epidemic."

Autism occurs in all parts of the world, in all races and social classes. Autism is three times more common in boys than in girls. However, in the United States it does occur much more often in boys than in girls; four out of every five people with autism are boys.

stereotypies Patterned repetitive movements, hand-wringing, hand flapping, finger-twisting, or complex whole-body movements and utterances that occur often in many individuals with AUTISTIC DISORDER. When engaged in stereotypies the individual is effectively "tuned out" from attending to events in the environment, but when stereotypies are reduced or suppressed, the individual can be induced to engage in productive learning activities.

stim An abbreviation for "self-stimulation," a term for behaviors (such as rocking) whose sole purpose appears to be to stimulate the autistic individual's senses. Many people with autism report that some "self-stims"—such as TOE WALKING, spinning, hand-flapping, screaming, or ECHOLALIA—seem to help calm them down, improve their concentration, or shut out an overwhelming sound.

Supplemental Security Income (SSI) In the past, a diagnosis of autism almost automatically qualified a child for SSI payments, provided the parents met the earnings and resources requirements of the SSI program. However, the government is now interpreting the law more strictly. In the new direction at the Social Security Administration (SSA), the regulations operate on the basis of function rather than diagnosis. Today, a child must have "marked and severe functional limitations" in order to be found disabled. If medication improves behavior, the child might not qualify under this heading.

In addition, the administration requires that a child with autism have "qualitative deficits in verbal and nonverbal communication and in imaginative activity." However, many children with autism communicate nonverbally in a satisfactory manner and engage in very imaginative activities. If this is the case, the child is not disabled, according to the SSA.

Parents should provide an honest but completely accurate description of how the child functions and demand that the school and the teacher do the same, asking them to make statements that show the severity of the disability. The child should be shown at a normal functioning level, not just how the child functions on a good day.

tactile perception   Perception through the sensory system of touch, in which direct physical contact is transmitted through the nervous system to the brain.

TEACCH   An acronym for "Treatment and Education of Autistic and related Communication-handicapped Children," a university based treatment program that helps parents act as co-therapists for their autistic children. The method emphasizes structuring the environment, employing one-on-one teaching, and using classrooms that provide visual cues on how to complete tasks (a red ball, for example, goes through a red circle). TEACCH also encourages children to be more independent by teaching them to use newly mastered skills in less-structured environments, such as mainstream classrooms.

This program was developed at the University of North Carolina/Chapel Hill in 1971 by developmental PSYCHOLOGIST Eric Schopler to provide a structured learning environment for children with autism as a way of improving their strengths and independence. The multidisciplinary program involves the family and community in an intensive treatment regimen, five hours a day, five days a week in a TEACCH classroom.

Although this popular intervention is supported by years of anecdotal data, very little scientific data exist on the outcomes of TEACCH. However, other researchers are studying ways to combine this method with others, such as the Young Autism Project (YAP), launched in 1970 by behavioral psychologist Ivar Lovaas, Ph.D., at the University of California at Los Angeles. The YAP relies exclusively on DISCRETE TRIAL TRAINING, which teaches autistic children thousands of individual behaviors, such as tying a shoe or eating with a fork, one at a time. Researchers at the University of Utah found that children receiving a combination of the two treatments (YAP training at school and TEACCH methods at home) showed three to four times better progress than did children who received only the school-based treatment.

theory of mind   A hypothesis that people with AUTISTIC DISORDER lack an awareness of the fact that others have beliefs, desires, and intentions that are different from their own. This awareness in non-autistic individuals starts developing at a relatively young age. Proponents of this theory believe that the autistic person does not readily develop theories about what is going on in other people's minds. Instead, autistic individuals' awareness of other people's mind is something that is developed intellectually through their own efforts. Adherents of this theory suggest that some or all of other typical characteristics of autism stem from this one main deficit.

toe walking   Walking on tiptoes is quite common in young children age three and younger; but toe walking in children five years and older is not normal and is a typical sign of AUTISTIC DISORDER. Some experts believe that a dysfunctional vestibular system, a common problem in autism, may be responsible for toe walking. The vestibular system provides the brain with feedback about the body's motion and position.

It may be possible to reduce or eliminate toe walking by stimulating the vestibular system by swinging the child on a glider swing.

Physical exercises may be able to stretch out, chair, or bench the tendon in order to reduce toe walking. Placing a cast on the person's leg to stretch out the tendon is another intervention used to stop toe walking. Typically, the cast is applied every two weeks for a total of six to eight weeks. However, the few longer-term studies of this procedure suggest it is not successful in stopping toe walking in the long term.

token economy A behavior therapy procedure in which tokens (such as coins or poker chips) are awarded for desired behavior. The tokens can then be exchanged for privileges or treats.

Tourette syndrome A neurological disorder characterized by tics, or rapid, sudden movements or vocalizations that occur involuntarily and repeatedly in a consistent fashion. Tourette syndrome may sometimes coexist with AUTISTIC DISORDER. To be diagnosed with Tourette syndrome, an individual must have multiple motor tics as well as one or more vocal tics over a period of more than one year. These need not all occur simultaneously, but in general the tics may occur many times a day, usually in brief, intense groupings, nearly every day or intermittently.

Common simple tics include eye blinking, shoulder jerking, picking movements, grunting, sniffing, and barking. Complex tics include facial grimacing, arm flapping, coprolalia (use of obscene words), palilalia (repeating one's own words) and echolalia (repeating another's words or phrases).

For individuals with Tourette, tics may vary over time in terms of their frequency and severity, as well as in type and location. In some cases, symptoms may disappear for a period of weeks or even months. Although there is an involuntary quality to the tics experienced by individuals with Tourette, most persons have some control over their symptoms, at least briefly, and even for hours at a time. However, suppressing them may simply postpone more severe outbursts.

Up to 20 percent of children have at least a transient tic disorder at some point. Once believed to be rare, Tourette syndrome is now known to be a more common disorder that represents the most complex and severe manifestation of the spectrum of tic disorders.

An abnormal metabolism of the neurotransmitters dopamine and SEROTONIN are linked to the disorder, which is genetically transmitted. Parents have a 50 percent chance of passing the gene on to their children. Girls with the gene have a 70 percent chance of displaying symptoms; boys with the gene have a 99 percent chance of displaying symptoms.

Symptoms and Diagnostic Path

Tourette is commonly associated not only with autistic disorder, but also with other problems, including attention deficit hyperactivity disorder (ADHD), anxiety, mood or panic disorders, obsessive-compulsive disorder (OCD), and behavior problems. In most children, Tourette syndrome has a fluctuating course. Anxiety, stress, and fatigue often intensify tics, which are usually significantly reduced during sleep or when the patient is focused on an activity. Psychoactive drugs, particularly cocaine and stimulants, have a tendency to worsen tics.

In most cases, tics peak in severity between ages nine and 11, but between 5 and 10 percent of patients continue to have unchanged or worsening symptoms into adolescence and adulthood. In this population, the likelihood of tics continuing for decades is substantial. Patients in their seventh, eighth, and ninth decades of life may have tics that have been present since childhood. In most older patients, the tics tend to become quite stable over time, although occasionally new tics will be acquired. There is no reliable way to predict which children will have a poorer prognosis.

The single most important component of managing the condition is to get an accurate diagnosis. In cases of Tourette syndrome, tics occur suddenly during normal activity, unlike tic occurrence in other movement disorders such as

- *chorea:* a pattern of nonrepetitive irregular movements
- *stereotypy:* frequent, repetitive behaviors performed for no *obvious reason* and with no functional purpose
- *dystonia:* a slow, constant repetitive behavior

The physician will want to rule out any secondary causes of tic disorders. A complete general physical examination, with specific attention to the neurologic part of the examination, is important. The thyroid-stimulating hormone (TSH) level should be measured in most patients, since tics may occur together with hyperthyroidism. A throat culture should be checked for group A beta-hemolytic streptococcus, especially if symptoms get worse or better with ear or throat infections. The evidence of strep infection with a single occurrence of worsening tics is not enough to make a diagnosis of streptococcus-induced, autoimmune-caused Tourette syndrome.

An electroencephalogram is useful only in patients in whom it is difficult to differentiate tics from manifestations of epilepsy. Imaging studies are not likely to be helpful, and the importance of other studies depends on symptoms. For example, a urine drug screen for cocaine and stimulants should be considered in the case of a teenager with sudden onset of tics and inappropriate behavior symptoms. A person with a family history of liver disease associated with a parkinsonian or hyperkinetic movement disorder should undergo a serum copper test to rule out Wilson's disease.

The basic workup is usually appropriate in a patient with a gradual onset of symptoms, a developmental progression of tics, and a family history of tics or OCD.

Treatment Options and Outlook

Applied behavioral analysis treatment programs using positive reinforcement appear to be most helpful in managing tic disorders. Target behaviors may be categorized into two groups: skill deficiencies (areas that initially require concentration to build social and academic skills) and behavior excesses (in which the goal is to help the patient decrease the frequency of these behaviors).

Drug treatment The goal in tic control is to use the lowest dosage of medication that will bring the patient's functioning to an acceptable level. This may result in only modest levels of tic reduction. The most common drug treatments are HALOPERIDOL, pimozide (Orap), RISPERIDONE (RISPERDAL), and CLONIDINE (CATAPRES). Guanfacine (Tenex) is not labeled for use in children under 12 years of age. Less often, CLONAZEPAM (KLONOPIN) may be prescribed.

For tics of mild to moderate severity, or in patients who are wary of drug side effects, an initial trial of clonidine or guanfacine may be tried. These medications are modestly effective in tic control and have a range of less specific benefits. Many children taking them may be less irritable or less impulsive, and manifestations of ADHD may improve as well.

Side effects may include sedation, weight gain, poor school performance, social anxiety (including refusal to go to school in children), and unusual body movements, including tardive dyskinesias, a potentially irreversible drug-caused movement disorder that may be difficult to distinguish from tics. When pimozide is used, baseline and follow-up electrocardiograms are recommended.

Most patients with Tourette syndrome require medication for up to two years. About 15 percent of patients require long-term medication for tic control. When tics appear to be stable and adequately controlled for a period of four to six months, a slow and gradual reduction in medication should follow. If tics increase, incremental increases in medication may be needed.

Because many patients with Tourette syndrome have other conditions, treatment for these conditions may be necessary. Treatment of ADHD with Tourette's has been controversial because of reports that stimulants, often prescribed to relieve symptoms of ADHD, hasten the onset or increase the severity of tics in some patients. This observation alone may not be a contraindication for stimulant treatment in patients with significant symptoms of ADHD. Stimulants alone may not substantially worsen the course or severity of the disorder. In some cases, it may be necessary to treat both the ADHD and the Tourette syndrome with a stimulant in combination with either clonidine or guanfacine, or with a neuroleptic agent. A trial of clonidine or guanfacine alone may be sufficient to adequately treat both conditions. When possible, multiple drug use should be avoided, especially in children.

Treatment of OCD with the class of antidepressants known as selective serotonin reuptake inhibitors (such as Prozac) may be effective. With these medications, there is often a significant delay between start of treatment and response, as long as four to six weeks. Behavior therapy is also effective in the treatment of OCD.

transition plan   A plan for the movement from one place or idea to another. In the context of autism, a transition plan refers to the change from school to adult life. For disabled students, this may require extra effort and planning for the individuals and their support teams. Transition legislation in the INDIVIDUALS WITH DISABILITIES ACT (IDEA) states that transition services and planning be written into the INDIVIDUALIZED EDUCATION PROGRAM (IEP) by the time a child is aged 14. (Some states require transition planning to begin at an age younger than 14.) IDEA defines transition services as a coordinated set of activities for a student that promotes movement from school to post-school activities, including postsecondary education, vocational training, employment, continuing and adult education, adult services, independent living, and community participation. A student receiving special education services in public schools meets regularly with family and school staff to address the IEP; once a student is in high school, these meetings should begin to plan for the transition from high school to adult life.

The contents of a transition plan should include

1. current levels of performance
2. interests and aptitudes
3. post-school goals
4. transition activities—specific steps to be taken (such as career/vocational counseling)
5. designation of responsible persons to oversee the transition after high school

Individualized Transition Plan

An individualized transition plan (ITP) may be written as a specific area within the IEP or as a separate document that is also agreed upon by school officials and the parents. Transition planning should be oriented to life after high school, not limited to what will be accomplished before leaving school, and should involve a master plan including long-range goals and a coordinated set of activities for each. A school system may work with agencies such as the local Department of Vocational Rehabilitation,

Social Security Administration, or independent and supported living centers that may provide training or direct services to help the school with a student's transition.

When thinking about transition from high school, the parents and family of the child should consider what the child likes to do and can do; the possibility of college, vocational education, or adult education; possible careers; transportation; where the child might live; financial outlook; health insurance; friendship needs; community help; special interests; religious affiliation; recreation; volunteer work.

The National Information Center for Children and Youth with Disabilities offers a transition summary series that helps families and students with disabilities focus on taking definite steps toward a successful transition, at http://www.nichcy.org.

A student's options after high school can be increased by a good transition plan during school and by being given the opportunity to experience different settings and develop work-appropriate skills. A good transition plan allows parents, school officials, and agency personnel to work together to make these opportunities available.

tuberous sclerosis complex (TSC)   A rare genetic disorder that causes benign brain tumors, EPILEPSY, severe learning disabilities, and very challenging behaviors; it occurs quite often in people with autism. The condition includes a wide variation in physical and intellectual abilities.

About a quarter to half of children with TSC also develop behaviors that lead to a diagnosis of autism, with another fourth having problems that lead to a diagnosis of AUTISM SPECTRUM DISORDERS (ASD). The rate of autism spectrum disorders in the general population is substantially lower (around 0.5 or 0.6 percent), so there is a substantial increase in autism in children with tuberous sclerosis. Although most autistic children with TSC also are mentally retarded, aspects of autism spectrum disorders can affect those with no learning problems. More than half of all children with TSC will also have attention deficit and overactive behaviors that could be diagnosed as attention deficit hyperactivity disorder (ADHD).

Tuberous sclerosis complex occurs in both sexes and in all races and ethnic groups and is often first recognized in children experiencing seizures and mental handicaps. However, the symptoms of TSC vary greatly and may often not appear until later in life. There is presently no cure, and there is no way to predict how severely or mildly an individual may be affected by TSC.

The condition is caused by mutations in one of two genes (TSC1 and TSC2), which produce abnormal growth of tissue in the brain and other organs, such as the skin or kidneys. Experts believe it is these "cortical tubers" that lead to the epilepsy, learning disability, autism, and attention deficit disorders so often seen in these patients.

In some genetic conditions such as this one, a mutation in one copy of the gene is enough to cause the condition. About a third of people with TSC inherit it from a parent who also has the condition. If a parent has TSC and passes on the copy of the gene with the mutation, then the child also will be affected. If the parent passes on the copy of the gene without the mutation, the child will not have TSC. Thus, there is a 50 percent chance with each pregnancy for a parent with TSC to have a child with TSC. This is true regardless of the sex of the parent or the sex of the child. In the remaining two-thirds of people with TSC, neither parent shows any symptoms or signs of TSC. Instead, one of the normal genes from one parent changes to the abnormal form, leading to a new occurrence of TSC in the child. Normally, these parents do not have another child with TSC because the mutation was sporadic, not inherited. However, some families have more than one child with TSC, even though neither parent showed symptoms or findings of TSC.

Research has discovered that more *inherited* cases of tuberous sclerosis complex are linked to a malfunctioning TSC1 gene, and more sporadic cases to a faulty TSC2 gene. In addition, the learning disability and epilepsy associated with growths in the brain known as cortical tubers are more frequent in people with TSC2 and less frequent in people with TSC1 mutations.

Scientists have also determined that a small number of physically unaffected parents of a child with TSC actually have TSC mutations in some of their cells. Because the mutation is limited to a small por-

tion of all of the body's cells, these individuals show no signs of TSC, but if a portion of the egg or sperm cells of a parent carries the TSC mutation, that parent can have more than one affected child, possibly at the same 50/50 chance that people with TSC have. A person who carries cells with TSC mutations in her egg or his sperm supply has what is called "germline mosaicism." The occurrence of germline mosaicism has led geneticists to estimate a recurrence risk ranging from 1 percent to 3 percent. At this time, there is no simple way to determine whether an unaffected parent of a child with TSC has germline mosaicism.

Some experts believe that the abnormalities in brain development that occur in tuberous sclerosis may interfere with the proper development of brain areas vital to the development of social communication skills. It could be that if cortical tubers that develop during brain development in children with tuberous sclerosis involve the temporal lobes, there is a higher chance that an autism spectrum disorder will develop. This is not suprising, because the temporal lobes process auditory information (especially speech sounds) as well as information about faces and facial expressions.

However, it appears that the presence of cortical tubers in the temporal lobes is not enough by itself to trigger autism. Instead, a higher risk of autism occurs if temporal lobe tubers occur with seizures in infancy. It could be that the tubers cause both the seizures as well as autism. Further research to try to determine which of these two explanations is correct is required, especially as it has such important implications for treatment.

First described in the 1880s, tuberous sclerosis complex affects only some organs in most individuals. Most people who are mildly affected by TSC lead active and productive lives, but TSC is a lifelong condition.

Symptoms and Diagnostic Path

Primary symptoms of TSC include tumors of the brain, heart, kidneys, skin, lungs, and eyes, along with mental retardation, seizures, autism, skin lesions, and pitted teeth. People with TSC may exhibit only a few or many of these symptoms. The presence of brain lesions is linked to the appearance of mental retardation and seizures, although only 60 percent of patients with TSC have seizures, and only 40 percent are mentally retarded. Brain involvement also has been linked to autism and behavioral disorders.

Since about 25 percent of people with TSC are autistic and another 25 percent show signs of autism spectrum disorder, including higher functioning autism or ASPERGER'S SYNDROME, behavior symptoms are common in this group and are one way to begin the diagnosis of TSC. Benign heart tumors, which can be picked up during prenatal ultrasound, are another early sign of TSC.

A physician will use an ultraviolet light to better visualize the white patches on the skin that characterize TSC and often are difficult to see, especially on infants and people with very pale skin. The entire body should be examined. Some of the skin signs may not be present at birth; the facial tumors do not usually appear until between the ages of three and five at the earliest, and the fibrous growths do not usually occur until much later in life.

Treatment Options and Outlook

There is no cure for TSC, but symptoms can be treated. Skin symptoms most often treated are facial tumors and fibrous growths. The facial tumors can be removed using dermabrasion or laser treatment when they are small, before they enlarge and become fibrous. They most likely will recur and need further treatment, but they will be milder than if left untreated. Epilepsy drugs can be used to treat epilepsy.

twirling   One type of repetitive movements typical in people with AUTISTIC DISORDER. Typical twirling movements seen in autism include twirling the hair, hands, or bodies. Experts call such behaviors STEREOTYPIES or self-stimulation.

See also SYMPTOMS OF AUTISM.

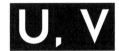

upledger cranio-sacral therapy See CRANIAL SACRAL THERAPY.

vaccines and autism The possible link between autism and vaccinations is a matter of considerable controversy. Of particular concern are many vaccinations that began to be administered in the 1980s, typically to children between ages one and two.

Some parents and experts believe that the measles-mumps-rubella (MMR) combination vaccine in particular is the culprit behind some cases of autism, pointing to evidence of measles virus detected in the gut, spinal fluid, and blood of these children. Some experts suspect thimerosal, a mercury-based preservative in childhood vaccines such as the MMR, may be the link. The number of vaccines given to children has risen over the last two decades, and most of those vaccines contained thimerosal, which is 50 percent mercury. These experts believe that the symptoms of mercury poisoning in children are very similar to the symptoms of autism. In response to these concerns, manufacturers of children's vaccines have removed thimerosal from many vaccines.

However, the National Institute of Child Health and Human Development (NICHD) argues there has been no conclusive, scientific evidence that any part of a vaccine, nor any combination of vaccines causes autism. The NICHD also points out that no conclusive data exists that any type of preservative (such as thimerosal) used during the manufacture of vaccines plays any role in causing autism.

Moreover, in a 2001 investigation by the Institute of Medicine, a committee concluded that the "evidence favors rejection of a causal relationship. . . . between MMR vaccines and autistic spectrum disorders (ASD)." The committee acknowledged, however, that they could not rule out the possibility that the MMR vaccine could contribute to ASD in a small number of children. While other researchers agree the data do not support a link between the MMR and autism, more research is clearly needed.

However, current scientific evidence does not support the hypothesis that MMR vaccine, or any combination of vaccines, causes the development of autism, including regressive forms of autism, according to the U.S. Centers for Disease Control and Prevention (CDC). The question about a possible link between MMR vaccine and autism has been extensively reviewed by independent groups of experts in the United States including the National Academy of Sciences, the Institute of Medicine, and the National Institute of Child Health and Human Development. These reviews have concluded that the available epidemiologic evidence does not support a causal link between MMR vaccine and autism.

The few existing studies that suggest a causal relationship between MMR vaccine and autism have generated media attention. However, these studies have "significant weaknesses" according to the CDC and are far outweighed by the epidemiologic studies that have consistently failed to show a relationship between MMR vaccine and autism.

Data from California have been used to illustrate an increase in cases of autism since the introduction of the MMR vaccine. However, claims that the number of cases of autism has been increasing since the introduction of the MMR are based on numbers, not rates, and do not account for population growth and changes in the composition of the population. In addition, changes in the diagnostic definition of autism were not taken into account. And as in other areas of the country, children with autism are currently being diagnosed at earlier ages, so there will be an increase in the number of reported cases.

The CDC concludes that there is no convincing evidence that vaccines such as the MMR cause long-term health effects. On the other hand, people can become ill and die from the diseases the vaccines prevent. Measles outbreaks have recently occurred in the United Kingdom and Germany after an increase in the number of parents who chose not to have their children vaccinated with the MMR vaccine.

Isolated reports about these vaccines causing long-term health problems may sound alarming, the CDC notes, but it maintains that careful review of the science reveals that these reports are isolated and not confirmed by scientifically sound research. Detailed medical reviews of health effects reported after receipt of vaccines have often proven to be unrelated to vaccines but rather have been related to other health factors. Because these vaccines are recommended widely to protect the health of the public, research on any serious hypotheses about their safety is important to pursue. This is why several studies are underway to investigate still unproven theories about vaccinations and severe side effects.

The National Immunization Program at the CDC, along with the American Academy of Pediatrics (AAP) and the American Academy of Family Physicians (AAFP), suggests that physicians follow the recommended childhood immunization schedule that is published every year. Physicians are advised to take careful family histories of all their patients to bring to light any factors that might influence their recommendations about the timing of vaccinations.

Some researchers and physicians have recommended an alternative vaccine schedule that involves delaying some vaccinations and separating the measles, mumps, and rubella vaccinations. Medical experts argue that a vaccine is not licensed unless it is considered safe and its benefits far outweigh perceived risks. For a vaccine to be included on the annual Recommended Childhood Immunization Schedule for the United States, it must first be approved by the Advisory Committee on Immunization Practices from the CDC, the AAP, and the AAFP. Scientists and physicians in these organizations carefully weigh the risks and benefits of newly developed vaccines, monitor the safety and

effectiveness of existing vaccines, and track cases of vaccine-preventable diseases.

The topic of vaccine safety became prominent during the mid 1970s when lawsuits were filed on behalf of those presumably injured by the diphtheria, pertussis, tetanus (DPT) vaccine. In order to reduce liability and respond to public health concerns, Congress passed the National Childhood Vaccine Injury Act (NCVIA) in 1986. Designed for citizens injured or killed by vaccines, this system provides a no-fault compensation alternative to suing vaccine manufacturers and providers. The act also created safety provisions to help educate the public about vaccine benefits and risks and to require doctors to report adverse events after vaccination as well as keep records on vaccines administered and health problems that occurred following vaccination. The act also created incentives for the production of safer vaccines.

Vineland Adaptive Behavior Scale-II An assessment tool that is one of the oldest measures of personal and social skills used for everyday living from birth to adulthood and that is used nearly exclusively around the world to assess the adaptive behavior of individuals with AUTISTIC DISORDER. This second edition of the assessment, updated in 2005, provides critical data for predicting autistic disorder and ASPERGER'S SYNDROME and for the diagnosis or evaluation of a wide range of disabilities, including MENTAL RETARDATION, developmental delays, functional skills impairment, and speech/language problems. The Vineland summarizes adaptive behavior in three areas: receptive, expressive, and written communication; personal, domestic, and community daily living issues; and socialization (interpersonal, play and leisure, and coping).

The Expanded Form of the Vineland was designed for program planning, and it is often used to measure the effectiveness of treatment and the development of social skills.

vitamins and autism While there are no vitamins that can correct the underlying neurological problems that seem to cause autism, some parents believe that adding certain vitamins or minerals to their autistic child's diet may help with behavioral issues. Over the past 10 years, there have been claims that adding essential vitamins such as B_6, B_{12}, magnesium, and cod liver oil, and removing gluten and casein from a child's diet may improve digestion, allergies, and sociability. Others believe that vitamin C may improve depression and ease symptoms in patients with autism. While many researchers and experts do not agree that these therapies are effective or scientifically valid, many parents and some physicians report improvement in people with autism with the use of individual or combined nutritional supplements. In any case most experts would agree that adding vitamins in appropriate amounts will not be harmful.

A few studies conducted in 2000 suggest that intestinal disorders and chronic gastrointestinal inflammation may slow the absorption of essential nutrients and disrupt immune system and metabolic functions that depend on these vitamins. Other studies have shown that some children with autism may have low levels of vitamins A, B_1, B_3, B_5, biotin, selenium, zinc, and magnesium, while others may have a higher copper-to-zinc ratio. This would suggest that people with autism should avoid copper and take extra zinc to boost their immune system. Other studies have indicated a need for more calcium.

The most common vitamin supplement recommended to treat autism is vitamin B, which plays an important role in producing enzymes needed by the brain. In 18 studies on the use of vitamin B and magnesium (which makes vitamin B more effective), almost half of the individuals with autism showed improvement, with fewer behavioral problems, better eye contact and attention, and improvements in learning. Other research studies have shown that cod liver oil supplements (rich in vitamins A and D) may improve eye contact and behavior of children with autism. Vitamin C may improve brain function and symptom severity in children with autism. A small Arizona study noted improvements in sleep and gastrointestinal problems with a multivitamin/mineral complex, as well as better language, eye contact, and behavior.

The Autism Society of America (ASA) recommends that parents considering adding vitamins or minerals to a child's diet should obtain a lab analysis of the child's current nutritional status. A blood test is the most accurate way to measure vitamin and mineral levels. The ASA also recommends parents consult an expert in nutritional therapy when planning on giving a child vitamins, since large doses of some vitamins and minerals may not be harmful and others can be toxic.

Vitamin supplements should then be added to the diet slowly, one by one, so that their effects can be observed for one to two months.

Wawro, Richard (1952–) An AUTISTIC SAVANT from Edinburgh, Scotland who is internationally known for his detailed oil wax crayon drawings of intense depth and color.

Diagnosed as severely retarded and autistic at the age of three, he exhibited an obsession for sameness, withdrawal, twirling, and spinning objects. Unable to speak until age 11, he required surgery for cataracts on both eyes during childhood.

He began drawing on a chalkboard at about the same time he was diagnosed, covering a tiny chalkboard with images. At age six, he was introduced to drawing with crayons. Six years later, experts were startled at his skill, describing his work as an "incredible phenomenon."

Like other savants, Wawro has an incredible memory for each picture, and can date them precisely in his mind. He draws from images seen only once, on television or in a book, but he often adds his own interpretations or improvisation. He seems especially fascinated with light, and his ability to capture light and shadow is striking.

At the completion of each picture, Richard takes it to his father for approval. Richard's mother died in 1979, but in spite of their closeness, Richard did not stop painting.

He had his first exhibition in Edinburgh at age 17; today, he is known worldwide and has sold more than 1,000 pictures in more than 100 exhibitions. One of his exhibitions was opened by then-minister of education Margaret Thatcher, who owns several of his pictures—as does Pope John Paul II.

An award-winning documentary about Richard Wawro (*With Eyes Wide Open*) opened in 1983. A videotape (*A Real Rainman: Portrait of an Autistic Savant*) was also produced.

Wild Boy of Aveyron Possibly the first documented case of a child with suspected AUTISTIC DIS-ORDER, Victor was a feral child found wandering naked in the woods near Saint Sernin sur Rance in southern France at the end of the 18th century. Captured while digging up vegetables from a tanner's garden, the boy could not speak but instead emitted a few weird cries, trying to hide himself from his captors. The next day, local gendarmes took the boy to a hospice in a nearby town, where intense debate centered on his origins and condition. Aged about 12, he had several scars, which suggested that he had been living in the wild for some time. He got his name from the character in a French play (*Victor, ou l'enfant de la forêt*—Victor, or the Child of the Forest).

Finally, Victor, now famed as the "wild boy of Aveyron," was given to sympathetic young doctor Jean-Marc Itard, who concluded that Victor was in fact an abandoned intelligent deaf-mute, who had somehow been able to survive on his own. Itard wanted to teach him to speak and civilize him, but he made little progress. Scientific debate about his condition was renewed from time to time, and the story of the wild boy was influential in the development of several theories of language learning and human evolution. Since then, some experts suspect he actually had autism.

Recent research into local and national archives in France suggests that Victor was probably abandoned by his family. Victor died at age 40 at an annex of the Paris Institution des Sourds-Muets (Paris Institute of Deaf-Mutes).

Williams syndrome A rare genetic disorder characterized by mild MENTAL RETARDATION and some types of autistic behavior, including developmental and language delays, poor gross motor skills, hypersensitivity to sounds, and PERSEVERATION (the multiple repetition of words or actions). The syndrome occurs when a portion of DNA material on chromosome 7 is missing, which happens in one out of 20,000 to 50,000 births.

Symptoms and Diagnostic Path

Symptoms vary among patients. Although they exhibit some autistic tendencies, children with Williams syndrome do not have the social problems so typical of individuals with autism. Although individuals with Williams syndrome may show competence in areas such as language, music, and interpersonal relations, their IQ is usually below average, and they are considered moderately to mildly retarded; they also may have developmental delay, learning disabilities, or attention deficit disorder.

Individuals with Williams syndrome seem to have a higher rate of musicality, than the general population. Among those with increased levels of musicality there are people with Williams syndrome who are musically gifted, but many others are not. It is a love of music, rather than musical giftedness, that appears to be a common trait among these individuals.

They also share additional physical symptoms such as cardiovascular problems, high blood pressure, low birth weight, slow weight gain, feeding problems, irritability during infancy, dental and kidney abnormalities, musculoskeletal problems, and high calcium levels. Children with Williams syndrome have distinctive elfin facial features, with almond-shaped eyes, oval ears, full lips, small chins, narrow faces, and broad mouths.

Treatment Options and Outlook

There is neither a cure for Williams syndrome nor a standard course of treatment; instead, treatment is aimed at easing symptoms. Individuals with Williams syndrome need regular monitoring for potential medical problems by a physician familiar with the disorder, as well as specialized services to help them make the most of their potential.

The prognosis for individuals with Williams syndrome varies. Some people may be able to master self-help skills, complete academic or vocational school, and live in supervised homes or on their own, while others may not progress to this level.

yeast A type of fungus that is normally present in the body. In certain conditions it can grow out of control, causing vaginal yeast infections or thrush. Some people believe that more severe symptoms of yeast overgrowth may trigger autism symptoms.

In particular, overgrowth of *Candida albicans* (a form of yeast) is associated with long-term antibiotic treatment, and it has been linked by some people to antibiotic treatment for continuous ear infections during infancy.

For this reason, some individuals advocate giving anti-yeast medications to children with autism in an effort to control symptoms. However, the benefits of this practice have not been proven in clinical studies.

APPENDIXES

Appendix I: Organizations

Appendix II: Helpful Web Sites

Appendix III: State Autism Organizations

Appendix IV: Autism Resources by State

Appendix V: Collaborative Programs of Excellence
in Autism

Appendix VI: Clinical Trials for Autistic Disorder

APPENDIX I
ORGANIZATIONS

ADVOCACY

Autism National Committee
P.O. Box 429
Forest Knolls, CA 94933
http://www.autcom.org

An autism advocacy organization dedicated to social justice for all citizens with autism, offering a shared vision and a commitment to positive approaches. The organization was founded in 1990 to protect and advance the human rights and civil rights of all persons with autism, pervasive developmental disorders, and related differences of communication and behavior. The organization welcomes the participation of all family members, people with autism/PDD, caring professionals, and other friends who wish to implement the right to self-determination by hearing and heeding the voices of people with autism. The group provides information, support, networking, advocacy, a strong voice in federal legislation and policy, a newsletter, conferences and trainings, a bookstore, a variety of unique publications, and an ongoing reappraisal of fundamental research and treatment. The Web site offers the most recent issue of their newsletter; updates on politics and judicial decisions; commentary by people with autism; information about developmental and relationship-based approaches to early intervention and education; coverage of issues affecting community living, home-owning, and consumer choice; advocacy for access to augmentative, assistive, and facilitated communication; plus in-depth book reviews and a bookstore.

Autism Network International
P.O. Box 35448
Syracuse, NY 13210

(315) 476-2462
http://www.ani.autistics.org

The only autistic-run national self-help and advocacy organization for autistic people, the network is dedicated to supporting people with autism, offering peer support, tips, problem solving, information, and referrals. ANI publishes a newsletter, arranges pen pals, and conducts advocacy activities. ANI members believe that the best advocates for autistic people are autistic people themselves and that supports for autistic people should be aimed at helping them to compensate, navigate, and function in the world. ANI provides a forum for autistic people to share information, peer support, and tips for coping and problem-solving, and advocates for appropriate services and civil rights for all autistic people. ANI also provides a social outlet for autistic people to explore and participate in autistic social experiences. In addition to promoting self-advocacy for high-functioning autistic adults, ANI works to improve the lives of autistic people who, whether because they are too young, or because they do not have adequate communication skills, are not able to advocate for themselves. ANI helps autistic people who are unable to participate directly by providing information and referrals for parents and teachers and by educating the public about autism. Services include a pen pal directory for autistic people and people with related developmental neurological abnormalities (hydrocephalus, Tourette syndrome, Williams syndrome). People who are able to correspond independently receive the full pen pal directory; people who need to have someone else help them with correspondence will receive a directory containing only other people who also receive assistance with correspondence. However, their information will still be included in the full directory, along with a notation that they use assisted communication, so that independent communicators who do not mind having a third party see their mail will be able to write to them.

ANI also offers an Internet discussion list open to autistic people, family members, and friends, as well as a speaker referral service for individuals and organizations wishing to engage autistic speakers for presentations or interviews. Only people with a formal diagnosis of autism, pervasive development disorder, or Asperger's syndrome may be included on the speaker list. Finally, the group offers a reference library of educational materials about autism, self-advocacy, and civil rights.

Autism Speaks
2 Park Avenue, 11th Floor
New York, NY 10016
(212) 252-8584
http://www.autismspeaks.org

An advocacy group dedicated to funding global biomedical research into the causes, prevention, treatments, and cure for autism; to raising public awareness about autism and its effects on individuals, families, and society; and to bringing hope to all who deal with the hardships of this disorder. The organization is committed to raising the funds necessary to support these goals. Autism Speaks aims to bring the autism community together as one strong voice to urge the government and private sector to listen to member concerns and take action to address this urgent global health crisis. Autism Speaks was formed by a merger between Autism Speaks and the National Alliance for Autism Research (NAAR) in 2006. The consolidation of the two charities is based on their joint commitment to accelerate and fund biomedical research into the causes, prevention, treatments and cure for autism spectrum disorders; to increase awareness of the nation's fastest growing developmental disorder; and to advocate for the needs of affected families.

ANGELMAN SYNDROME

Angelman Syndrome Foundation
3015 E. New York Street, Suite A2265
Aurora, IL 60504
(800) 432-6435 or (630) 978-4245

A foundation that provides information on diagnosis, treatment, management of Angelman syndrome, and offers support and advocacy through education, information exchange, and research. The group also offers local contacts and a newsletter.

APRAXIA

Childhood Apraxia of Speech Association (CASANA)
1151 Freeport Road, #243
Pittsburgh, PA 15238
(412) 767-6589
http://www.apraxia-kids.org/about/CASANA/index.html

A nonprofit organization whose mission is to strengthen the support systems in the lives of children with apraxia of speech so that each child is afforded their best opportunity to learn to talk. The association provides electronic and print information to families, professionals, policymakers, and other members of the public and supports parents and professionals. The association works to improve public policy and services for children affected by the disorder, provides training opportunities for families and professionals, encourages research into childhood apraxia, and co-sponsors a biennial scientific research symposium.

ASPERGER'S DISORDER

Asperger Syndrome Coalition of the United States (ASC-US)
7 MAAP Services, Inc.
P.O. Box 524
Crown Point, IN 46307
(904) 745-6741
http://maapservices.org

A national nonprofit support and advocacy organization for Asperger's syndrome and related disorders that is committed to providing the most up-to-date and comprehensive information on the condition.

AUDITORY TRAINING

Center for the Study of Autism
P.O. Box 4538
Salem, OR 97302

(503) 643-4121
http://www.autism.org

The Center for the Study of Autism (CSA) provides information about autism to parents and professionals, and conducts research on the usefulness of various therapeutic interventions, including those on auditory integration training, Temple Grandin's Hug Box, visual training, irlen lenses, intelligence testing, and Asperger's syndrome. Much of the center's research is undertaken in collaboration with the Autism Research Institute in San Diego. The Center for the Study of Autism provides information to parents and professionals through workshops, conferences, and articles. Its Web site offers detailed information on autism and all its aspects, along with videos, articles, and Web casts.

Society for Auditory Intervention Techniques (SAIT)

P.O. Box 4538
Salem, OR 97302
http://www.sait.org

Society dedicated to the enhancement of the quality of life for individuals with autism through auditory integration training (AIT) and other auditory-based interventions. SAIT distributes information about auditory integration training (AIT) and other auditory-based interventions to professionals and parents. The organization establishes policies, training, and equipment standards, offers guidelines for practitioners, and promotes professional and ethical standards. The organization also provides information to practitioners and others regarding standard procedures, promotes networking and sharing of information, and advises and evaluates research on the efficacy of AIT and other auditory-based interventions.

AUTISM

Association for Science in Autism Treatment

389 Main Street, Suite 202
Malden, MA 02148
(781) 397-8943
http://www.asatonline.org

A national, nonprofit organization formed by a group of parents and professionals concerned about the care and treatment of individuals with autistic disorder.

ASAT is dedicated to disseminating accurate, scientifically valid information about autism and its treatment options and committed to science as the most objective, time-tested, and reliable approach to discerning between safe, effective treatments and those that are harmful or ineffective. They educate professionals and the public about state-of-the-art, valid treatments for people with autism and support certification to ensure everyone with autism receives treatment from practitioners who have met minimum standards of competency. The association also forms interactive, supportive partnerships with universities to develop accredited educational programs for autism practitioners and improves standards of care for people with autism.

Autism Research Institute

4182 Adams Avenue
San Diego, CA 92116
(619) 281-7165
http://www.autismwebsite.com/ARI/index.htm

This nonprofit organization was established in 1967 by Dr. Bernie Rimland, primarily devoted to conducting and disseminating research on the causes of autism and on methods of preventing, diagnosing, and treating autism and other severe behavioral disorders of childhood. The Center for the Study of Autism in Oregon is an affiliate of the Autism Research Institute. Established in 1967, the San Diego–based nonprofit ARI is world headquarters for research and information on autism and related disorders, and the epicenter of a rapidly growing movement that maintains that autism can be treated effectively through intensive behavior modification and a variety of individualized biomedical treatments. ARI provides free and low-cost information to parents, professionals and the media by mail and on its Web site. A publication list of available books, tapes, videos and articles is available at the ARI Web site and by mail.

Autism Society of America (ASA)

7910 Woodmont Avenue, Suite 300
Bethesda, MD 20814-3067

(301) 657-0881 or (800) 3-AUTISM
http://www.autism-society.org

A nonprofit organization that, through advocacy, public awareness, education, and research, seeks to promote opportunities for persons within the autism spectrum and their families to be fully included, participating members of their communities. Founded in 1965 by a small group of parents, the society is the leading source of information and referral on autism and for decades has been the largest collective voice representing the autism community. Members are connected through a volunteer network of more than 240 chapters in 50 states.

Autism Society of America Foundation
7910 Woodmont Avenue, Suite 300
Bethesda, MD 20814
(800) 3AUTISM, ext. 127 or
    (301) 657-0881, ext. 127
http://www.autism-society.org.foundation/
    foundation.html

A fund-raising organization founded in 1996 by the Autism Society of America, the largest and oldest organization representing people with autism. The ASAF has implemented action on several autism research priorities, developing up-to-date statistics; developing a national registry of individuals and families with autism who are willing to participate in research studies; and implementing a system to identify potential donors of autism brain tissue for research purposes and facilitating the donation process. In addition, the foundation contributes money for applied and biomedical research in the causes of and treatment approaches to autism.

Cure Autism Now (CAN)
5455 Wilshire Boulevard, Suite 2250
Los Angeles, CA 90036-4272
(888) 828-8476
http://www.cureautismnow.org

Cure Autism Now (CAN) is an organization of parents, clinicians, and leading scientists committed to accelerating the pace of biomedical research in autism through raising money for research projects, education and outreach. Founded by parents of

children with autism in 1995, the organization has grown from a kitchen-table effort to the largest provider of support for autism research and resources in the country. The organization's primary focus is to fund essential research through a variety of programs designed to encourage innovative approaches toward identifying the causes, prevention, treatment and a cure for autism and related disorders. Since its founding, Cure Autism Now has committed more than $25 million in research, the establishment and ongoing support of the Autism Genetic Resource Exchange (AGRE), and numerous outreach and awareness activities aimed at families, physicians, governmental officials and the general public. Cure Autism Now believes that, with enough determination, money and manpower, answers are found sooner rather than later.

Doug Flutie Jr. Foundation for Autism
P.O. Box 767
Framingham, MA 01701
http://www.dougflutiejrfoundation.org

Nonprofit foundation designed to help financially disadvantaged families with an autistic member fund education and research, and to serve as a communications center for new programs and services developed for individuals with autism. NFL quarterback Doug Flutie Sr. and his wife Laurie started "Dougie's Team" in 1998 to honor their son Doug Jr., who was diagnosed with autism at age three, and to help other families facing childhood autism through support and education. The Fluties began raising funds for autism in 1998; in 2000, they established the Doug Flutie Jr. Foundation for Autism, Inc. as an independent foundation to continue this work. Since 1998, the Fluties have helped raise more than $5 million for autism through corporate and individual donations, fund-raisers, and endorsement promotions featuring Doug and Doug Jr., as well as through sales of Flutie Flakes and other related items.

The foundation awards annual grants to nonprofit organizations that provide services for children with autism and to organizations that conduct research on the causes and effects of autism.

In addition, fund-raising events are held throughout the year, including the Full Court Charity Challenge, Marino 5K Road Race, and the Doug Flutie Jr. Celebrity Golf Classic. Funds are generated through sponsorships, registration fees, and live and silent auctions that are held in conjunction with the events. Past grants have funded summer camp scholarships for children with developmental disabilities, a music therapy program, an after-school program, scholarships for parents to attend educational autism conferences, equipment for occupational and physical therapy, recreational programs, a pediatrician awareness program and many other programs that serve children with autism.

Families for Early Autism Treatment
P.O. Box 255722
Sacramento, CA 95865
http://www.feat.org

A nonprofit organization of parents, educators, and other professionals dedicated to providing education, advocacy, and support for the northern California autism community. It is designed to help families with children diagnosed with autism spectrum disorder, including autism, pervasive developmental disorder, or Asperger's syndrome. It offers a network of support where families can meet each other and discuss issues surrounding autism and treatment options. FEAT offers a quarterly newsletter, a library, and parent resource meetings designed to provide information to families whose children have been diagnosed with autism and to provide access to a network of families who can be supportive. Throughout the year, FEAT has parties, field trips, and fund-raising events.

Indiana Resource Center for Autism
2853 E. 10th Street
Bloomington, IN 47408-2696
(812) 855-6508
http://www.iidc.indiana.edu/irca/fmain1.html

A clinic that conducts outreach training and consultations, engages in research, and develops information on behalf of individuals across the autism spectrum, including autism, Asperger's syndrome, and other pervasive developmental disorders. The center provides communities,

organizations, agencies, and families with the knowledge and skills to support children and adults in typical early intervention, school, community, work, and home settings. The Indiana Resource Center for Autism does not promote one method or a single approach; instead, IRCA staff strive to address the specific needs of the individual by providing information and training on a variety of strategies and methods.

COMMUNICATION

American Sign Language Teachers Association
P.O. Box 92445
Rochester, NY 14692-9998
http://www.aslta.org

The American Sign Language Teachers Association—ASLTA is the only national organization dedicated to the improvement and expansion of the teaching of ASL and deaf studies at all levels of instruction. Founded in 1975 to meet the increasing need for ASL teachers, ASLTA is an individual membership organization of more than 1,000 ASL and deaf studies educators from elementary through graduate education as well as agencies. The organization offers position papers on class size, class meeting frequency, guidelines for hiring American Sign Language teachers, and maintains a Code of Ethics, as well as offering certification. It also offers information about ASL, a store, a newsletter, and an annual conference, and advocates for legislation recognizing ASL as a language. It also promotes the hiring of certified teachers of ASL.

American Speech-Language-Hearing Association (ASHA)
10801 Rockville Pike
Rockville, MD 20852
(800) 498-2071 (voice mail) or (301) 897-5700 (TTY)
http://www.asha.org

The American Speech-Language Hearing Association is the professional, scientific, and credentialing association for more than 12,000 audiologists, speech-language pathologists, and speech, language and hearing scientists. Audiologists specialize in preventing and assessing hearing disorders as well as providing audiologic treatment including hearing aids. Speech-language pathologists identify, assess, and treat speech and language problems including swallowing disorders. The Web site offers lots of information, a referral line, summer camps, publications, newsletters, insurance information.

International Society for Augmentative and Alternative Communication
49 The Donway West, Suite 308
Toronto, ON M3C 3M9
Canada
(416) 385-0351
http://www.isaac-online.org/en/home.html

ISAAC is an international society that works to improve the life of every child and adult with speech difficulties. ISAAC started in 1983, and today has members in 50 countries use communication aids, their families, therapists, teachers, doctors, researchers, and people who make communication aids, such as electronic talking boxes, computers, books and boards with pictures or letters, or sign language. ISAAC supports and encourages the best possible communication methods for people who find communication difficult. Some people need to use communication aids because they are born with disabilities like cerebral palsy. Other people get disabilities when they are older because they have an accident or an illness. All these people have a "vision" that everyone in the world who could communicate more easily by using augmentative and alternative communication (AAC), will be able to do so.

DEVELOPMENTAL DISABILITIES

American Association on Mental Retardation
444 N. Capitol Street, NW, Suite 846
Washington, DC 20001
(800) 424-3688 or (202) 387-1968
http://www.aamr.org

National organization providing information, services, and support, plus advocacy.

Association of University Centers on Disabilities (American Association of University Affiliated Programs for Persons with Developmental Disabilities)
1010 Wayne Avenue, Suite 920
Silver Spring, MD 20910
(301) 588-8252
http://www.aauap.org

AAMR is a nonprofit association that promotes progressive policies, sound research, effective practices, and universal human rights for people with intellectual and developmental disabilities. AAMR is dedicated to achieving full societal inclusion and participation of people with intellectual and developmental disabilities, advocates for equality, individual dignity and other human rights, and tries to expand opportunities for choice and self-determination. The group also tries to influence positive attitudes and public awareness by recognizing the contributions of people with intellectual disabilities and promotes genuine accommodations to expand participation in all aspects of life. The association helps families and other caregivers to provide support in the community and works to increase access to quality health, education, vocational, and other human services and supports. It is also interested in advancing basic and applied research to prevent or minimize the effects of intellectual disability and to enhance the quality of life, cultivating and providing leadership in the field, and seeking a diversity of disciplines, cultures, and perspectives. Finally, the association tries to enhance skills, knowledge, rewards and conditions of people working in the field, encourage promising students to pursue careers in the field of disabilities, and establish partnerships and strategic alliances with organizations that share our values and goals.

The Arc (formerly Association for Retarded Citizens)
1010 Wayne Avenue, Suite 650
Silver Spring, MD 20910
(301) 565-3842
http://www.thearc.org

The Arc is the grassroots national organization of and for people with mental retardation and related developmental disabilities and their families, with more than 140,000 members affiliated through approximately 1,000 state and local chapters across the nation. It advocates for the rights and full participation of all children and adults with intellectual and developmental disabilities. Together with a network of members and affiliated chapters, the group improves systems of supports and services; connects families; inspires communities and influences public policy. The Arc also is devoted to promoting and improving supports and services for people with mental retardation and their families, and fosters research and education regarding the prevention of mental retardation in infants and young children.

It was founded in 1950 by a small group of parents and other concerned individuals because at that time, little was known about the condition of mental retardation or its causes, and there were virtually no programs and activities in communities to assist in the development and care of children and adults with mental retardation and to help support families. In the early days the association worked to change the public's perception of children with mental retardation and to educate parents and others regarding the potential of people with mental retardation. The Arc also worked to procure services for children and adults who were denied day care, preschool, education and work programs.

Voice of the Retarded

5005 Newport Drive, Suite 108
Rolling Meadows, IL 60008
(847) 253-6020
http://www.vor.org

A national organization that advocates for a full range of quality residential options and services. This includes home, community residences, congregate and large facilities. VOR opposes efforts that eliminate options for persons with mental retardation, medically fragile conditions and challenging behaviors. VOR advocates that the final determination of what is appropriate depends on the unique abilities and needs of the individual and desires of the family and guardians. VOR watches and acts when legal actions in any one state threaten residential choice, guardianship

issues or raise other nationally significant, precedent setting legal issues. VOR members include families, organizations and professionals who support high quality care with adequate funding and legal options.

DIET

Autism Network for Dietary Intervention

P.O. Box 335
Pennington, NJ 08534
http://www.autismndi.com

A nonprofit organization dedicated to providing continued support for families implementing a special gluten- and casein-free diet. The network's activities are based on the belief that many cases of autism are caused by an immune system dysfunction that affects the body's ability to break down certain proteins and combat yeasts and bacteria. ANDI was established by parent researchers Lisa Lewis and Karyn Seroussi to help families around the world get started on and maintain the diet.

Feingold Association of the United States

P.O. Box 6550
Alexandria, VA 22306
(703) 768-FAUS or (800) 321-3287
e-mail: help@feingold.org
http://www.feingold.org

    AND

554 East Main Street, Suite 301
Riverhead, NY 11901
(631) 369-9340
http://www.feingold.org

A nonprofit organization of families, educators, and health professionals dedicated to helping children and adults apply proven dietary techniques for better behavior, learning, and health. The association was founded by parents who supported the work of pediatrician Ben F. Feingold, M.D., chief of allergy at Kaiser-Permanente Medical Center in San Francisco during the 1960s. Dr. Feingold used an elimination diet that excluded aspirin and foods believed to contain salicylate compounds, as well as synthetic colorings and flavorings, to help children with behavior problems and autism who had not been helped by medical interventions. In May 1976 parent volunteers established a national organization to support the work of the many local Feingold diet groups. The association conducts extensive research with manufacturers to identify foods and nonfood items that are free of the offending additives. They publish books listing thousands of acceptable brand name products that are readily available in most supermarkets. This information is updated 10 times a year through the association's newsletter, *Pure Facts.*

DISABILITIES

American Association of People with Disabilities
1629 K Street NW, Suite 503
Washington, DC 20006
(800) 840-8844 or (202) 457-0046
http://www.aapd-dc.org

AAPD is the largest national nonprofit cross-disability member organization in the United States, dedicated to ensuring economic self-sufficiency and political empowerment for the more than 56 million Americans with disabilities. AAPD works in coalition with other disability organizations for the full implementation and enforcement of disability nondiscrimination laws, particularly the Americans with Disabilities Act (ADA) of 1990 and the Rehabilitation Act of 1973. Members include people with disabilities in America, plus families and friends. The organization leverages the numbers of people with disabilities and their families and friends to access economic and other benefits to form an organization which will be a positive private-sector force to achieve the goal of full inclusion in American society. AAPD was founded after five key leaders from the disability community (who were instrumental in drafting, advocating for and passage of the landmark civil rights law, the Americans with Disabilities Act) met to organize a national, nonpartisan organization that can and will represent 54 million Americans with disabilities.

Association for the Severely Handicapped (TASH)
29 W. Susquehanna Avenue, Suite 210
Baltimore, MD 21204
(410) 828-8274
http://www.tash.org

An international advocacy association of people with disabilities, their families, and others, with 38 chapters throughout the world. It actively promotes the full inclusion and participation of those with disabilities and seeks to eliminate physical and social obstacles that interfere with quality of life. The Association for the Severely Handicapped (TASH) focuses on those people with disabilities who are most at risk for being excluded from the mainstream, are perceived by traditional service systems as being most challenging, are most likely to have their rights abridged, and are most likely to be at risk for living, working, playing, and/or learning in segregated environments. TASH creates opportunities for collaboration among families, self-advocates, professionals, policymakers and other advocates; advocates for equity, opportunities, social justice, and rights; provides information and supports excellence in research that translates to excellence in practice. TASH also promotes individualized, quality supports, and works toward the elimination of institutions, congregate living settings, segregated schools/classrooms, sheltered work environments, and other segregated services in favor of quality, individualized, inclusive supports. TASH also supports legislation, litigation and public policy and promotes communities in which no one is segregated and everyone belongs.

Children's Defense Fund
25 E. Street NW
Washington, DC 20001
(202) 628-8787
http://www.childrensdefense.org

The mission of the Children's Defense Fund is to leave no child behind and to ensure every child a healthy start, a head start, a fair start, a safe start, and a moral start in life and successful passage to adulthood with the help of caring families and communities. CDF provides a strong, effective voice for all the children of America who cannot vote, lobby, or speak for themselves. They pay particular attention to the needs of poor and minority children and those with disabilities. CDF educates the nation about the needs of children and encourages preventive investment before they get sick or into trouble, drop out of school, or suffer family breakdown. CDF began in 1973 and is a private, nonprofit organization supported by foundation and corporate grants and individual donations, and has never taken government funds.

Commission on Mental and Physical Disability Law American Bar Association

740 15th Street NW
Washington, DC 20005
(202) 662-1570
http://www.abanet.org/disability

This ABA-affiliated group is committed to justice for those with physical disabilities and maintains resources and references for helping the disability community. The Commission's mission is to promote the ABA's commitment to justice and the rule of law for persons with mental, physical, and sensory disabilities and to promote their full and equal participation in the legal profession. Since 1973, the ABA's Commission on Mental and Physical Disability has been the primary entity within the ABA that focuses on the law-related concerns of persons with mental and physical disabilities. The Commission's members include lawyers and other professionals, many of whom have disabilities.

Disability Rights Advocates

449 15th Street, Suite 303
Oakland, CA 94612
(510) 451-8644
http://www.dralegal.org

Nonprofit civil rights organization for people with disabilities. This nonprofit civil rights law firm is dedicated to protecting and advancing the civil rights of people with disabilities. DRA advocates for disability rights through high-impact litigation, as well as research and education, and does not charge clients for services. DRA's mission is to ensure dignity, equality, and opportunity for people with all types of disabilities throughout the United States and worldwide. DRA's national advocacy work includes high-impact class action litigation on behalf of people with all types of disabilities, including mobility, hearing, vision, learning and psychological disabilities. Through negotiation and litigation, DRA has made thousands of facilities throughout the country accessible and has enforced access rights for millions of people with disabilities in many key areas of life, including education, employment, transportation and health care. DRA also engages in nonlitigation advocacy throughout the country, including research and education projects focused on opening up access to schools, the professions and health care.

Disability Rights Education and Defense Fund, Inc.

2212 Sixth Street
Berkeley, CA 94710
(510) 644-2555
http://www.dredf.org

A national law and policy center dedicated to protecting and helping people with disabilities through legislation, litigation, advocacy, technical help, and education. Founded in 1979 by people with disabilities and parents of children with disabilities, the Disability Rights Education and Defense Fund, Inc. (DREDF) is a national law and policy center dedicated to protecting and advancing the civil rights of people with disabilities through legislation, litigation, advocacy, technical assistance, and education and training of attorneys, advocates, persons with disabilities, and parents of children with disabilities.

Family Resource Center on Disabilities (FRCD)

20 East Jackson Boulevard, Room 300
Chicago, IL 60604
(800) 952-4199 or (312) 939-3513
http://www.frcd.org

Coalition of parents, professionals, and volunteers dedicated to improving services for all children with disabilities. Formerly known as the Coordinating Council for Handicapped Children, FRCD was organized in 1969 by parents, professionals, and volunteers who sought to improve services for all children with disabilities. In 1976, the Family Resource Center on Disabilities (FRCD) became one of five pilot programs to operate a parent center funded by the U.S. Department of Education, Office of Special Education Programs (then known as the Bureau of Education for the Handicapped). Today, there are approximately 80 federally funded Parent Centers throughout the United States. During its 30-year existence FRCD has answered more than 200,000 requests for information, training, and support services.

National Dissemination Center for Children with Disabilities (NICHCY)

P.O. Box 1492
Washington, DC 20013
(800) 695-0285
http://www.nichcy.org

This national information and referral center provides information on disabilities and disability-related issues for families, educators, and other professionals with a special focus on children from birth to age 22. The association provides information on specific disabilities, early intervention, special education and related services, individualized education programs, family issues, disability organizations, professional associations, education rights, and transition to adult life. The group also offers referrals, information services, and materials in English and Spanish.

National Institute for People with Disabilities

460 West 34th Street
New York, NY 10001
(212) 563-7474
http://www.yai.org

Since its inception in 1957, YAI/National Institute for People with Disabilities Network has been a national leader in the provision of services, education and training in the field of developmental and learning disabilities. The YAI/NIPD Network has always been in the forefront of education and training in the field of disabilities. The Web site offers information, clubs, newsletters, information on careers, training materials, and a national conference.

National Library Service for the Blind and Physically Handicapped

1291 Taylor Street, NW
Washington, DC 20011
(202) 707-5100; 888-657-7323; (202) 707-0744 (TDD)
http://www.loc.gov/nls

Through a national network of cooperating libraries, NLS administers a free library program of braille and audio materials circulated to eligible borrowers in the United States by postage-free mail. The talking-book program was established by an act of Congress in 1931 to serve blind adults. It was expanded in 1952 to include children, in 1962 to provide music materials, and again in 1966 to include individuals with other physical impairments that prevent the reading of standard print. Any resident of the United States or American citizen living abroad who is unable to read or use standard print materials as a result of a temporary or permanent visual or physical limitation may receive service.

National Organization on Disability (N.O.D.)

910 16th Street NW, Suite 600
Washington, DC 20006
(202) 293-5960
http://www.nod.org

National disability network group concerned with all disabilities of all ages. The mission of the National Organization on Disability is to expand the participation and contribution of America's 54 million men, women and children with disabilities in all aspects of life. By raising disability awareness through programs and information, together we can work toward closing the participation gaps. Programs include the Community Partnership Program, National Partnership Program, CEO Council, Emergency Preparedness Program, Religion and Disaiblity Program, and the World Committee on disability. N.O.D. also awards a number of competitions for disability-friendly communities and nations.

National Parent Network on Disabilities

1130 17th Street NW, Suite 400
Washington, DC 20036

(202) 463-2299
http://www.npnd.org

A nonprofit organization dedicated to empowering parents of children with disabilities. Located in Washington, D.C., the group provides information on the activities of all three branches of government that affect people with disabilities. The primary activities include supporting legislation that will improve the lives and protect the rights of all disabled persons. Members include individuals and family members, as well as national, state, and local organizations that represent the interests of individuals with disabilities.

Protection and Advocacy
100 Howe Avenue, Suite 185-N
Sacramento, CA 95825
(800) 776-5746
http://www.pai-ca.org

Nonprofit agency that provides legal assistance to those with physical, developmental, and psychiatric disabilities. Services include information and referral to other help, peer and self-advocacy training, representation in administrative and judicial proceedings, investigation of abuse and neglect, and legislative advocacy.

Sibling Support Project
Children's Hospital and Medical Center
P.O. Box 5371 CL-09
Seattle, WA 98105
(206) 368-0371
http://www.thearc.org/siblingsupport

The Sibling Support Project, believing that disabilities, illness, and mental health issues affect the lives of all family members, seeks to increase the peer support and information opportunities for brothers and sisters of people with special needs and to increase parents' and providers' understanding of sibling issues. It trains local service providers on how to create community-based peer support programs for young siblings; hosts workshops, listservs, and Web sites for young and adult siblings; and increases parents' and providers' awareness of siblings' unique, lifelong, and ever-changing concerns through workshops, Web sites, and written materials.

World Institute on Disability (WID)
510 16th Street, Suite 100
Oakland, CA 94612
(510) 763-4100
http://www.wid.org

Nonprofit public policy center dedicated to independence and inclusion of people with disabilities. World Institute on Disability is a nonprofit research, public policy and advocacy center dedicated to promoting the civil rights and full societal inclusion of people with disabilities. WID's work focuses on four areas: employment and economic development; accessible health care and personal assistance services; inclusive technology design; and international disability and development. More than half of the Board of Directors and staff are people with disabilities and are respected national leaders in the disability field as well as in industry, government and social services. Since its founding in 1983 by Ed Roberts, Judy Heumann, and Joan Leon, WID has earned a reputation for groundbreaking research and public education on issues important to people with disabilities. WID brings a diverse disability perspective and provides comprehensive analyses crucial to improving public policy and civil rights for people with disabilities.

EDUCATION

Association on Higher Education and Disability (AHEAD)
P.O. Box 540666
Waltham, MA 02454
(781) 788-0003
http://www.ahead.org

Organization of professionals committed to full participation in higher education for those with disabilities, offering education and training. AHEAD is a professional association committed to full participation of persons with disabilities in postsecondary education. As an international resource, AHEAD values diversity, personal growth and development, and creativity; promotes leadership and exemplary practices; and provides professional development and disseminates information. AHEAD also addresses current and emerging issues with respect to disability, education, and accessibility to achieve universal access. Since 1977, AHEAD has delivered quality training to higher education personnel through conferences, workshops, publications and consultation. AHEAD members represent a diverse network of professionals who actively address disability issues on their campuses and in the field of higher education.

National Association for the Education of Young Children (NAEYC)
1509 16th Street, NW
Washington, DC 20036
(202) 232-8777 or (800) 424-2460
http://www.naeyc.org

The National Association for the Education of Young Children (NAEYC) is a national membership organization that focuses on children from birth to age eight. It sponsors an annual conference, publishes a bimonthly journal, and has a catalog of books, brochures, videos, and posters. It is dedicated to improving the well-being of all young children, with particular focus on the quality of educational and developmental services for all children from birth through age eight. Founded in 1926, NAEYC is the world's largest organization working on behalf of young children with nearly 100,000 members, a national network of over 300 local, state, and regional affiliates, and a growing global alliance of other organizations. Membership is open to all individuals who share a desire to serve and act on behalf of the needs and rights of all young children.

National Association of Private Special Education Centers (NAPSEC)
1522 K Street NW, Suite 1032
Washington, DC 20005
(202) 408-3338
http://www.napsec.org

The National Association of Private Special Education Centers (NAPSEC) is a nonprofit association that represents private special education centers and their leaders. The group promotes high-quality programs for individuals with disabilities and their families and advocates for access to the continuum of alternative placements and services. NAPSEC represents about 300 programs nationally, and more than 500 at the state level through the Council of Affiliated State Associations. NAPSEC programs provide special education for both privately and publicly placed individuals. The majority of the membership serves publicly placed individuals who are funded through the Individuals with Disabilities Education Act (IDEA). Ten percent of the membership provide services to privately placed individuals only and receive no federal funding.

National Center on Accelerating Student Learning
Vanderbilt Kennedy Center
Peabody Box 328, Vanderbilt University
Nashville, TN 37203
(615) 343-4782

The National Center on Accelerating Student Learning (CASL) is designed to accelerate learning for students with disabilities in the early grades and thereby to provide a solid foundation for strong achievement in the intermediate grades and beyond. CASL is a five-year collaborative research effort supported by the U.S. Department of Education's Office of Special Education Programs (OSEP). Participating institutions are Teachers College of Columbia University and Vanderbilt University.

National Center on Educational Outcomes
University of Minnesota
350 Elliott Hall
75 East River Road
Minneapolis, MN 55455
(612) 626-1530
http://education.umn.edu/nceo

The National Center on Educational Outcomes provides national leadership in the participation of students with disabilities in national and state assessments, standards-setting efforts, and graduation requirements. It was established in 1990 to provide national leadership in designing and building educational assessments and accountability systems that appropriately monitor educational results for all students, including students with disabilities and students with limited English proficiency. Since its establishment, NCEO has been working with states and federal agencies to identify important outcomes of education for students with disabilities and examining the participation of students in national and state assessments, including the use of accommodations and alternate assessments. It also has evaluated national and state practices in reporting assessment information on students with disabilities, and conducts directed research in the area of assessment and accountability.

Parent Advocacy Coalition for Educational Rights (PACER)

8161 Normandale Boulevard
Minneapolis, MN 55437
(952) 838-9000
http://www.pacer.org

This parent-to-parent organization has lots of resources for parents of children with disabilities, including training programs for parents and youth, technical assistance, and advocacy. The mission of PACER Center is to expand opportunities and enhance the quality of life of children and young adults with disabilities and their families, based on the concept of parents helping parents. Through its ALLIANCE and other national projects, PACER responds to thousands of parents and professionals each year. From California to Minnesota to New York, PACER resources make a difference in the lives of 6.5 million children with disabilities nationwide. With assistance to individual families, workshops, materials for parents and professionals, and leadership in securing a free and appropriate public education for all children, PACER's work affects and encourages families in Minnesota and across the nation.

FRAGILE X SYNDROME

National Fragile X Foundation

P.O. Box 190488
San Francisco, CA 94119
(925) 938-9300
http://www.fragilex.org

Nonprofit organization that provides advocacy, consultation, information, research, newsletters, referrals, and education. Founded in 1984, the National Fragile X Foundation unites the Fragile X community to enrich lives through educational and emotional support, promote public and professional awareness, and advance research toward improved

treatments and a cure for Fragile X. It offers free telephone consultation, basic information, and medical and genetic services referral. The association is an educational and legislative advocate and operates 100 regional service chapters nationally and internationally. It also offers family assistance grants and research grants, and local, national, and international conference sponsorship. A newsletter and educational resources (books, audio, video) are available for a fee.

GENETIC ISSUES

Autism Genetic Resource Exchange

Research Program
5455 Wilshire Boulevard, Suite 715
Los Angeles, CA 90036
(866) 612-2473 or (323) 931-6577
http://www.agre.org

Nonprofit organization created by Cure Autism Now (CAN) to advance genetic research in autism spectrum disorders. The goal of AGRE is to facilitate more rapid progress in the identification of the genetic underpinnings of autism and autism spectrum disorders by making this information available to the scientific community. This substantial collection, which has now grown to almost 700 multiplex and simplex families, has clearly moved the field in that direction. AGRE is a DNA repository and family registry, housing a database of genotypic and phenotypic information that is available to the entire scientific community. In this 6th edition, there are 142 new pedigrees. As they become available, additional family pedigrees will be posted on the online catalog which, based on the expanding nature of the resource, provides the most up-to-date availability of pedigrees and biomaterials. Cell lines have been established for the majority of families in this collection and serum is available on a subset of the subjects until stocks are depleted. Most AGRE families have had extensive evaluations by a variety of pediatricians, psychiatrists, and other neurodevelopmental specialists.

American Hyperlexia Association

194 W. Spangler, Suite B
Elmhurst, IL 60126

(630) 415-2212
http://www.hyperlexia.org

A nonprofit organization comprised of parents and relatives of children with hyperlexia, speech and language professionals, education professionals, and other concerned individuals. AHA is dedicated to the advancement of the education and general welfare of children with hyperlexia, and encourages research related to hyperlexia. The association also tries to help families of children with hyperlexia get appropriate services. Note: the AHA has been inactive since late 2004. However, their Web site remains available as a source of information on this subject.

INTERNATIONAL

Autisme France
1209 Chemin des Campelières
06254 Mougine Cedex
France
http://autisme.france.free.fr

Autisme France was created in 1989 by parents of autistic chidren who were experiencing problems in encouraging their development. Today, thanks to its partners and affiliated organizations, Autisme France is providing a movement of hope and solidarity. Autisme France edits a newsletter three times a year, *La lettre d'Autisme France* and presents the latest information on its Web site along with practical advice and helpful research.

Autism Society Canada
Box 22017, 1670 Heron Road
Ottawa, ON K1V OC2
Canada
(613) 789-8943
http://www.autismsocietycanada.ca

Nonprofit group founded in 1976 by a group of Canadian parents in an effort to encourage the formation of autism societies in all provinces and territories and to address the national autism issues. Today, the ASC is the only national autism charitable organization committed to advocacy, public education, information and referral, and provincial development support. Its goal, through collaboration with Canadian governments, is to reduce the impact of autism spectrum disorders (ASD) on individuals and their families, minimize its lost, and maximize individual potential. The ASC provides information, encourages research, communicates with government, agencies, and other organizations on behalf of those affected by ASD, and promotes conferences and workshops.

National Autistic Society of Great Britain
393 City Road
London ECIVING
http://www.nas.org.uk

The National Autistic Society champions the rights and interests of all people with autism and ensures they and their families receive quality services appropriate to their needs. Their Web site includes information about autism and Asperger's syndrome, along with information about the NAS and its services and activities. The National Autistic Society runs a range of nonprofit schools and colleges for students of all ages with widely varying needs, including more able students and those with high support needs arising out of challenging behaviors. The society also provides a wide range of residential and day services for adults with autistic spectrum disorders, including residential and day provision in urban and rural settings offering flexible, specialized support to individuals with varying needs. The aim of all services is to offer access to as full, enjoyable and meaningful a life as possible to each individual.

MENTAL RETARDATION

See DEVELOPMENTAL DISABILITIES.

MUSIC THERAPY

American Musical Therapy Association
8455 Colesville Road, Suite 1000
Silver Spring, MD 20910
(301) 589-3300
http://www.musictherapy.org

The mission of the American Music Therapy Association is to advance public awareness of the benefits of music therapy and increase access to quality music therapy services in a rapidly changing world. Founded in 1998, AMTA's purpose is the progressive development of the therapeutic use of music in rehabilitation, special education, and community settings. Predecessors to the American Music Therapy Association included the National Association for Music Therapy and the American Association for Music Therapy. AMTA is committed to the advancement of education, training, professional standards, credentials, and research in support of the music therapy profession.

RESEARCH

Autism Research Institute

4182 Adams Avenue
San Diego, CA 92116
(619) 281-7165
www.autismwebsite.com/ari/index.htm

A nonprofit organization devoted to conducting and publicizing its research into the causes of autism and on methods of preventing, diagnosing, and treating autism and other severe behavioral disorders of childhood. The institute provides this information to parents and professionals throughout the world.

ARI was established in 1967 by Bernard Rimland, Ph.D., an international authority on autism and the father of a high-functioning autistic son. Dr. Rimland is the author of *Infantile Autism,* the founder of the Autism Society of America, and was chief technical advisor on *Rain Man,* a film that featured an adult with autism.

ARI's data bank contains more than 35,000 detailed case histories of autistic children from more than 60 countries. The organization publishes the Autism Research Review International, a quarterly newsletter covering biomedical and educational advances in autism research.

Center for the Study of Autism

P.O. Box 4538
Salem, OR 97302
(503) 643-4121

The Center for the Study of Autism (CSA) provides information about autism to parents and professionals, and conducts research on the usefulness of various therapeutic interventions, including those on auditory integration training, Temple Grandin's Hug Box, visual training, Irlen lenses, intelligence testing, and Asperger's syndrome. Much of the center's research is undertaken in collaboration with the Autism Research Institute in San Diego. The Center for the Study of Autism provides information to parents and professionals through workshops, conferences, and articles. Its Web site offers detailed information on autism and all its aspects, along with videos, articles, and Web casts.

Cure Autism Now (CAN) Foundation

5455 Wilshire Boulevard, Suite 2250
Los Angeles, CA 90036
(888) 828-8476
http://www.canfoundation.org

An organization of parents, clinicians, and scientists committed to accelerating the pace of biomedical research in autism by raising money for research projects, education, and outreach. Founded in 1995 by parents of children with autism, the organization's primary focus is to fund essential research through a variety of programs designed to encourage innovative approaches toward identifying the causes, prevention, treatment, and a cure for autism and related disorders. CAN has grown to be the largest private funder of autism research and resources in the country. This funding includes support for pilot research grants, young investigator awards, bridge grants, targeted research projects and the establishment and ongoing support of the world's first collaborative gene bank for autism; the Autism Genetic Resource Exchange (AGRE).

Since its founding, Cure Autism Now has committed more than $20 million in support of the AGRE, as well as helping fund numerous outreach and awareness activities aimed at families, physicians, governmental officials, and the general public. CAN has also helped triple the number of scientists working in the field of autism and motivated passage of the Children's Health Act of 2000.

RETT DISORDER

International Rett Disorder Association
9121 Piscataway Road, Suite 2B
Clinton, MD 20735
(800) 818-7388 or (301) 856-3334
http://www.rettdisorder.org

A support group for parents of children with
Rett disorder, founded by parents in early 1984
and dedicated to better understanding of this
disorder. Members include parents, relatives,
doctors, therapists, researchers, and friends
interested in providing a better future for girls
with Rett disorder. IRSA supports medical research
to determine the cause and find a cure for Rett
disorder, increases public awareness of the
condition, and provides information and support to
families of affected children.

Rett Disorder Research Foundation (RDRF)
4600 Devitt Drive
Cincinnati, OH 45246
(513) 874-3020
http://www.rsrf.org

The RDRF was founded in late 1999 by a
small but passionate group of parents who
were concerned by the lack of research being
conducted on Rett disorder. Today RDRF is the
world's leading private funder of Rett research,
funding 82 projects at 57 of the world's premier
institutions totaling approximately $8.8 million.
RDRF organizes the only annual scientific
meeting devoted to Rett disorder, and each June
RDRF convenes more than 100 researchers and
clinicians from around the world for a three
day Rett disorder symposium. As a volunteer
organization, RDRF has raised millions since its
inception. The foundation directs 97 percent
of each dollar donated directly to program
services. RDRF's mission is to fund, promote and
accelerate biomedical research for the treatment
and cure of Rett disorder.

SENSORY INTEGRATION

Sensory Integration International (SII)
P.O. Box 5339
Torrance, CA 90510-5339

(310) 320-9986 or (310) 533-8338
http://www.sensoryint.com

Sensory Integration International is a nonprofit, tax-exempt corporation concerned with
the impact of sensory integrative problems on
people's lives. Its goal is to improve quality of life
for persons with sensory processing disorders,
advocating early intervention to prevent
sensory inefficiencies that have the potential
of contributing to debilitating social or health
conditions. SII promotes education about the
impact of inadequate sensory processing and
its relationship to health and one's occupation.
SII was founded by a group of occupational
therapists dedicated to helping people with
disabilities through the application of knowledge
from the neurobehavioral sciences. The
organization has focused its efforts on research
and professional education in the area of learning
disabilities, with emphasis on the pioneering
work of Dr. A. Jean Ayres, but now promotes
evaluation of other treatment approaches
and theoretical models that address sensory
integration throughout the life span in a variety
of diagnostic groups. Membership includes
occupational therapists, physical therapists,
parents, educators, speech therapists, physicians,
nurses, psychologists, and other health-care and
childcare professionals.

SPECIAL EDUCATION

See EDUCATION.

TREATMENT

Association for the Advancement
of Behavior Therapy
305 Seventh Avenue, 16th Floor
New York, NY 10001-6008
(212) 647-1890
http://www.aabt.org/staff

A professional interdisciplinary organization
concerned with applying behavioral and cognitive
sciences to understanding human behavior and
developing interventions to enhance the human
condition. ABCT is a not-for-profit organization

of more than 4,500 mental health professionals and students who utilize and/or are interested in empirically based behavior therapy or cognitive behavior therapy.

Association for Behavior Analysis

1219 South Park Street
Kalamazoo, MI 49001
(269) 492-9310
htpp://www.abainternational.org

The Association develops and supports the growth and vitality of behavior analysis through research, education and practice. It serves as an advocate for and facilitator of research, and develops, improves, and disseminates best practices in the recruitment, training, and professional development of behavior analysts. The association focuses on the practice of behavior analysis (including certification, continuing education, code of ethics, practice standards, legislation and public policy, third party payments), and produces convention and conference programs and scholarly journals.

Autism Treatment Center of America Son-Rise Program

2080 South Undermountain Road
Sheffield, MA 01257
(413) 229-2100
http://www.autismtreatmentcenter.org

The Autism Treatment Center of America is the worldwide teaching center for The Son-Rise Program, a unique treatment for children and adults challenged by autism, autism spectrum disorders, pervasive developmental disorder (PDD), Asperger's syndrome, and other developmental difficulties. During the last 25 years, the center has worked with more than 22,000 parents and professionals from around the world teaching them a system of treatment and education featuring love and positive reinforcement.

Division TEACCH

CB 7180
100 Renee Lynne Court
University of North Carolina
Chapel Hill, NC 27599

(919) 966-2174
http://www.teacch.com/teacch.htm

Division TEACCH works to enable individuals with autism to function as meaningfully and as independently as possible, to provide services throghout North Carolina to individuals with autism and their families, and to provide information, integrate clinical services, and disseminate information about the theory of the TEACCH method. TEACCH was developed in the early 1970s by Eric Schopler, to focus on the person with autism and the development of a program around the person's skills, and interests. In 1972, the state created the Division for the Treatment and Education of Autistic and Related Communication Handicapped Children. Located in the psychiatry department at the University of North Carolina at Chapel Hill, the program (named Division TEACCH) was the first statewide, comprehensive community-based program dedicated to improving the understanding and services for autistic and communciation handicapped children and their families.

Interdisciplinary Council On Developmental and Learning Disorders

4938 Hampden Lane, Suite 800
Bethesda, MD 20814
(301) 656-2667
htpp://www.icdl.com

Organization founded by psychiatrist Stanley Greenspan that includes a multidisciplinary network of professionals who believe in individualizing assessment and treatment approaches based on a child's specific functional developmental profile. The group's aim is to support families of children with developmental and/or learning disorders by providing resource information and opportunities for communication and to promote floor time (the Developmental, Individual-Difference, Relationship-Based intervention model). The group also advocates for sound public policies that support children with developmental and/or learning disorders and their families.

APPENDIX II
HELPFUL WEB SITES

APRAXIA

Apraxia-Kids
http://www.apraxia-kids.org

ASPERGER'S DISORDER

Asperger's Connection
http://www.ddleadership.org/aspergers/index.
html

Asperger's Disorder Home Page
http://www.aspergers.com

AUTISM AND AUTISTIC DISORDER

The Autism Autoimmunity Project
http://www.taap.info

Autism-PDD Resources Network
http://www.autism-pdd.net

Autism Resources on the Internet
http://www.autism.org/links.html

Independent LIving on the Autistic Spectrum Mailing List
http://www.inlv.demon.nl

CAMPS

Courage Camps
http://www.couragecamps.org

Kids Camps
http://www.kidscamps.com

DISABILITIES

Americans with Disabilities Act Home Page
http://www.usdoj.gov/crt/ada/adahom1.htm

EDUCATION

Education Overview
http://www.autism-society.org/site/PageServer?
pagename=EducationOverview

National Early Childhood Technical Assistance Center
http://www.nectac.org

APPENDIX III
STATE AUTISM ORGANIZATIONS

ALABAMA

Autism Society of Alabama
3100 Lorna Road, Suite 132
Birmingham, AL 35216-5450
(877) 428-8476
http://www.autism-alabama.org

North Alabama Chapter: Autism Society of America
P.O. Box 2902
Huntsville, AL 35804-2902
(256) 424-7910

ARIZONA

Autism Society of Greater Phoenix
P.O. Box 10543
Phoenix, AZ 85064-0543
(480) 940-1093
http://www.phxautism.org

Pima County (AZ) Chapter: ASA
P.O. Box 44156
Tucson, AZ 85733-4156
(520) 770-1541
http://www.tucsonautism.org

ARKANSAS

Arkansas Chapter, Autism Society of America
2001 Pershing Circle, F-13
North Little Rock, AR 72114-1841
(501) 682-9930

CALIFORNIA

California Chapter: Autism Society of America
P.O. Box 8600
Long Beach, CA 90808-0600
(800) 700-0037
http://www.geocities.com/HotSprings/Chalet/1782

Central California Chapter: Autism Society of America
P.O. Box 13213
Fresno, CA 93794-3213
(559) 227-8991
http://www.asaccc.org

Coachella Valley (CA) Chapter ASA
P.O. Box 3605
Palm Desert, CA 92255-1052
(760) 779-0012
http://coachellavalleyautism.org

Greater Long Beach/South Bay Chapter: ASA
8620 Portafino Place
Whittier, CA 90603-1038
(562) 943-3335

Kern Autism Network: ASA
9501 Lokern Road
McKittrick, CA 93251-9746

Los Angeles Chapter: Autism Society of America
P.O. Box 8600
Long Beach, CA 90808-0600
(562) 804-5556

Northern California, Autism Society of
976 Mangrove Avenue
Chico, CA 95926-3950
(530) 897-0900

North San Diego County (CA) Chapter ASA
P.O. Box 131161
Carlsbad, CA 92013-1161
(760) 479-1420
http://www.nccasa.com

**Orange County Chapter, Autism Society
 of America**
5591 Yuba Avenue
Westminster, CA 92683-2843
(714) 799-7500
http://www.asaoc.org

**San Diego Chapter, Autism Society
 of America**
P.O. Box 420908
San Diego, CA 92142-0908
(619) 298-1981
http://www.sd-autism.org

**San Francisco Bay Chapter, Autism Society
 of America**
1360 Sixth Avenue
Belmont, CA 94002-3818
(650) 637-7772
http://sfautismsociety.virtualave.net

**San Gabriel Valley Chapter, Autism Society
 of America**
P.O. Box 1755
Glendora, CA 91740-1755
(626) 580-8927

Santa Barbara (CA) Chapter
P.O. Box 630
Carpinteria, CA 93014-0630
(805) 560-3762
http://www.asasb.org

Tulare County (CA) Chapter ASA
4125 W. Noble Avenue, #209
Visalia, CA 93277-1662
(559) 747-2126

**Ventura County Chapter, Autism Society
 of America**
P.O. Box 2690
Ventura, CA 93002-2690

(818) 207-0135
http://www.VCAS.info

COLORADO

Boulder County (CO) Chapter ASA
194 Mesa Court
Louisville, CO 80027-9401
(720) 272-8231
http://www.autismboulder.org

**Colorado Chapter, Autism Society of
 America**
701 S. Logan Street, Suite 103
Denver, CO 80209-4169
(720) 214-0794
http://www.autismcolorado.org

Pikes Peak (CO) Chapter ASA
1813 Chapel Hills Drive
Colorado Springs, CO 80920-3714
(719) 630-7072

CONNECTICUT

Autism Society of Connecticut - ASCONN
P.O. Box 1404
Guilford, CT 06437
(888) 453-4975
http://www.autismsocietyofct.org

Natchaug Region (CT) Chapter ASA
95 Bolton Branch Road
Coventry, CT 06238-1002
(860) 742-5195

**South Central Connecticut Chapter,
 Autism Society of America**
20 Washington Avenue
North Haven, CT 06473-2343
(203) 235-7629

WASHINGTON, D.C.

**District of Columbia Chapter, Autism Society
 of America**
5167 Seventh Street NE
Washington, DC 20011-2624
(202) 561-5300

DELAWARE

Autism Society of Delaware, Inc.
5572 Kirkwood Highway
Wilmington, DE 19808
(302) 472-2638
http://www.delautism.org

FLORIDA

Autism Association of Northeast Florida

Helps those concerned with autism spectrum disorder to utilize current resources and to promote awareness, advocacy, and education within the community.

Orlando Hispanic Autism Parent Support Group

Nuestra Misión: Mantener informada a la comunidad sobre los recursos en el área central de Florida.

Broward County (FL) Chapter ASA
P.O. Box 450476
Sunrise, FL 33345-0476
(954) 577-4141

Emerald Coast (FL) Chapter ASA
916 Lido Circle East
Niceville, FL 32578-4403
(850) 897-2252

Florida Chapter, Autism Society of America
P.O. Box 970646
Pompano Beach, FL 33097-0646
(954) 349-2820
http://www.autismfl.com

Greater Orlando (FL) Chapter ASA
4743 Hearthside Drive
Orlando, FL 32837-5445
(407) 855-0235
http://www.asgo.org

Gulf Coast Chapter, Autism Society of America
P.O. Box 21105
Saint Petersburg, FL 33742-1105

(727) 786-8075
http://web.tampabay.rr.com/autism

Jacksonville (FL) Chapter ASA
1526 University Boulevard West, #235
Jacksonville, FL 32217-2006
(904) 680-5104

Manasota (FL) Chapter ASA
P.O. Box 18934
Sarasota, FL 34276-1934
(941) 426-9059
http://www.manasotaautism.com

Marion County (FL) Chapter ASA
P.O. Box 65
Reddick, FL 32686-0065
(352) 591-3120

Miami-Dade County (FL) Chapter, Autism Society of America
P.O. Box 831405
Miami, FL 33283-1405
(305) 969-3900
e-mail: rlpvega@aol.com

Palm Beaches Chapter, Autism Society of America
901 NW Fourth Avenue
Boca Raton, FL 33432
(561) 688-9010

Panhandle (FL) Chapter, Autism Society of America
4148 N. Cambridge Way
Milton, FL 32571-7368
(850) 995-0003
http://www.autismpensacola.org

South Florida Chapter, Autism Society of America
21212 Harbor Way, Apartment 143
Miami, FL 33180-3524
(305) 681-0407

Southwest Florida Chapter, Autism Society of America
1259 Shannondale Drive
Fort Myers, FL 33913
(239) 768-0723

GEORGIA

Central Georgia Chapter, Autism Society of America
523 Pinecrest Road
Macon, GA 31204-1764
(478) 745-4994

The Greater Georgia Chapter, Autism Society of America
2971 Flowers Road South, Suite 140
Atlanta, GA 30341
(770) 451-0954
http://www.asaga.com

Northeast Georgia Chapter, Autism Society of America
P.O. Box 48366
Athens, GA 30604-8366
(706) 208-0066
http://negac-autsoc.tripod.com

HAWAII

Autism Society of Hawaii
P.O. Box 2995
Honolulu, HI 96802-2995
(808) 228-0122
http://www.autismhawaii.org

IDAHO

Panhandle (ID) Chapter ASA
P.O. Box 3393
Post Falls, ID 83877
(208) 676-8884

Treasure Valley (ID) Chapter ASA
7842 Rainbow Place
Nampa, ID 83687-9404
(208) 336-5676
http://www.asatvc.org

ILLINOIS

Autism Society of Illinois
2200 South Main Street, Suite 317
Lombard, IL 60148-5366
(630) 691-1270
http://www.autismillinois.org

Central Illinois Chapter ASA (ASACIC)
P.O. Box 8781
Springfield, IL 62791
(877) 311-7703
http://www.asacic.org

Chicago Southside (IL) Chapter ASA
21363 Old North Church Road
Frankfort, IL 60423

Far West Suburban Illinois Chapter ASA
P.O. Box 9166
Downers Grove, IL 60515
(630) 969-1094

Kankakee Valley (IL) Chapter ASA
318 Meadows Road North
Bourbonnais, IL 60914
(815) 933-3467

Metropolitan Chicago (IL) Chapter ASA
1550 W. 88th Street, #202A
Chicago, IL 60620
(773) 233-4210

Northeast Illinois Chapter, Autism Society of America
707 Crossland Drive
Grayslake, IL 60030-1697
(847) 543-4502
http://www.livingwithautism.com

North Suburban Illinois Chapter ASA
199 Shadowbend Drive
Wheeling, IL 60090-3151
(847) 541-9969

Northwest Suburban IL Chapter Autism Society of America
2200 Kensington Drive
Schaumburg, IL 60194
(847) 885-8006
http://www.autismillinois.com

Southern Illinois Chapter ASA
P.O. Box 822
O'Fallon, IL 62269
(618) 530-7894
http://www.asosi.org

Southwest Suburban Cook County (IL) Chapter ASA
4533 W. 90th Place
Hometown, IL 60456-1052
(708) 424-8565

INDIANA

Central Indiana Chapter of Autism Society of America
P.O. Box 50534
Indianapolis, IN 46250
(317) 578-9940
http://www.centralindianaautism.netfirms.com

East Central Chapter of the Autism Society of America
2008 West 12th Street
Anderson, IN 46016
(765) 642-8520

Elkhart Indiana Chapter of Autism Society of America
624 South 10th Street
Goshen, IN 46526
(574) 533-3376

Indiana Chapter, ASA State Chapter
P.O. Box 8502
Bloomington, IN 47407-8502
(812) 332-7236
http://www.autismindiana.org

Northwest Indiana Chapter, Autism Society of America
13908 Delaware Street
Crown Point, IN 46307
(219) 662-2668

South Central Chapter of the Autism Society of America
7044 North Purcell Drive
Bloomington, IN 47408
(812) 876-1251
http://www.geocities.com/bloomingtonautism

South Central Indiana Chapter ASA
8245 Patricksburg Road
Spencer, IN 47460-6332
(812) 876-1251

Southwest Indiana Chapter of Autism Society of America
1020 Brandon Avenue
Jasper, IN 47546
(812) 634-9614

State Chapter Autism Society of Indiana
207 N. Pennsylvania Street, #300
Indianapolis, IN 46204
(260) 493-6050
http://www.autismindiana.org

IOWA

East Central Iowa Chapter, Autism Society of America
3928 Terrace Hill Drive NE
Cedar Rapids, IA 52402

Iowa Chapter, Autism Society of America
4549 Waterford Drive
West Des Moines, IA 50265
(888) 722-4799
http://www.autismia.org

Quad Cities Chapter, Autism Society of America
P.O. Box 472
Bettendorf, IA 52722
(888) 722-4799
http://www.autismqc.org

Siouxland (IA) Chapter ASA
3016 Cass Avenue
Salix, IA 51052-8078
(712) 943-7847

KANSAS

Johnson County (KS) Chapter ASA
P.O. Box 3122
Shawnee Mission, KS 66203-0122
(913) 897-1234
http://www.asjck.org

Kansas Chapter, Autism Society of America
2250 N. Rock Road, Suite 118-254
Wichita, KS 67226-2325

(316) 943-1191
http://www.ask.hostrack.net

KENTUCKY

ASK/Autism Society of Kentuckiana
P.O. Box 90
Pewee Valley, KY 40056
(502) 222-4706
http://www.ask-lou.org

Bluegrass (KY) Chapter ASA
243 Shady Lane
Lexington, KY 40503-2034
(859) 278-4991
http://www.geocities.com/
    autismsocietyofthebluegrass

Purchase Area (KY) Chapter ASA
4125 Roettger Drive
Kevil, KY 42053-8879
(270) 442-6126

Western Kentucky Chapter ASA
P.O. Box 1647
230 Second Street, Suite 206
Henderson, KY 42419
(270) 826-0510

LOUISIANA

Acadian Society for Autistic Citizens
202 Sandalwood Drive
Lafayette, LA 70507-3726
(337) 236-6658
http://www.lastateautism.org/acadian

Bayou (LA) Chapter ASA
P.O. Box 3361
Morgan City, LA 70381-3367
(985) 395-4403

**Greater New Orleans Chapter, Autism
    Society of America**
P.O. Box 74632
Metairie, LA 70033-4632
(504) 464-5733

**Louisiana Chapter, Autism Society
    of America**
4425 Annunciation Street
New Orleans, LA 70115-1523

(800) 955-3760
http://www.lastateautism.org

**Northeast Louisiana Chapter, Autism Society
    of America**
P.O. Box 4762
Monroe, LA 71211-4762
(318) 343-7698
http://www.autismnela.org

Northwest Louisiana Chapter ASA
625 Red Chute Lane
Bossier City, LA 71112-9713
(318) 747-1662
e-mail: nwlac3@yahoo.com

**Southwest Louisiana Chapter, Autism
    Society of America**
P.O. Box 1805
Lake Charles, LA 70602
(337) 855-2068

MAINE

Maine Chapter: Autism Society of America
72B Main Street
Winthrop, ME 04364-1406
(800) 273-5200
http://www.asmonline.org

MARYLAND

Anne Arundel County (MD) Chapter ASA
P.O. Box 1304
Millersville, MD 21108
(410) 923-8800
http://www.aaccasa.org

**Baltimore-Chesapeake Chapter, Autism
    Society of America**
P.O. Box 10822
Parkville, MD 21234-0822
(410) 655-7933
http://www.bcc-asa.org

Frederick County (MD) Chapter ASA
11127 Innsbrook Way
Ijamsville, MD 21754-9058

Harford County (MD) Chapter ASA
1315 Vanderbilt Road
Bel Air, MD 21014
(410) 836-7177, ext. 617

Howard County (MD) Chapter ASA
7231 Cadence Court
Columbia, MD 21046
(410) 760-5595
http://www.howard-autism.org

Montgomery County Chapter, Autism Society of America
4125 Queen Mary Drive
Olney, MD 20832-2109
(301) 652-3912
http://www.autismmontgomerycounty.com

Prince George's County Chapter, Autism Society of America
P.O. Box 633
Bowie, MD 20718-0633
(301) 627-4820

Washington County (MD) Chapter ASA
721 Georgia Avenue
Hagerstown, MD 21740
(240) 420-3692

MASSACHUSETTS

Massachusetts Chapter, Autism Society of America
47 Walnut Street
Wellesley Hills, MA 02481
(781) 237-0272, ext. 17
http://www.geocities.com/asamasschapter

MICHIGAN

The Autism Society of America Macomb / St. Clair Chapter
P.O. Box 182186
Shelby Twp., MI 48318-2186
(586) 447-2235
http://www.macombasa.org

Autism Society of Michigan
6035 Executive Drive, Suite 109
Lansing, MI 48911
(517) 882-2800
http://www.autism-mi.org

NEW JERSEY

The New Jersey Center for Outreach and Services for the Autism Community, Inc.
1450 Parkside Avenue, Suite 22
Ewing, NJ 08638
(609) 883-8100
http://www.njcosac.org/cosaccontactus

NEW YORK

GRACE (Getting Resources for Autistic Children's Equality) Foundation of New York
6581 Hylan Boulevard
Staten Island, NY 10309
(718) 605-7500
http://www.graceofny.org

NORTH DAKOTA

FMFEAT (Fargo Moorhead Families for Early Autism Treatment)
P.O. Box 1325
Fargo, ND 58107
e-mail: fmfeat@yahoo.com
http://fmfeat.tripod.com

OHIO

Autism Society of Northwest Ohio
4848 Dorr Street
Toledo, OH 43615
(419) 578-ASNO (2766)
Fax: (419) 536-5038
http://www.asno.org

PENNSYLVANIA

Autism Society of Berks County, Pennsylvania
P.O. Box 6683
Wyomissing, PA 19610
(610) 736-3739
http://www.autismsocietyofberks.org

TEXAS

**Autism Society of Greater Tarrant
    County**
P.O. Box 161516
Fort Worth, TX 76161
(817) 390-2829
http://www.asgtc.org

**Dallas Asperger Network for Information
    Support and Help**
3409 Ashington Lane
Plano, TX 75023
(972) 491-3365
http://www.aspergerinfo.org

UTAH

Autism Society of Utah
Utah Parent Center
2290 East 4500 South, Suite 110
Salt Lake City, UT 84117-4428
(801) 272-1051 or (800) 468-1160

WISCONSIN

Autism Society of Wisconsin
P.O. Box 165
Two Rivers, WI 54241
(888) 428-8476
http://www.asw4autism.org

APPENDIX IV
AUTISM RESOURCES BY STATE

ALABAMA

CLIENT ASSISTANCE PROGRAM

Department of Rehabilitation Services
P.O. Box 11586
Montgomery, AL 36111-0586
(334) 281-2276 (V/TTY) or (800) 228-3231
    (V/TTY in AL)

OFFICE OF STATE COORDINATOR OF VOCATIONAL EDUCATION FOR STUDENTS WITH DISABILITIES

Special Needs Programs, Department of Education
Gordon Persons Building
P.O. Box 302101
Montgomery, AL 36130-2101
(334) 242-9108

PARENT TRAINING AND INFORMATION PROJECT

Special Education Action Committee, Inc. (SEAC)
P.O. Box 161274
Mobile, AL 36616-2274
(334) 478-1208 or (800) 222-7322 (in AL)

PROGRAMS FOR CHILDREN WITH DISABILITIES: AGES THREE THROUGH FIVE

Dept. of Education, Div. of Special Education Services
P.O. Box 302101
Montgomery, AL 36130-2101
(334) 242-8114 or (800) 392-8020 (in AL)

PROGRAMS FOR CHILDREN WITH SPECIAL HEALTH CARE NEEDS

Alabama Department of Rehabilitation Services
Children's Rehabilitation Service
2129 East South Boulevard, P.O. Box 11586
Montgomery, AL 36111-0586
(334) 281-8780 or (800) 846-3697
http://www.rehab.state.al.us

PROGRAMS FOR INFANTS AND TODDLERS WITH DISABILITIES: AGES BIRTH THROUGH TWO

Alabama's Early Intervention System
Department of Rehabilitation Services
2129 East South Boulevard, P.O. Box 11586
Montgomery, AL 36111-0586
(334) 281-8780
http://www.rehab.state.al.us

PROTECTION AND ADVOCACY AGENCY

Alabama Disabilities Advocacy Program (ADAP)
526 Martha Parham West
The University of Alabama
P.O. Box 870395
Tuscaloosa, AL 35487-0395
(800) 826-1675; (205) 348-4928;
    (205) 348-9484 (TTY)

STATE DEPARTMENT OF EDUCATION: SPECIAL EDUCATION

Dept. of Education, Div. of Special Education Services
P.O. Box 302101
Montgomery, AL 36130-2101
(334) 242-8114 or (800) 392-8020 (in AL)

STATE DEVELOPMENTAL DISABILITIES PLANNING COUNCIL

Alabama Developmental Disabilities Planning Council

RSA Union Building
100 N. Union Street
P.O. Box 301410
Montgomery, AL 36130-1410
(334) 242-3973 or (800) 232-2158

STATE MENTAL HEALTH REPRESENTATIVE FOR CHILDREN AND YOUTH

Alabama Department of Mental Health

RSA Union Building
P.O. Box 301410
Montgomery, AL 36130-1410
(334) 242-3218

STATE MENTAL RETARDATION PROGRAM

Department of Mental Health/Mental Retardation

RSA Union Building
100 N. Union Street
P.O. Box 301410
Montgomery, AL 36130-1410
(334) 242-3701

STATE VOCATIONAL REHABILITATION AGENCY

Department of Rehabilitation Services

2129 East South Boulevard, P.O. Box 11586
Montgomery, AL 36111-0586
(334) 281-8780
e-mail: webinfo@rehab.state.al.us
http://www.rehab.state.al.us/vr.html

TECHNOLOGY-RELATED ASSISTANCE STAR (STATEWIDE TECHNOLOGY ACCESS AND RESPONSE FOR ALABAMIANS WITH DISABILITIES)

2125 East South Boulevard

P.O. Box 20752
Montgomery, AL 36120-0752

(334) 613-3480; (334) 613-3519 (TTY);
(800) 782-7656 (in AL)

ALASKA

HEALTH-CARE PROGRAM FOR CHILDREN WITH SPECIAL NEEDS

State of Alaska

Section of Maternal, Child, and Family Health
1231 Gambell Street
Anchorage, AK 99501-4627
(907) 269-3460

OFFICE OF STATE COORDINATOR OF VOCATIONAL EDUCATION FOR STUDENTS WITH DISABILITIES

Office of Adult and Vocational Education

800 West 10th Street, Suite 200
Juneau, AK 99801-1894
(907) 465-8729

PARENT TRAINING AND INFORMATION PROJECT

P.A.R.E.N.T.S., Inc.

4743 E. Northern Lights Boulevard
Anchorage, AK 99508
(907) 337-7678 (V/TTY) or (800) 478-7678
(in AK)
http://www.parentsinc.org

PROGRAMS FOR CHILDREN WITH DISABILITIES AGES THREE THROUGH FIVE

Office of Special Services and Supplemental Programs

Department of Education
801 West 10th Street, Suite 200
Juneau, AK 99801-1894
(907) 465-2972

PROGRAMS FOR CHILDREN WITH SPECIAL HEALTH-CARE NEEDS

Special Needs Services Unit

1231 Gambell Street

Anchorage, AK 99501-4627
(907) 269-3460

PROGRAMS FOR INFANTS AND TODDLERS WITH DISABILITIES: AGES BIRTH THROUGH TWO

State of Alaska Department of Health and Social Services
Special Needs Services Unit
1231 Gambell Street
Anchorage, AK 99501-4627
(907) 269-3460

PROTECTION AND ADVOCACY AGENCY

Disability Law Center of Alaska
615 East 82nd, Suite 101
Anchorage, AK 99518
(907) 344-1002
e-mail: disablaw@anc.ak.net

STATE DEPARTMENT OF EDUCATION: SPECIAL EDUCATION

Office of Special Education/Alaska Department of Education
801 West 10th Street, Suite 200
Juneau, AK 99801-1894
(907) 465-2972

STATE DEVELOPMENTAL DISABILITIES PLANNING COUNCIL

Governor's Council on Disabilities and Special Education
P.O. Box 240249
Anchorage, AK 99524-0249
(907) 269-8990

STATE MENTAL HEALTH REPRESENTATIVE FOR CHILDREN AND YOUTH

Child and Adolescent Mental Health
Division of Mental Health/Developmental
　Disabilities
Department of Health and Social Services
P.O. Box 110620
Juneau, AK 99811-0620
(907) 465-3370 or (907) 465-2225 (TTY)

STATE MENTAL RETARDATION PROGRAM

Developmental Disabilities Section
Division of Mental Health/Developmental
　Disabilities
Department of Health and Social Services
Pouch 110620
Juneau, AK 99811-0620
(907) 465-3372 or (907) 465-2225 (TTY)

STATE VOCATIONAL REHABILITATION AGENCY

Division of Vocational Rehabilitation
801 West 10th Street, M.S. 0581
Juneau, AK 99801
(907) 274-5630 or (907) 274-5605

TECHNOLOGY-RELATED ASSISTANCE

Rose Foster, Information and Referral
Assistive Technologies of Alaska
1016 W. Sixth Avenue, #105
Anchorage, AK 99507-1068
(907) 563-0146 (V/TTY) or (800) 770-0138
　(V/TTY)
http://www.labor.state.ak.us/at/index.htm

UNIVERSITY-AFFILIATED PROGRAM

University of Alaska Anchorage
Center for Human Development
2330 Nichols Street
Anchorage, AK 99508
(907) 272-8270

ARIZONA

OFFICE OF STATE COORDINATOR OF VOCATIONAL EDUCATION FOR STUDENTS WITH DISABILITIES

Division of Vocational Education, Department of Education
1535 West Jefferson, Bin 60
Phoenix, AZ 85007
(602) 542-3450

PARENT TRAINING AND INFORMATION PROJECT

Pilot Parent Partnerships
4750 N. Black Canyon Highway, Suite 101
Phoenix, AZ 85017-3621
(602) 242-4366 or (800) 237-3007 (in AZ)
http://ade.state.az.us

PROGRAMS FOR CHILDREN WITH DISABILITIES: AGES THREE THROUGH FIVE

Exceptional Student Services, Department of Education
1535 West Jefferson
Phoenix, AZ 85007
(602) 542-3852
e-mail: lbusenb@mail1.ade.state.az.us
http://ade.state.az.us

PROGRAMS FOR INFANTS AND TODDLERS WITH DISABILITIES: AGES BIRTH THROUGH TWO

Interagency Coordinating Council for Infants and Toddlers
Department of Economic Security
1717 West Jefferson
P.O. Box 6123 (801-A-6)
Phoenix, AZ 85005
(602) 542-5577

PROGRAMS FOR CHILDREN AND YOUTH WHO ARE DEAF OR HARD OF HEARING

Arizona Council for the Hearing Impaired
1400 Washington Street, Room 126
Phoenix, AZ 85007
(602) 542-3323 (V/TTY) or (800) 352-8161 (V/TTY)

Arizona State Schools for the Deaf and the Blind
1200 W. Speedway Boulevard
P.O. Box 87010
Tucson, AZ 85754

PROGRAMS FOR CHILDREN WITH SPECIAL HEALTH-CARE NEEDS

Office of Children with Special Health Care Needs
Department of Health
1740 W. Adams
Phoenix, AZ 85007
(602) 542-1860

PROTECTION AND ADVOCACY AGENCY

Arizona Center for Disability Law
3839 N. Third Street, #209
Phoenix, AZ 85012
(602) 274-6287
http://www.acdl.com

STATE DEPARTMENT OF EDUCATION: SPECIAL EDUCATION

Exceptional Student Services, Department of Education
1535 West Jefferson
Phoenix, AZ 85007
(602) 542-3084

STATE DEVELOPMENTAL DISABILITIES PLANNING COUNCIL

Governor's Council on Developmental Disabilities
1717 West Jefferson Street
Site Code (074Z)
Phoenix, AZ 85007
(602) 542-4049

STATE DEVELOPMENTAL DISABILITIES PROGRAM

Department of Economic Security
Division of Developmental Disabilities
P.O. Box 6123, Site Code (791A)
Phoenix, AZ 85005
(602) 542-0419

STATE MENTAL HEALTH AGENCY

Division of Behavioral Health Services
Department of Health Services
2122 E. Highland Avenue

Phoenix, AZ 85016
(602) 381-8999

STATE MENTAL HEALTH REPRESENTATIVE FOR CHILDREN AND YOUTH

Division of Behavioral Health Services
Department of Health Services
2122 E. Highland Avenue, Suite 100
Phoenix, AZ 85016
(602) 381-8998

STATE VOCATIONAL REHABILITATION AGENCY

Rehabilitation Services Bureau 930A
Department of Economic Security
1789 West Jefferson 2NW
Phoenix, AZ 85007
(602) 542-3332

TECHNOLOGY-RELATED ASSISTANCE

Arizona Technology Access Program (AZTAP)
Institute for Human Development
Northern Arizona University
P.O. Box 5630
Flagstaff, AZ 86011
(520) 523-7035; (520) 523-1695 (TTY);
    (800) 477-9921
http://www.nau.edu/ihd/aztap.html

UNIVERSITY-AFFILIATED PROGRAM

Institute for Human Development
Northern Arizona University
P.O. Box 5630
Flagstaff, AZ 86011
(520) 523-4791
 http://www.nau.edu/ihd

ARKANSAS

CLIENT ASSISTANCE PROGRAM

Advocacy Services, Inc.
1100 N. University, Suite 201

Little Rock, AR 72207
(501) 296-1775 or (800) 482-1174

FOCUS, INC.
305 West Jefferson Avenue
Jonesboro, AR 72401
(870) 935-2750

OFFICE OF STATE COORDINATOR OF VOCATIONAL EDUCATION FOR STUDENTS WITH DISABILITIES

Department of Workforce Education
Three Capitol Mall, Luther S. Hardin Building
Little Rock, AR 72201-1083
(501) 682-1800

PARENT TRAINING AND INFORMATION PROJECT

Arkansas Disability Coalition
2801 Lee Avenue, Suite B
Little Rock, AR 72205
(501) 614-7020 (V/TTY) or (800) 223-1330 (V/TTY)
e-mail: adc@cei.net

PROGRAMS FOR CHILDREN WITH DISABILITIES: AGES THREE THROUGH FIVE

Preschool Programs, Special Education, Dept. of Educ.
#4 Capitol Mall, Room 105-C
Little Rock, AR 72201-1071
(501) 682-4225

PROGRAMS FOR CHILDREN WITH SPECIAL HEALTH-CARE NEEDS

Children's Medical Services
Department of Human Services
P.O. Box 1437, Slot #256
Little Rock, AR 72203-1437
(501) 682-2277

PROGRAMS FOR INFANTS AND TODDLERS WITH DISABILITIES: AGES BIRTH THROUGH TWO

Div. of Developmental Diseases Services, Dept. of Human Services
P.O. Box 1437, Donaghey Plaza North
Fifth Floor, Slot 2520

Little Rock, AR 72203-1437
(501) 682-8676

PROTECTION AND ADVOCACY AGENCY

Advocacy Services, Inc.
1100 N. University, Suite 201
Little Rock, AR 72207
(501) 296-1775 or (800) 482-1174 (V/TTY)
http://www.advocacyservices.org

STATE AGENCY FOR THE VISUALLY IMPAIRED

Department of Human Services
Division of Services for the Blind
522 Main Street, Suite 100
P.O. Box 3237
Little Rock, AR 72203
(501) 682-5463 or (800) 960-9270

STATE DEPARTMENT OF EDUCATION: SPECIAL EDUCATION

Special Education Unit, Department of Education
Special Education Building C, Room 105
#Four Capitol Mall
Little Rock, AR 72201-1071
(501) 682-4225

STATE DEVELOPMENTAL DISABILITIES PLANNING COUNCIL

Governor's Developmental Disabilities Council
Freeway Medical Tower
5800 West 10th, Suite 805
Little Rock, AR 72204
(501) 661-2589

STATE DEVELOPMENTAL DISABILITIES PROGRAM

Division of Developmental Disabilities Services
Dept. of Human Services
P.O. Box 1437, Slot #2500
7th and Main Streets, Fifth Floor
Little Rock, AR 72203-1437
(501) 682-8662

STATE MENTAL HEALTH AGENCY

Arkansas Division of Mental Health Services
4313 West Markham Street
Little Rock, AR 72205
(501) 686-9164

STATE MENTAL HEALTH REPRESENTATIVE FOR CHILDREN AND YOUTH

Division of Mental Health Services
4313 West Markham Street
Little Rock, AR 72205-4096
(501) 686-9166

STATE VOCATIONAL REHABILITATION AGENCY

Department of Workforce Education
Arkansas Rehabilitation Services
1616 Brookwood Drive
P.O. Box 3781
Little Rock, AR 72203-3781
(501) 296-1616

TECHNOLOGY-RELATED ASSISTANCE

Arkansas Increasing Capabilities Access Network
2201 Brookwood, Suite 117
Little Rock, AR 72202
(501) 666-8868 (V/TTY) or (800) 828-2799 (in AR)

CALIFORNIA

CLIENT ASSISTANCE PROGRAM

Client Assistance Program
830 K Street Mall, Second Floor
Sacramento, CA 95814
(916) 322-5066; (800) 952-5544 (V);
   (800) 598-3273 (TTY)

OFFICE OF STATE COORDINATOR OF VOCATIONAL EDUCATION FOR STUDENTS WITH DISABILITIES

Department of Education
721 Capitol Mall

Sacramento, CA 95814
(916) 657-2451

PARENT TRAINING AND INFORMATION PROJECTS

Disability Rights Education and Defense Fund, Inc. (DREDF)
2212 Sixth Street
Berkeley, CA 94710
(510) 644-2555

Exceptional Parents Unlimited
4120 North First Street
Fresno, CA 93726
(209) 229-2000

MATRIX, A Parent Network and Resource Center
94 Galli Drive
Novato, CA 94949
(415) 884-3535
http://www.volunteersolutions.org/marin/org/1333572.html

Northern California Coalition for Parent Training
Information (NCC)
Parents Helping Parents
3041 Olcott Street
Santa Clara, CA 95054-3222
(408) 727-5775
http://www.php.com

Parents Helping Parents—San Francisco
594 Monterey Boulevard
San Francisco, CA 94127
(415) 841-8820

Support for Families of Children with Disabilities
2601 Mission Street, Suite 710
San Francisco, CA 94110
(415) 282-7494

Team of Advocates for Special Kids (TASK)
100 West Cerritos Avenue
Anaheim, CA 92805-6546
(714) 533-TASK

Team of Advocates for Special Kids (TASK), San Diego
4550 Kearny Villa Road

San Diego, CA 92123
(619) 874-2386 or (619) 874-2375
http://www.taskca.org

PROGRAMS FOR CHILDREN WITH DISABILITIES: AGES THREE THROUGH FIVE

Special Education Div./California Dept. of Education
515 L Street, Suite 270
Sacramento, CA 95814
(916) 445-4623
http://www.cde.ca.gov/spbranch/sed/index.htm

PROGRAMS FOR CHILDREN WITH SPECIAL HEALTH-CARE NEEDS

State Children's Medical Services Branch
Department of Health Services
714 P Street, Room 350
Sacramento, CA 95814
(916) 654-0832

PROGRAMS FOR CHILDREN AND YOUTH WHO ARE DEAF OR HARD OF HEARING

State Office of Deaf Access
Department of Social Services
744 P Street, MS 19-91
Sacramento, CA 95814
(916) 229-4573 or (916) 229-4577 (TTY)
e-mail: deaf.access@dss.ca.gov

PROGRAMS FOR INFANTS AND TODDLERS WITH DISABILITIES: AGES BIRTH THROUGH TWO

Prevention and Children Services Branch
Department of Developmental Services
1600 Ninth Street, Room #310
Sacramento, CA 95814
(916) 654-2773

PROTECTION AND ADVOCACY AGENCY

Protection and Advocacy, Inc.
100 Howe Avenue, Suite 185N
Sacramento, CA 95825
(916) 488-9950 or (800) 776-5746 (in CA)
http://www.pai-ca.org

STATE DEPARTMENT OF EDUCATION: SPECIAL EDUCATION

Special Education, Department of Education
515 L Street, Suite 270
Sacramento, CA 95814
(916) 445-4729
http://www.cde.ca.gov/spbranch/sed/index.htm

STATE DEVELOPMENTAL DISABILITIES PLANNING COUNCIL

State Council on Developmental Disabilities
2000 O Street, Room 100
Sacramento, CA 95814
(916) 322-8481

STATE EDUCATION AGENCY RURAL REPRESENTATIVE

Special Education Division
CA Department of Education
515 L Street, Suite 270
Sacramento, CA 95814
(916) 327-3505

STATE MENTAL HEALTH AGENCY

Department of Mental Health
1600 Ninth Street
Sacramento, CA 95814
(916) 654-2309

STATE MENTAL HEALTH REPRESENTATIVE FOR CHILDREN AND YOUTH

Systems of Care, Department of Mental Health
1600 Ninth Street, Room 250
Sacramento, CA 95814
(916) 654-3551

STATE MENTAL RETARDATION PROGRAM

Dept. of Developmental Services, Health and Welfare Agency
1600 Ninth Street, Second Floor
Sacramento, CA 95814
(916) 654-1897

STATE VOCATIONAL REHABILITATION AGENCY

Department of Rehabilitation
830 K Street Mall, Room 307
Sacramento, CA 95814
(916) 445-3971

TECHNOLOGY-RELATED ASSISTANCE

California Assistive Technology System
CA Department of Rehabilitation
830 K Street
Sacramento, CA 95814
(916) 324-3062 (V/TTY) or (800) 390-2699 (V/TTY, in CA)

UNIVERSITY-AFFILIATED PROGRAM

Center for Child Development and Developmental Disabilities
Children's Hospital LA
USC-University Affiliated Program
P.O. Box 54700, MS #53
Los Angeles, CA 90054-0700
(213) 669-2300

University of California at Los Angeles, UAP
760 Westwood Plaza
Los Angeles, CA 90024
(310) 825-0470

COLORADO

CLIENT ASSISTANCE PROGRAM

Contact PROTECTION AND ADVOCACY AGENCY
(800) 288-1376 (in CO)

OFFICE OF STATE COORDINATOR OF VOCATIONAL EDUCATION FOR STUDENTS WITH DISABILITIES

CO Community College and Occupational Educ. System
1391 North Speer Boulevard, Suite 600
Denver, CO 80204-2554
(303) 595-1577

PARENT TRAINING AND INFORMATION PROJECT

PEAK Parent Center, Inc.
6055 Lehman Drive, Suite 101
Colorado Springs, CO 80918
(719) 531-9400 or (800) 284-0251

PROGRAMS FOR CHILDREN WITH DISABILITIES: AGES THREE THROUGH FIVE

Department of Education/Prevention Initiatives
201 East Colfax Avenue, Room 305
Denver, CO 80203
(303) 866-6712

PROGRAMS FOR CHILDREN WITH SPECIAL HEALTH-CARE NEEDS

Health Care Program For Children with Special Needs (HCP)
CO Department of Public Health
and Environment
4300 Cherry Creek Drive South
Denver, CO 80246
(303) 692-2370

PROGRAMS FOR INFANTS AND TODDLERS WITH DISABILITIES: AGES BIRTH THROUGH TWO

Early Childhood Initiatives
State Department of Education
201 East Colfax, Room 305
Denver, CO 80203
(303) 866-6709

PROTECTION AND ADVOCACY AGENCY

The Legal Center for People with Disabilities and Older People
455 Sherman Street, Suite 130
Denver, CO 80203
(303) 722-0300
(800) 288-1376 (in CO only)

STATE DEVELOPMENTAL DISABILITIES PLANNING COUNCIL

Colorado Developmental Disabilities Planning Council
777 Grant Street, Suite 304
Denver, CO 80203
(303) 894-2345

STATE EDUCATION AGENCY RURAL REPRESENTATIVE

Special Education/Department of Education
201 East Colfax
Denver, CO 80203
(303) 866-6681

STATE MENTAL HEALTH AGENCY

Mental Health Services
3824 West Princeton Circle
Denver, CO 80236
(303) 866-7400

STATE MENTAL HEALTH REPRESENTATIVE FOR CHILDREN AND YOUTH

Mental Health Services, Department of Human Services
3824 West Princeton Circle
Denver, CO 80236
(303) 866-7406

STATE MENTAL RETARDATION PROGRAM

Developmental Disabilities Services
3824 West Princeton Circle
Denver, CO 80236
(303) 866-7450

STATE VOCATIONAL REHABILITATION AGENCY

Division of Vocational Rehabilitation
Department of Human Services
110 16th Street, Second Floor
Denver, CO 80202
(303) 620-4153

TECHNOLOGY-RELATED ASSISTANCE

Colorado Assistive Technology Project (CATP)
The Pavillion
1919 Ogden, A036-Box B140
Denver, CO 80218
(303) 864-5100 (V); (303) 864-5110 (TTY);
(800) 255-3477 (CO only)

UNIVERSITY-AFFILIATED PROGRAM

Colorado UAP
University of CO Health Sciences Center, Kempe Center
1825 Marron Street
Denver, CO 80218
(303) 864-5261

CONNECTICUT

CLIENT ASSISTANCE PROGRAM

Contact PROTECTION AND ADVOCACY AGENCY

PARENT-TO-PARENT

Parent-to-Parent Network of CT
Connecticut Children's Medical Center
282 Washington Street
Hartford, CT 06106
(860) 545-9021

PARENT TRAINING AND INFORMATION PROJECT

Connecticut Parent Advocacy Center (CPAC)
338 Main Street
Niantik, CT 06357
(860) 739-3089 or (800) 445-2722 (in CT)
http://members.aol.com/cpacinc/cpac.htm

PROGRAMS FOR CHILDREN AND YOUTH WHO ARE DEAF OR HARD OF HEARING

Connecticut Commission on the Deaf and Hearing Impaired
1245 Farmington Avenue

West Hartford, CT 06107
(860) 561-0196 (V/TTY)

PROGRAMS FOR CHILDREN WITH DISABILITIES: AGES THREE THROUGH FIVE

Bureau of Early Childhood Education and Social Services
CT Department of Education
25 Industrial Park Road
Middletown, CT 06457
(860) 638-4211

PROGRAMS FOR CHILDREN WITH SPECIAL HEALTH CARE NEEDS

CT Department of Public Health
410 Capitol Avenue, MF #911MAT
P.O. Box 340308
Hartford, CT 06134-0308
(860) 509-8074

Easter Seals Camp Hemlocks
P.O. Box 198
Hebron, CT 06248-0198
(860) 228-9496, ext. 200 or (860) 228-2091 (TTY)
http://www.easterealscamphemlocks.org

PROGRAMS FOR INFANTS AND TODDLERS WITH DISABILITIES: AGES BIRTH THROUGH TWO

State Birth to Three System
Department of Mental Retardation
460 Capitol Avenue
Hartford, CT 06106
(860) 418-6147

PROTECTION AND ADVOCACY AGENCY

Office of Protection and Advocacy for Persons with Disabilities
60 B Weston Street
Hartford, CT 06120-1551
(860) 297-4300; (800) 842-7303 (in CT);
(860) 566-2102 (TTY)
http://www.ct.gov/opapd/site/default.asp

STATE AGENCY FOR THE LEGALLY BLIND AND VISUALLY IMPAIRED

Board of Education and Services for the Blind (BESB)
184 Windsor Avenue
Windsor, CT 06109
(860) 602-4000
http://www.besb.state.ct.us

STATE DEPARTMENT OF EDUCATION: SPECIAL EDUCATION

Bureau of Special Education and Pupil Services
Connecticut Dept. of Education
25 Industrial Park Road
Middletown, CT 06457-1520
(860) 638-4265

STATE DEPARTMENT OF SOCIAL SERVICES

Bureau of Rehabilitation Services
Department of Social Services
10 Griffin Road, North
Windsor, CT 06095
(860) 298-2003

STATE DEVELOPMENTAL DISABILITIES PLANNING COUNCIL

Council on Developmental Disabilities
460 Capitol Avenue
Hartford, CT 06106-1308
(860) 418-6157 or (860) 418-6172 (TTY)

STATE MENTAL HEALTH AGENCY

Department of Mental Health and Addiction Services
410 Capitol Avenue
Hartford, CT 06106
(860) 418-7000

STATE MENTAL HEALTH REPRESENTATIVE FOR CHILDREN

Department of Children and Families
505 Hudson Street
Hartford, CT 06106
(860) 550-6528
http://www.state.ct.us/dcf

STATE MENTAL RETARDATION PROGRAM

Department of Mental Retardation
460 Capitol Avenue
Hartford, CT 06106
(860) 418-6000
http://www.dmr.state.ct.us

STATE TRANSITION COORDINATOR

Bureau of Special Education
Connecticut Department of Education
Room 369
P.O. Box 2219
Hartford, CT 06145-2219
(860) 713-6910
http://www.state.ct.us/sde/deps/special/#contact

TECHNOLOGY-RELATED ASSISTANCE

Bureau of Rehabilitation Services
DSS/BRS
25 Sigourney Street, 11th Floor
Hartford, CT 06106
(860) 424-4881; (800) 537-2549;
 (860) 424-4839 (TTY)

UNIVERSITY-AFFILIATED PROGRAM

A.J. Pappanikou Center for Developmental Disabilities
263 Farmington Avenue, MC6222
Farmington, CT 06030
(860) 679-1500 or (866) 623-1315
http://www.uconnucedd.org

WECAHR (WESTERN CONNECTICUT ASSOCIATION FOR HUMAN RIGHTS)

11 Lake Avenue Ext.
Danbury, CT 06811
(203) 792-3540
http://www.wecahr.org

DELAWARE

CLIENT ASSISTANCE PROGRAM

Client Assistance Program, United Cerebral Palsy, Inc.
254 East Camden-Wyoming Avenue

Camden, DE 19934
(302) 698-9336

OFFICE OF STATE COORDINATOR
OF VOCATIONAL EDUCATION
FOR STUDENTS WITH DISABILITIES

**Vocational Technology Education and School
to Work Transition**
Department of Education
P.O. Box 1402
Dover, DE 19903
(302) 739-4638

OTHER STATE AGENCIES FOR PERSONS
WITH DISABILITIES

**Governor's Advisory Council for Exceptional
Citizens (GACEC)**
George V. Massey Station
516 West Loockerman Street
Dover, DE 19904
(302) 739-4553
http://denver.state.de.us/gov/gacecweb.nsf?open

State Council for Persons with Disabilities
Margaret M. O'Neill Building
P.O. Box 1401
Dover, DE 19903
http://www2.state.de.us/scpd

PARENT TRAINING AND INFORMATION
PROJECTS

**Parent Information Center of Delaware, Inc.
(PIC)**
5570 Kirkwood Highway
Orchard Commons Business Center
Wilmington, DE 19808
(302) 999-7394 or (888) 547-4412
http://www.picofdel.org

PROGRAMS FOR CHILDREN AND YOUTH
WHO ARE DEAF OR HARD OF HEARING

**Delaware Office for the Deaf and Hard
of Hearing**
Division of Vocational Rehabilitation
Department of Labor Building
4425 North Market Street, 3rd Floor
Wilmington, DE 19802
(302) 761-8275 (V/TTY) or (302) 761-8336 (TTY)

PROGRAMS FOR CHILDREN
WITH DISABILITIES:
AGES THREE THROUGH FIVE

**Exceptional Children and Early Childhood
Group**
Department of Education
401 Federal Street, Suite 2
Dover, DE 19901-3639
(302) 739-5471
http://www.doe.state.de.us/Exceptional_Child/
ececehome.htm

PROGRAMS FOR CHILDREN
WITH SPECIAL HEALTH CARE NEEDS

Family Health Services
Division of Public Health
P.O. Box 637, Jesse Cooper Building
Dover, DE 19903
(302) 739-3111

PROGRAMS FOR INFANTS
AND TODDLERS WITH DISABILITIES:
AGES BIRTH THROUGH TWO

Management Services Division
Health and Social Services, Second Floor,
Room 204
1901 North DuPont Highway
New Castle, DE 19720
(302) 577-4647

PROTECTION AND ADVOCACY
AGENCY

Disabilities Law Program
Community Service Building
100 West 10th Street, Suite 801
Wilmington, DE 19801
(302) 575-0660
http://www.declasi.org/dis.html

REGIONAL ADA TECHNICAL
ASSISTANCE AGENCY

TransCen, Inc.
451 Hungerford Drive, Suite 700
Rockville, MD 20850
(301) 424-2002
http://transcen.org

STATE AGENCY FOR THE VISUALLY IMPAIRED

Division for the Visually Impaired (DVI)
Health and Social Services
1901 N. DuPont Highway, Biggs Building
New Castle, DE 19720
(302) 255-9800
http://www.dhss.delaware.org/dhss/dvi/index.html

STATE DEPARTMENT OF EDUCATION: SPECIAL EDUCATION

Exceptional Children and Early Childhood Group
Department of Education
401 Federal Street, Suite 2
Dover, DE 19901-3639
(302) 739-5471
http://www.doe.state.de.us/Exceptional_Child/ececehome.htm

STATE DEVELOPMENTAL DISABILITIES PLANNING COUNCIL

Delaware Developmental Disabilities Planning Council
Margaret M. O'Neill Building, Second Floor
410 Federal Street, Suite 2
Dover, DE 19901
(302) 739-3333
http://www.state.de.us/ddc/default.htm

STATE DIVISION OF VOCATIONAL REHABILITATION

Delaware Division of Vocational Rehabilitation
4425 North Market Street
P.O. Box 9969
Wilmington, DE 19809-0969
(302) 761-8275 or (302) 761-8336 (TTY)

STATE MENTAL HEALTH AGENCY

Division of Alcoholism, Drug Abuse and Mental Health
Department of Health and Social Services
1901 North DuPont Highway
New Castle, DE 19720
(302) 577-4461

STATE MENTAL HEALTH REPRESENTATIVE FOR CHILDREN

Division of Child Mental Health Services
Department of Services for Children, Youth, and Their Families
1825 Faulkland Road
Wilmington, DE 19805-1195
(302) 633-2600

STATE MENTAL RETARDATION PROGRAM

Division of Mental Retardation
Department of Health and Social Services
Jesse Cooper Building
P.O. Box 637/Federal Street
Dover, DE 19903
(302) 739-4386

TECHNOLOGY-RELATED ASSISTANCE

Delaware Assistive Technology Initiative (DATI)
University of Delaware
Alfred I. duPont Hospital for Children
P.O. Box 269
Wilmington, DE 19899-0269
(302) 651-6790; (302) 651-6794 (TTY); (800) 870-DATI

UNIVERSITY-AFFILIATED PROGRAM

University of Delaware
Center for Disabilities Studies
A University Affiliated Program
166 Graham Hall
Newark, DE 19716
(302) 831-6974
http://www.udel.edu/cds

FLORIDA

CLIENT ASSISTANCE PROGRAM

Contact PROTECTION AND ADVOCACY AGENCY

OFFICE OF STATE COORDINATOR OF VOCATIONAL EDUCATION FOR STUDENTS WITH DISABILITIES

Division of Workforce Development
Department of Education, Turlington Building
325 W. Gaines Street, Suite 714
Tallahassee, FL 32399-0400
(850) 487-3164
http://www.firn.edu/doe

PARENT TRAINING AND INFORMATION PROJECTS

Family Network on Disabilities of Florida, Inc.
2735 Whitney Road
Clearwater, FL 33760
(813) 523-1130 or (800) 825-5736
http://fndfl.org

PROGRAMS FOR CHILDREN AND YOUTH WHO ARE DEAF OR HARD OF HEARING

Deaf and Hard of Hearing Services Program
Division of Vocational Rehabilitation
2002 Old Saint Augustine Road, Building A
Tallahassee, FL 32399-0696
(850) 488-2867 (V/TTY)
http://www.rehabworks.org

PROGRAMS FOR CHILDREN WITH DISABILITIES: AGES THREE THROUGH FIVE

Office of Early Intervention and School Readiness
Division of Public Schools and Community
  Education
Department of Education
325 West Gaines Street, Suite 325
Tallahassee, FL 32399-0400
(850) 488-6830

PROGRAMS FOR CHILDREN WITH SPECIAL HEALTH CARE NEEDS

Children's Medical Services Programs
Department of Health and Rehabilitative Services
1309 Winewood Boulevard, Building 6, Room 130
Tallahassee, FL 32399-0700
(850) 487-2690

PROGRAMS FOR INFANTS AND TODDLERS WITH DISABILITIES: AGES BIRTH THROUGH TWO

Children's Medical Services
Department of Health
1317 Winewood Boulevard, Building 6, Room 130
Tallahassee, FL 32399-0700
(850) 487-2690
http://www.cms-kids.com

PROTECTION AND ADVOCACY AGENCY

Advocacy Center for Persons with Disabilities
2671 Executive Center Circle West, Suite 100
Tallahassee, FL 32301-5029
(850) 488-9071 or (800) 346-4127 (TTY)
(800) 342-0823 or (800) 350-4566 (Spanish- and
  Creole-speaking clients)
http://www.advocacycenter.com

REGIONAL ADA TECHNICAL ASSISTANCE AGENCY

Southeast Disability and Business Technical Assistance Center (SEDBTAC), Region Four
Center for Assistive Technology
Georgia Institute of Technology
490 Tenth Street
Atlanta, GA 30318
(800) 949-4232 (V/TTY)
http://www.sedbtac.org

STATE AGENCY FOR VISUAL IMPAIRMENTS

Division of Blind Services
Department of Education
1320 Executive Center Drive
Room 100, Atkins Building
Tallahassee, FL 32399-2050
(850) 245-0300
http://www.state.fl.us/dbs

STATE DEPARTMENT OF EDUCATION: SPECIAL EDUCATION

Bureau of Instructional Support and Community Services
Division of Public Schools and Community
  Education

Department of Education
325 West Gaines Street, Suite 614
Tallahassee, FL 32399-0400
(850) 488-1570

STATE DEVELOPMENTAL DISABILITIES PLANNING COUNCIL

Florida Developmental Disabilities Council
124 Marriott Drive, Suite 203
Tallahassee, FL 32301-2981
(850) 488-4180

STATE DEVELOPMENTAL SERVICES

Department of Children and Families
Developmental Services Program Office
1317 Winewood Boulevard, Building 3, Room 325
Tallahassee, FL 32399-0700
(850) 488-4257
e-mail: Charles_Kimber@dcf.state.fl.us
http://www.state.fl.us/cf_web

STATE DIVISION OF VOCATIONAL REHABILITATION

Division of Vocational Rehabilitation
Department of Labor and Employment Security
2002 Old St. Augustine Road, Building A
Tallahassee, FL 32399-0696
(850) 488-6210

STATE EDUCATION AGENCY RURAL REPRESENTATIVE

Instructional Programs
Division of Public Schools and Community
    Education
Department of Education
Florida Education Center, Room 514
Tallahassee, FL 32399
(850) 488-2601

STATE MENTAL HEALTH AGENCY

Mental Health Programs Office
Department of Children and Families
1317 Winewood Boulevard
Tallahassee, FL 32399-0700
(850) 488-8304
http://www.dcf.state.fl.us/mentalhealth

STATE MENTAL HEALTH REPRESENTATIVE FOR CHILDREN AND YOUTH

Children's Mental Health Program
Mental Health Programs Office
1317 Winewood Boulevard
Tallahassee, FL 32399-0700
(850) 487-2920
http://www.dcf.state.fl.us/mentalhealth

TECHNOLOGY-RELATED ASSISTANCE

Florida Alliance for Assistive Service and Technology (FAAST)
325 John Knox Road, Building B
Tallahassee, FL 32303
(850) 487-3278
http://www.faast.org

UNIVERSITY-AFFILIATED PROGRAM

Mailman Center for Child Development
University of Miami School of Medicine
P.O. Box 016820 (D-820)
Miami, FL 33101
(305) 243-6801
http://pediatrics.med.miami.
    edu/mailman/mailman

GEORGIA

CLIENT ASSISTANCE PROGRAM

Client Assistance Program
123 North McDonough Street
Decatur, GA 30030
(404) 373-2040 or (800) 822-9727 (in GA)
http://www.vocrehabga.org/lev3j.html

COUNCIL ON DEVELOPMENTAL DISABILITIES FOR GEORGIA

Governor's Council on Developmental Disabilities
2 Peachtree Street, N.W., Third Floor,
    Suite 3-210
Atlanta, GA 30303-3142
(404) 657-2126 or (888) 275-4233
http://www.gcdd.org

**OFFICE OF STATE COORDINATOR
OF VOCATIONAL EDUCATION
FOR STUDENTS WITH DISABILITIES**

Department of Education
Vocational Education Special Needs Unit
1752 Twin Towers East
Atlanta, GA 30334
(404) 657-8324

PARENT-TO-PARENT

Parent to Parent of Georgia, Inc.
3805 Presidential Parkway, Suite 207
Atlanta, GA 30340
(770) 451-5484 or (800) 229-2038
http://www.parenttoparentofga.org

**PARENT TRAINING AND INFORMATION
PROJECT**

**Parents Educating Parents and Professionals
for All Children (PEPPAC)**
6613 East Church Street, Suite 100
Douglasville, GA 30134
(770) 577-7771

**PROGRAMS FOR CHILDREN
WITH DISABILITIES: AGES THREE
THROUGH FIVE**

Preschool Special Education
GA Department of Education
1870 Twin Towers East
Atlanta, GA 30334-5060
(404) 657-9955

**PROGRAMS FOR CHILDREN WITH SPECIAL
HEALTH-CARE NEEDS**

Child and Adolescent Health Unit
GA Department of Resources
Two Peachtree Street, Seventh Floor, Room 7-312
Atlanta, GA 30303
(404) 657-2712

**PROGRAMS FOR INFANTS AND TODDLERS
WITH DISABILITIES: AGES BIRTH
THROUGH TWO**

Babies Can't Wait (BCW) Program
Division of Public Health

Two Peachtree Street, Room 7-315
Atlanta, GA 30303-3166
(404) 657-2726

PROTECTION AND ADVOCACY AGENCY

Georgia Advocacy Office, Inc. (GAO)
150 Ponce de Leon Avenue, Suite 430
Decatur, GA 30030
(404) 885-1234 or (800) 537-2329 (in GA)
http://www.thegao.org

**REGIONAL ADA TECHNICAL
ASSISTANCE AGENCY**

**Southeast Disability and Business Technical
Assistance Center**
(SEDBTAC), Region Four
Center for Assistive Technology and Environmental Access
Georgia Institute of Technology
490 10th Street
Atlanta, GA 30318
(800) 949-4232
http://www.sedbtac.org

**STATE DEPARTMENT OF EDUCATION:
SPECIAL EDUCATION**

Division for Exceptional Students
GA Department of Education
1870 Twin Towers East
Atlanta, GA 30334
(404) 656-3963

**STATE EDUCATION AGENCY RURAL
REPRESENTATIVE**

Division for Exceptional Students
GA Department of Education
1870 Twin Towers East
Atlanta, GA 30334
(404) 656-3963

STATE MENTAL HEALTH AGENCY

**Division of Mental Health/ Mental
Retardation/ Substance Abuse**
Department of Human Resources
Two Peachtree Street, N.W., 22nd Floor
Atlanta, GA 30303

(404) 657-2252
http://www.2.state.ga.us/Departments/DHR

STATE MENTAL HEALTH REPRESENTATIVE FOR CHILDREN AND YOUTH

Division of Mental Health/ Mental Retardation/ Substance Abuse
Department of Human Resources
Two Peachtree Street, N.W., 22nd Floor
Atlanta, GA 30303-3142
(404) 657-2273

STATE MENTAL RETARDATION PROGRAM

Division of Mental Health/ Mental Retardation/ Substance Abuse
Department of Human Resources
Two Peachtree Street, N.W., 22nd Floor
Atlanta, GA 30303-3142
(404) 657-6087

STATE VOCATIONAL REHABILITATION AGENCY

Department of Human Resources
Division of Rehabilitation Services
Two Peachtree Street, N.W., Room 35-403
Atlanta, GA 30303-3166
(404) 657-3053

TECHNOLOGY-RELATED ASSISTANCE

Georgia Tools for Life/Georgia Department of Labor
Vocational Rehabilitation Program
1700 Century Circle B-4
Atlanta, GA 30345
(404) 657-3082; (800) 497-8665;
    (404) 657-3085 (TTY)
http://www.gatfl.org

UNIVERSITY-AFFILIATED PROGRAM

University Affiliated Program of GA for Persons with Developmental Disabilities
The University of Georgia
850 College Station Road
Athens, GA 30602-4806
(706) 542-3457

HAWAII

DEVELOPMENTAL DISABILITIES PLANNING COUNCIL

State Planning Council on Developmental Disabilities
919 Ala Moana Boulevard, #113
Honolulu, HI 96814
(808) 586-8100

OFFICE OF STATE DIRECTOR OF VOCATIONAL EDUCATION

Office of the State Director for Career and Technical Education
University of Hawaii
Lower Campus Road
Lunalilo Freeway Portable 1
Honolulu, HI 96822-2489
(808) 956-7461
http://www.hawaii.edu/cte

PROGRAMS FOR CHILDREN AND YOUTH WHO ARE DEAF OR HARD OF HEARING

HI State Coordinating Council on Deafness
919 Ala Moana Boulevard, Room 101
Honolulu, HI 96814
(808) 586-8131 (V/TTY) or (808) 586-8130 (TTY)

PROGRAMS FOR CHILDREN WITH DISABILITIES: AGES THREE THROUGH FIVE

Special Education Section
Department of Education
3430 Leahi Avenue
Honolulu, HI 96815
(808) 733-4840

PROGRAMS FOR CHILDREN WITH SPECIAL HEALTH-CARE NEEDS

Children with Special Health Needs Branch
Department of Health
741 Sunset Avenue
Honolulu, HI 96816
(808) 733-9070
http://www.hawaii.gov/health/family-childhealth/
    cshcn/index.html

**PROGRAMS FOR INFANTS AND TODDLERS
WITH DISABILITIES: AGES BIRTH
THROUGH TWO**

Zero-to-Three Hawaii Project
Department of Health
1600 Kapiolani Boulevard, Suite 1401
Honolulu, HI 96814
(808) 957-0066

PROTECTION AND ADVOCACY AGENCY

Protection and Advocacy Agency
1580 Makaloa Street, Suite 1060
Honolulu, HI 96814
(808) 949-2922 or (800) 882-1057 (in HI)

**STATE DEPARTMENT OF EDUCATION:
SPECIAL EDUCATION**

Special Education Section
HI Department of Education
3430 Leahi Avenue
Honolulu, HI 96815
(808) 733-4990

**STATE EDUCATION AGENCY RURAL
REPRESENTATIVE**

**Office of Accountability and School
Instructional Services**
P.O. Box 2360
Honolulu, HI 96804
(808) 586-3316

STATE MENTAL HEALTH AGENCY

Adult Mental Health Division
1250 Punchbowl #256
Honolulu, HI 96813
(808) 586-4434
http://www.amhd.org

**STATE MENTAL HEALTH
REPRESENTATIVE FOR CHILDREN**

Child and Adolescent Mental Health Division
Department of Health
3627 Kilauea Avenue, Suite 101
Honolulu, HI 96816
(808) 733-9333
http://www.hawaii.gov/health/mental-health/camhd

STATE MENTAL RETARDATION PROGRAM

Developmental Disabilities Division
P.O. Box 3378
Honolulu, HI 96801
(808) 586-5840

**STATE VOCATIONAL
REHABILITATION AGENCY**

Division of Vocational Rehabilitation
Department of Human Services
1000 Bishop Street, Room 605
Honolulu, HI 96813
(808) 586-5355

UNIVERSITY-AFFILIATED PROGRAM

**Hawaii University Affiliated Program for
Developmental Disabilities**
University of Hawaii at Manoa
1776 University Avenue, UA 4-6
Honolulu, HI 96822
(808) 956-5009

IDAHO

**PARENT TRAINING INFORMATION
PROJECT**

Idaho Parents Unlimited Inc. (IPUL)
600 North Curtis Road, Suite 145
Boise, ID 83706
(208) 342-5884 (V/TTY) or (800) 242-4785
    (in ID)
http://www.ipuidaho.org

**PROGRAMS FOR CHILDREN
AND YOUTH WHO ARE DEAF
OR HARD OF HEARING**

**Idaho Council for the Deaf and Hard of
Hearing**
1720 Westgate Drive, Suite A
Boise, ID 83704
(208) 334-0879 (V); (208) 334-0803 (TTY);
    (800) 433-1323 (Voice-in ID only);
    (800) 433-1361 (TTY-in ID only)
http://www2.state.id.us/cdhh/cdhh1.htm

PROGRAMS FOR CHILDREN WITH DISABILITIES: AGES THREE THROUGH FIVE

Contact STATE DEPARTMENT OF EDUCATION: SPECIAL EDUCATION

PROGRAMS FOR CHILDREN WITH SPECIAL HEALTH-CARE NEEDS

Children's Special Health Program
Bureau of Clinical and Preventive Services
Idaho Department of Health and Welfare
P.O. Box 83720
Boise, ID 83720-0036
(208) 334-5962
http://www.healthandwelfare.idaho.gov

PROGRAMS FOR INFANTS AND TODDLERS WITH DISABILITIES: AGES BIRTH THROUGH TWO

Infant Toddler Program
Bureau of Developmental Disabilities
Department of Health and Welfare
450 West State Street
Boise, ID 83720-0036
(208) 334-5514
http://www.idahochild.org

PROTECTION AND ADVOCACY AGENCY

Comprehensive Advocacy, Inc.
4477 Emerald Street, Suite B-100
Boise, ID 83706
(208) 336-5353 or (800) 632-5125
http://users.moscow.com/co-ad

REGIONAL ADA ASSISTIVE TECHNOLOGY AGENCY WA

State Governor's Committee on Disability Issues and Employment
Idaho Department of Labor
317 West Main Street
Boise, ID 83735
(360) 334-6264 (V/TTY)

STATE AGENCY FOR THE BLIND AND VISUALLY IMPAIRED

Commission for the Blind and Visually Impaired (ICBVI)
341 West Washington Street
Boise, ID 83702
(208) 334-3220

STATE DEPARTMENT OF EDUCATION: SPECIAL EDUCATION

Special Education Section
Idaho Department of Education
P.O. Box 83720
Boise, ID 83720-0027
(208) 332-6910
http://www.sde.state.id.us/SpecialEd

STATE DEVELOPMENTAL DISABILITIES COUNCIL

Idaho State Council on Developmental Disabilities
802 West Bannock, Suite 308
Boise, ID 83702-5840
(208) 334-2178
http://www2.state.id.us/icdd

STATE DIVISION OF VOCATIONAL EDUCATION

State Division of Professional Technical Education
P.O. Box 83720
Boise, ID 83720-0095
(208) 334-3216

STATE EDUCATION AGENCY RURAL REPRESENTATIVE

Department of Education
650 West State Street
Boise, ID 83720-0001
(208) 334-2165

STATE MENTAL HEALTH AGENCY

Bureau of Mental Health and Substance Abuse
Division of Family and Community Service

Department of Health and Welfare
P.O. Box 83720
Boise, ID 83720-0036
(208) 334-6500

STATE MENTAL HEALTH
REPRESENTATIVE FOR CHILDREN

Division of Family and Community Services
Department of Health and Welfare
P.O. Box 83720
Boise, ID 83720-0036
(208) 334-5525

STATE MENTAL RETARDATION
PROGRAM

Bureau of Developmental Disabilities
Division of Family and Community Services
Department of Health and Welfare
P.O. Box 83720
Boise, ID 83720-0036

STATE VOCATIONAL
REHABILITATION AGENCY

Division of Rehabilitation
P.O. Box 83720
Boise, ID 83720-0096
(208) 334-3390 (V/TTY) or (208) 334-5512

TECHNOLOGY-RELATED ASSISTANCE

Idaho Assistive Technology Project
129 W. Third Street
Moscow, ID 83843
(800) 432-8324 (V/TTY) or (208) 885-3573
http://www.ets.uidaho.edu/icdd

UNIVERSITY-AFFILIATED
PROGRAM

ID Center on Developmental Disabilities
University Affiliated Program/University
    of Idaho
129 W. Third Street
Moscow, ID 83843
(208) 885-3559
http://www.ets.uidaho.edu/icdd

ILLINOIS

CLIENT ASSISTANCE PROGRAM

Illinois Client Assistance Program
100 North First Street, First Floor West
Springfield, IL 62702-5197
(217) 782-5374 (V/TTY)

OFFICE OF STATE COORDINATOR
OF VOCATIONAL EDUCATION
FOR STUDENTS WITH DISABILITIES

Illinois State Board of Education
100 North First Street, C-418
Springfield, IL 62777-0001
(217) 782-3370

PARENT-TO-PARENT

Family Resource Center on Disabilities
20 East Jackson Boulevard, Suite 900
Chicago, IL 60604
(312) 939-3513 or (800) 952-4199

PARENT TRAINING AND INFORMATION
PROJECTS

Charlotte Des Jardins, Director
Family Resource Center on Disabilities
20 East Jackson Boulevard, Room 900
Chicago, IL 60604
(312) 939-3513; (312) 939-3519 (TTY);
    (800) 952-4199

Family T.I.E.S. Network
830 S. Spring Street
Springfield, IL 62704
(800) 865-7842; (217) 544-5809 (V);
    (217) 544-5826 (TTY)

National Center for Latinos with Disabilities
1921 S. Blue Island Avenue
Chicago, IL 60608
(312) 666-3393 or (312) 666-1788 (TTY)

PROGRAMS FOR CHILDREN AND YOUTH
WHO ARE DEAF OR HARD OF HEARING

**Division of Services for Persons who are Deaf
    or Hard of Hearing**
Department of Rehabilitation Services

100 West Randolph Street, Suite 8-100
Chicago, IL 60601
(312) 814-2939 or (312) 814-3040 (TTY)

PROGRAMS FOR CHILDREN WITH DISABILITIES: AGES THREE THROUGH FIVE

Center for Educational Innovation and Reform
Department of Early Childhood Education
100 North First Street, E-230
Springfield, IL 62777-0001
(217) 524-4835

PROGRAMS FOR CHILDREN WITH SPECIAL HEALTH-CARE NEEDS

Division of Specialized Care for Children
University of Illinois at Chicago
P.O. Box 19481
2815 West Washington, Suite 300
Springfield, IL 62794-9481
(217) 793-2340

PROGRAMS FOR INFANTS AND TODDLERS AGES BIRTH THROUGH TWO

Help Me Grow
Bureau of Part H/Early Intervention
Dept. of Human Services
P.O. Box 19429
Springfield, IL 62794-9429
(217) 782-1981 or (800) 323-4769 (in IL)

PROTECTION AND ADVOCACY AGENCY

Equip for Equality, Inc.
11 East Adams, Suite 1200
Chicago, IL 60603
(312) 341-0022

REGIONAL ADA TECHNICAL ASSISTANCE AGENCY

University of IL/Chicago
Institute on Disability and Human Development
1640 West Roosevelt Road (MC/626)
Chicago, IL 60608-6902
(312) 413-1407 (V/TTY)

STATE DEPARTMENT OF EDUCATION: SPECIAL EDUCATION

Center for Educational Innovation and Reform
Program Compliance
100 North First Street, E-228
Springfield, IL 62777-0001
(217) 782-5589

Special Education Coordination
Illinois State Board of Education
100 North First Street
Springfield, IL 62777-0001
(217) 782-3371

STATE DEVELOPMENTAL DISABILITIES PLANNING COUNCIL

Illinois Planning Council on Developmental Disabilities
830 S. Spring Street
Springfield, IL 62704
(217) 782-9696 (V/TTY)

STATE EDUCATION AGENCY RURAL REPRESENTATIVE

Dept. of Rural Education, IL State Board of Education
123 South Tenth Street, Suite 200
Mt. Vernon, IL 62864
(618) 244-8383

STATE MENTAL HEALTH AGENCY

Division of Disability and Behavior Health Services
Department of Human Services
100 S. Grand Avenue West
Springfield, IL 62765
(217) 785-1469

STATE MENTAL HEALTH REPRESENTATIVE FOR CHILDREN

Department of Human Services
400 Stratton Building
Springfield, IL 62765
(217) 782-7555

STATE MENTAL RETARDATION PROGRAM

Department of Human Services
416 Stratton Building
Springfield, IL 62765
(217) 524-0453

STATE VOCATIONAL REHABILITATION AGENCY

Office of Rehabilitation Services
Department of Human Services
P.O. Box 19429
Springfield, IL 62794-9429
(217) 785-0218 (V) or (217) 782-5734 (TTY)

TECHNOLOGY-RELATED ASSISTANCE

Illinois Assistive Technology Project
One W. Old State Capitol Plaza, Suite 100
Springfield, IL 62701
(217) 522-7985(V/TTY) or (800) 852-5110
    (V/TTY, in IL)

UNIVERSITY-AFFILIATED PROGRAM

Institute on Disability and Human Development
University of Illinois at Chicago
1640 West Roosevelt Road
Chicago, IL 60608
(312) 413-1647 (V) or (312) 413-0453 (TTY)

INDIANA

DEVELOPMENTAL DISABILITIES PLANNING COUNCIL

Governor's Planning Council on Developmental Disabilities
143 West Market Street, Suite 404
Indianapolis, IN 46204
(317) 722-5555 (V) or (317) 722-5563 (TTY)

OFFICE OF STATE COORDINATOR OF VOCATIONAL EDUCATION FOR STUDENTS WITH DISABILITIES

Program Improvement and Modernization
325 West Washington Street

Indianapolis, IN 46204
(317) 232-1829

PARENT-TO-PARENT

Indiana Parent Information Network, Inc.
4755 Kingsway Drive, Suite 105
Indianapolis, IN 46205-1545
(317) 257-8683
http://www.ai.org/ipin

PARENT TRAINING AND INFORMATION PROJECT IN*SOURCE

809 North Michigan Street
South Bend, IN 46601-1036
(219) 234-7101; (219) 234-7101 (TTY);
    (800) 332-4433 (in IN)

PROGRAMS FOR CHILDREN AND YOUTH WHO ARE DEAF OR HARD OF HEARING

Deaf and Hard of Hearing Services
Division of Disability, Aging, and Rehabilitative
    Services
402 West Washington Street, Room W-453
P.O. Box 7083
Indianapolis, IN 46207-7083
(317) 232-1143 (V/TTY) or (800) 962-8408
    (V/TTY, in IN)

PROGRAMS FOR CHILDREN WITH DISABILITIES: AGES THREE THROUGH FIVE

Division of Special Education, Department of Education
State House, Room 229
Indianapolis, IN 46204-2798
(317) 232-0570

PROGRAMS FOR CHILDREN WITH SPECIAL HEALTH-CARE NEEDS

Children's Special Health Care Services
Division of Family and Children
Two N. Meridian Street, Section 7-B
Indianapolis, IN 46204
(317) 233-5578

PROGRAMS FOR INFANTS AND TODDLERS WITH DISABILITIES: AGES BIRTH THROUGH TWO

Indiana Family and Social Services Administration
Division of Families and Children/Bureau of Child Development
402 West Washington Street, Room W-386
Indianapolis, IN 46204
(317) 232-2429 or (317) 232-7948 (Fax)

PROTECTION AND ADVOCACY AGENCY

Indiana Protection and Advocacy Services
4701 N. Keystone Avenue
Indianapolis, IN 46205
(317) 722-5555; (800) 622-4845;
    (800) 838-1131 (TTY)

STATE DEPARTMENT OF EDUCATION: SPECIAL EDUCATION

Division of Special Education, Dept. of Education
State House, Room 229
Indianapolis, IN 46204-2798
(317) 232-0570
http://ideanet.doe.state.in.us/exceptional

STATE DIVISION OF VOCATIONAL REHABILITATION

Indiana Family and Social Services Administration
Vocational Rehabilitation Services
Division of Disability, Aging, and Rehabilitative Services
402 W. Washington Street, Room W453
P.O. Box 7083
Indianapolis, IN 46207-7083
(317) 232-1319 or (800) 545-7763, ext. 1319

STATE MENTAL HEALTH AGENCY

Indiana Family and Social Services Administration
Division of Mental Health, Family and Social Services Administration
402 West Washington Street, Room W353
Indianapolis, IN 46204-2739
(317) 232-7845

STATE MENTAL HEALTH REPRESENTATIVE FOR CHILDREN

Indiana Family and Social Services Administration
Childrens Services Bureau
Division of Mental Health
402 West Washington Street, Room W353
Indianapolis, IN 46204-2739
(317) 232-7934

STATE MENTAL RETARDATION PROGRAM

Indiana Family and Social Services Administration
Division of Disability, Aging and Rehabilitative Services
Bureau of Developmental Disabilities Services
402 West Washington Street
Indianapolis, IN 46204-2739
(317) 232-7933

TECHNOLOGY-RELATED ASSISTANCE

ATTAIN (Accessing Technology Through Action in Indiana)
1815 N. Meridian Street, Suite 200
Indianapolis, IN 46202
(800) 528-8246 (in IN); (317) 921-8766 (in Marion County); (800) 743-3333 (TTY)

UNIVERSITY-AFFILIATED PROGRAM

Indiana Institute on Disability and Community
Indiana University, Bloomington
2853 East 10th Street
Bloomington, IN 47408-2601
(812) 855-6508 or (812) 855-9396 (TTY)
http://www.isdd.indiana.edu

Riley Child Development Center
Indiana University School of Medicine
James Whitcomb Riley Hospital for Children
702 Barnhill Drive, Room 5837
Indianapolis, IN 46202-5225
(317) 274-8167

IOWA

CLIENT ASSISTANCE PROGRAM

Dept. Human Rights
Client Assistance Program
Capitol Complex, Lucas Building
Des Moines, IA 50319
(515) 281-3957 or (800) 652-4198 (V/TTY)

DEVELOPMENTAL DISABILITIES PLANNING COUNCIL

Governor's Developmental Disabilities Council
617 E. Second Street
Des Moines, IA 50309
(515) 281-9083

OFFICE OF STATE COORDINATOR OF VOCATIONAL EDUCATION FOR STUDENTS WITH DISABILITIES

Bureau of Community Colleges/Department of Education
Grimes State Office Building
Des Moines, IA 50319-0146
(515) 281-3866

PARENT TRAINING AND INFORMATION CENTER

SEEK Parent Center
406 SW School Street, Suite 207
Ankeny, IA 50021
(515) 956-0155 or (888) 431-4332

PROGRAMS FOR CHILDREN AND YOUTH WHO ARE DEAF OR HARD OF HEARING

Deaf Services Commission of Iowa
Iowa Department of Human Rights
Lucas State Office Building
Des Moines, IA 50319-0090
(515) 281-3164 (V/TTY)

PROGRAMS FOR CHILDREN WITH DISABILITIES: AGES THREE THROUGH FIVE

Bureau of Family and Community Services
Grimes State Office Building
Des Moines, IA 50319-0146
(515) 281-5433

PROGRAMS FOR CHILDREN WITH SPECIAL HEALTH-CARE NEEDS

Iowa Child Health Specialty Clinics
247 Hospital School
100 Hawkins Drive
Iowa City, IA 52242-1011
(319) 356-1118 or (319) 356-3715

PROGRAMS FOR INFANTS AND TODDLERS WITH DISABILITIES: AGES BIRTH THROUGH TWO

Iowa's System of Early Intervention Services
Grimes State Office Building
Des Moines, IA 50319-0146
(515) 281-7145

PROTECTION AND ADVOCACY AGENCY

Iowa Protection and Advocacy Services, Inc.
3015 Merle Hay Road, Suite Six
Des Moines, IA 50310
(515) 278-2502; (515) 278-0571 (TTY);
   (800) 779-2502

REGIONAL ADA TECHNICAL ASSISTANCE AGENCY

University of Missouri/Columbia
4812 Santanna Circle
Columbia, MO 65203
(573) 882-3600
http://www.idir.net/~adabbs

STATE AGENCY FOR THE VISUALLY IMPAIRED

Iowa Department for the Blind
524 Fourth Street
Des Moines, IA 50309-2364
(515) 281-1333 or (515) 281-1355 (TTY)
(515) 281-1263 (fax)

STATE DEPARTMENT OF EDUCATION: SPECIAL EDUCATION

Bureau of Family and Community Services
Department of Education

Grimes State Office Building
Des Moines, IA 50319-0146
(515) 281-5735
http://www.state.ia.us/educate

STATE DEVELOPMENTAL DISABILITIES PROGRAM

Division of Mental Health and Developmental Disabilities
Iowa Department of Human Services
Hoover State Office Building
1305 E. Walnut
Des Moines, IA 50319-0114
(515) 281-5126

STATE DIVISION OF VOCATIONAL REHABILITATION

Division of Vocational Rehabilitation Services/Department of Education
510 East 12th Street
Des Moines, IA 50319
(515) 281-4311

STATE EDUCATION AGENCY RURAL REPRESENTATIVE

Bureau of Children, Family and Community Services
Department of Education
Grimes State Office Building
Des Moines, IA 50319-0146
(515) 281-5735

STATE MENTAL HEALTH AGENCY

Division of Mental Health/Developmental Disabilities, Dept. of Human Services
Hoover State Office Building
1305 E. Walnut
Des Moines, IA 50319-0114
(515) 281-5126

STATE MENTAL HEALTH REPRESENTATIVE FOR CHILDREN

Division of Mental Health/Developmental Disabilities
Department of Human Services
Hoover State Office Building

Des Moines, IA 50319-0114
(515) 281-6086

TECHNOLOGY-RELATED ASSISTANCE

Iowa Program for Assistive Technology
Iowa University Affiliated Program
100 Hawkins Drive
Iowa City, IA 52242-1011
(800) 331-3027 (V/TTY) or (319) 356-0550
http://www.uiowa.edu/infotech

UNIVERSITY-AFFILIATED PROGRAM

Iowa University Affiliated Program
Division of Developmental Disabilities
University Hospital School
The University of Iowa
Iowa City, IA 52242
(319) 353-6390
http://www.uiowa.edu/uhs

KANSAS

CLIENT ASSISTANCE PROGRAM

Client Assistance Program
2914 SW Plass Ct., Suite B
Topeka, KS 66611-1925
(785) 266-8193 or (800) 432-2326

OFFICE OF STATE COORDINATOR OF VOCATIONAL EDUCATION FOR STUDENTS WITH DISABILITIES

Technical Education Team
Kansas State Department of Education
120 Southeast 10th Avenue
Topeka, KS 66612
(785) 296-2221

PARENT TRAINING AND INFORMATION CENTER

Families Together, Inc.
3340 W. Douglas, Suite 102
Wichita, KS 67203

(316) 945-7747; (888) 815-6364 (Wichita);
(800) 264-6343 (Topeka); (888) 820-6364
(Garden City); (800) 499-9443 (Spanish)
http://www.kansas.net/~family

PROGRAMS FOR CHILDREN AND YOUTH WHO ARE DEAF OR HARD OF HEARING

KS Commission for the Deaf and Hard of Hearing
3640 SW Topeka Boulevard, Suite 150
Topeka, KS 66611
(785) 267-6100 (V/TTY)or (800) 432-0698
(V/TTY, in KS)
http://www.ink.org/public/srs/KCDHH.html

PROGRAMS FOR CHILDREN WITH DISABILITIES: AGES THREE THROUGH FIVE

Student Support Services
Kansas State Department of Education
120 East 10th Avenue
Topeka, KS 66612-1182
(785) 296-7454

PROGRAMS FOR CHILDREN WITH SPECIAL HEALTH-CARE NEEDS

Services for Children with Special Health Care Needs
Department of Health and Environment
Landon State Office Building, 10th Floor
900 S.W. Jackson
Topeka, KS 66612
(785) 296-1316 or (800) 332-6262

PROGRAMS FOR INFANTS AND TODDLERS WITH DISABILITIES: AGES BIRTH THROUGH TWO

Infant-Toddler Services
State Department of Health and Environment
Landon State Office Building
900 S.W. Jackson, 10th Floor
Topeka, KS 66612-1290
(785) 296-6135

PROTECTION AND ADVOCACY AGENCY

Kansas Advocacy and Protective Services
3218 Kimball Avenue

Manhattan, KS 66503
(785) 776-1541 or (800) 432-8276

REGIONAL ADA TECHNICAL ASSISTANCE AGENCY

ADA Project
University of Missouri/Columbia
4812 Santanna Circle
Columbia, MO 65203
(573) 882-3600 (V/TTY)

STATE DEPARTMENT OF EDUCATION: SPECIAL EDUCATION

Student Support Services
Kansas State Department of Education
120 East 10th Avenue
Topeka, KS 66612
(785) 291-3097

STATE DEVELOPMENTAL DISABILITIES PLANNING COUNCIL

Kansas Council on Developmental Disabilities
Docking State Office Building, Room 141
915 SW Harrison Avenue
Topeka, KS 66612-1570
(785) 296-2608

STATE DEVELOPMENTAL DISABILITIES PROGRAM

Developmental Disabilities Services
Docking State Office Building, Fifth Floor North
Topeka, KS 66612-1570
(785) 296-3561

STATE DIVISION OF VOCATIONAL REHABILITATION

Rehabilitation Services
Department of Social and Rehabilitation Services
3640 SW Topeka Boulevard, Suite 150
Topeka, KS 66611
(785) 267-5301

STATE EDUCATION AGENCY RURAL REPRESENTATIVE

Student Support Services
State Board of Education

120 East 10th Avenue
Topeka, KS 66612
(913) 291-3097

STATE MENTAL HEALTH AND DEVELOPMENTAL DISABILITIES COMMISSION

Mental Health and Developmental Disabilities
Dept. of Social and Rehabilitation Services
Docking State Office Building
915 SW Harrison Street, Fifth Floor North
Topeka, KS 66612-1570
(913) 296-3773

STATE MENTAL HEALTH REPRESENTATIVE FOR CHILDREN AND YOUTH

Child and Adolescent Mental Health Programs
Docking State Office Building, Fifth Floor North
Topeka, KS 66612-1570
(785) 296-7272

TECHNOLOGY-RELATED ASSISTANCE

Assistive Technology for Kansans Project
2601 Gabriel
P.O. Box 738
Parsons, KS 67357
(316) 421-8367 (V/TTY); (316) 421-0954 (fax)

UNIVERSITY-AFFILIATED PROGRAM

Span Institute
University of Kansas
1052 Robert Dole Human Development Center
Lawrence, KS 66045
(785) 864-4295

University of Kansas Medical Center, Kansas City
4001 Miller Building, 3901 Rainbow Boulevard
Kansas City, Kansas 66106-7335
(913) 588-5943

KENTUCKY

CLIENT ASSISTANCE PROGRAM

Client Assistance Program
209 St. Clair, Fifth Floor

Frankfort, KY 40601
(502) 564-8035 or (800) 633-6283 (in KY)

DIRECTIONS DISABILITY LINK

Ask Us, Inc.
201 Burley Avenue
Lexington, KY 40503-1009
(606) 233-9370

DIVISION OF SECONDARY VOCATIONAL EDUCATION

Special Vocational Programs
Capitol Plaza Tower, Room 2114
500 Mero Street
Frankfort, KY 40601
(502) 564-3775
http://www.kde.state.ky.us

PARENT-TO-PARENT

Parent Outreach: Parents Supporting Parents
1146 South Third Street
Louisville, KY 40203
(502) 584-1239

PARENT TRAINING AND INFORMATION PROJECT

Paulette Logsdon, Director
Kentucky Special Parent Involvement Network (KY-SPIN)
2210 Goldsmith Lane, Suite 118
Louisville, KY 40218
(502) 456-0923 or (800) 525-7746

PROGRAMS FOR CHILDREN AND YOUTH WHO ARE DEAF OR HARD OF HEARING

Kentucky Commission on the Deaf and Hard of Hearing
632 Versailles Road
Frankfort, KY 40601
(502) 573-2604 (V/TTY) or (800) 372-2907 (V/TTY, in KY)
http://www.state.ky.us/agencies/kcdhh

PROGRAMS FOR CHILDREN WITH DISABILITIES: AGES THREE THROUGH FIVE

Office of Learning Program Development
500 Mero Street, Capitol Plaza Tower, 16th Floor
Frankfort, KY 40601
(502) 564-7056
http://www.kde.state.ky.us

PROGRAMS FOR CHILDREN WITH SPECIAL HEALTH-CARE NEEDS

Commission for Children with Special Health Care Needs
982 Eastern Parkway
Louisville, KY 40217-1566
(502) 595-4459 or (800) 232-1160

PROGRAMS FOR INFANTS AND TODDLERS WITH DISABILITIES: AGES BIRTH THROUGH TWO

Infant and Toddler Program
Department of Mental Health and Mental Retardation Services
100 Fair Oaks Lane, 4E-E
Frankfort, KY 40621-0001
(502) 564-7700

PROTECTION AND ADVOCACY AGENCY

Department for Public Advocacy, Protection and Advocacy Division
100 Fair Oaks Lane, Third Floor
Frankfort, KY 40601
(502) 564-2967 or (800) 372-2988 (V/TTY, in KY)

STATE AGENCY FOR THE VISUALLY IMPAIRED

Department for the Blind
P.O. Box 757
Frankfort, KY 40602-0757
(502) 564-4754

STATE DEPARTMENT OF EDUCATION: SPECIAL EDUCATION

Division of Exceptional Children's Services
Kentucky Department of Education
Capitol Plaza Tower, Eighth Floor

500 Mero Street
Frankfort, KY 40601
(502) 564-4970
http://www.kde.state.ky.us

STATE DEVELOPMENTAL DISABILITIES PLANNING COUNCIL

Kentucky Developmental Disabilities Planning Council
Dept. For Mental Health/Mental Retardation Services
100 Fair Oaks Lane, 4E-F
Frankfort, KY 40621-0001
(502) 564-7842

STATE DIVISION OF VOCATIONAL REHABILITATION

Department of Vocational Rehabilitation
Cabinet for Workforce Development
209 St. Clair
Frankfort, KY 40601
(502) 564-4440

STATE EDUCATION AGENCY RURAL REPRESENTATIVE

Department of Education
500 Mero Street, Capitol Plaza Tower, Eighth Floor
Frankfort, KY 40601
(502) 564-4970

STATE MENTAL HEALTH AGENCY

Department for Mental Health/Mental Retardation Services
Cabinet for Health Services
100 Fair Oaks Lane
Frankfort, KY 40601-0001
(502) 564-4527

STATE MENTAL HEALTH REPRESENTATIVE FOR CHILDREN AND YOUTH

Children and Youth Services Branch
Department for Mental Health and Mental Retardation Services
100 Fair Oaks Lane, 4W-C

Frankfort, KY 40621-0001
(502) 564-7610

STATE MENTAL RETARDATION PROGRAM

Division of Mental Retardation/ Department for
Mental Health and Mental Retardation Services
100 Fair Oaks Lane, 4E-E
Frankfort, KY 40621-0001
(502) 564-7702

TECHNOLOGY-RELATED ASSISTANCE

Kentucky Assistive Technology Service (KATS) Network
Charles McDowell Center
8412 Westport Road
Louisville, KY 40242
(800) 327-5287 or (502) 327-0022
http://www.katsnet.org

UNIVERSITY-AFFILIATED PROGRAM

Human Development Institute
University Affiliated Facility
University of Kentucky
126 Mineral Industries Building
Lexington, KY 40506-0051
(606) 257-1714

LOUISIANA

CLIENT ASSISTANCE PROGRAM

Client Assistant Program
Advocacy Center for the Elderly and Disabled
225 Baronne Street, Suite 2112
New Orleans, LA 70112-2112
(504) 522-2337

OFFICE OF STATE COORDINATOR OF VOCATIONAL EDUCATION FOR STUDENTS WITH DISABILITIES

Department of Education/Office of Vocational Education
P.O. Box 94064
Baton Rouge, LA 70804-9064
(504) 342-5250

PARENT-TO-PARENT

Parent-to-Parent of Louisiana, Family Support Program
200 Henry Clay Avenue
New Orleans, LA 70118
(800) 299-9511, extension 4268

PARENT TRAINING AND INFORMATION PROJECT

Project PROMPT
4323 Division Street, Suite 110
Metairie, LA 70002-3179
(504) 888-9111 or (800) 766-7736 (in LA)

PROGRAMS FOR CHILDREN WITH DISABILITIES: AGES THREE THROUGH FIVE

Preschool Programs, Office of Special Education Services
Department of Education
P.O. Box 94064
Baton Rouge, LA 70804-9064
(504) 763-3555

PROGRAMS FOR CHILDREN WITH SPECIAL HEALTH-CARE NEEDS

Handicapped Children's Services
Office of Public Health
Department of Health and Human Resources
P.O. Box 60630, Room 607
New Orleans, LA 70160
(504) 568-5055

PROGRAMS FOR INFANTS AND TODDLERS WITH DISABILITIES: AGES BIRTH THROUGH TWO

Office of Special Education Services/ Dept. of Education
P.O. Box 94064
Baton Rouge, LA 70804-9064
(504) 763-3540

PROTECTION AND ADVOCACY AGENCY

Advocacy Center for the Elderly and Disabled
225 Baronne Street, Suite 2112
New Orleans, LA 70112-2112
(504) 522-2337 or (800) 960-7705 (in LA)

STATE DEPARTMENT OF EDUCATION: SPECIAL EDUCATION

Office of Special Educational Services
Louisiana State Department of Education
P.O. Box 94064
Baton Rouge, LA 70804-9064
(504) 342-3633

STATE DEVELOPMENTAL DISABILITIES PLANNING COUNCIL

Developmental Disabilities Council
P.O. Box 3455
Baton Rouge, LA 70821-3455
(504) 342-6804 or (800) 922-DIAL (in LA)

STATE DIVISION OF VOCATIONAL REHABILITATION

Dept. of Social Services/LA Rehabilitation Services
8225 Florida Boulevard
Baton Rouge, LA 70806-4834
(504) 925-4131

STATE EDUCATION AGENCY RURAL REPRESENTATIVE

Department of Education
Special Education
P.O. Box 599
Rayville, LA 71269

STATE MENTAL HEALTH AGENCY

Office of Human Services, Dept. of Health and Hospitals
P.O. Box 4049 - BIN #12
Baton Rouge, LA 70821-4049
(504) 342-9238

STATE MENTAL HEALTH REPRESENTATIVE FOR CHILDREN AND YOUTH

Office of Mental Health
Department of Health and Hospitals
P.O. Box 4049 - Bin #12
Baton Rouge, LA 70821-4049
(504) 342-9524

STATE MENTAL RETARDATION PROGRAM

Office for Citizens with Developmental Disabilities
Box 3117, Bin 21
Baton Rouge, LA 70821-3117
(504) 342-0095

STATE UNIVERSITY AFFILIATED PROGRAM

Human Development Center
Louisiana State University Medical Center
1100 Florida Avenue, Building 138
New Orleans, LA 70119
(504) 942-8200

TECHNOLOGY-RELATED ASSISTANCE

Louisiana Assistive Technology Access Network
P.O. Box 14115
Baton Rouge, LA 70898
(504) 925-9500 or (800) 270-6185 (V/TTY)

MAINE

CLIENT ASSISTANCE PROGRAM

C.A.R.E.S., Inc.
Four C Winter Street
Augusta, ME 04330
(207) 622-7055 or (800) 773-7055

OFFICE OF STATE COORDINATOR OF VOCATIONAL EDUCATION FOR STUDENTS WITH DISABILITIES

Programs for the Handicapped and Disadvantaged
Division of Program Services and Finance
Department of Education
23 State House Station
Augusta, ME 04333-0023
(207) 287-5854

PARENT TRAINING AND INFORMATION PROJECT

Maine Parent Federation/SPIN
P.O. Box 2067

Augusta, ME 04338-2067
(207) 582-2504 or (800) 870-7746 (in ME)

PROGRAMS FOR CHILDREN WITH DISABILITIES: AGES THREE THROUGH FIVE

Child Development Services
State House, Station #146
Augusta, ME 04333
(207) 287-3272

PROGRAMS FOR CHILDREN WITH SPECIAL HEALTH-CARE NEEDS

Coordinated Care Services for Children with Special Health Needs
Department of Human Services
151 Capitol Street, State House, Station #11
Augusta, ME 04333
(207) 287-5139

PROTECTION AND ADVOCACY AGENCY

Maine Advocacy Services
32 Winthrop Street, P.O. Box 2007
Augusta, ME 04338-2007
(207) 626-2774 or (800) 452-1948 (TTY, in ME)

STATE DEPARTMENT OF EDUCATION: SPECIAL EDUCATION

Division of Special Education, Dept. of Education
State House, Station #23
Augusta, ME 04333-0023
(207) 287-5950

STATE DEVELOPMENTAL DISABILITIES PLANNING COUNCIL

ME Developmental Disabilities Council
139 State House Station, Nash Building
Capitol and Sewall Streets
Augusta, ME 04333-0139
(207) 287-4213

STATE EDUCATION AGENCY RURAL REPRESENTATIVE

Division of Special Education
Department of Education

State House, Station #23
Augusta, ME 04333-0023
(207) 287-5950

STATE MENTAL HEALTH AGENCY

Department of Mental Health, Mental Retardation and Substance Abuse Services
411 State Office Building, Station #40
Augusta, ME 04333
(207) 287-4223

STATE MENTAL HEALTH REPRESENTATIVE FOR CHILDREN AND YOUTH

Division of Children with Special Needs
Department of Mental Health, Mental Retardation and Substance Abuse Services
411 State Office Building, Station #40
Augusta, ME 04333
(207) 287-4250

STATE MENTAL RETARDATION PROGRAM

Mental Retardation Services
Department of Mental Health, Mental Retardation and Substance Abuse Services
411 State Office Building, Station #40
Augusta, ME 04333
(207) 287-4200 or (207) 287-4242

STATE VOCATIONAL REHABILITATION AGENCY

Office of Rehabilitation Services/Division of Vocational Rehabilitation
Department of Labor
35 Anthony Avenue
Augusta, ME 04333-0150
(207) 624-5300

TECHNOLOGY-RELATED ASSISTANCE

Maine Consumer Information and Technology Training Exchange
Maine CITE Coordinating Center
Education Network of Maine
46 University Drive
Augusta, ME 04330
(207) 621-3195 (V/TTY)

UNIVERSITY-AFFILIATED PROGRAM

Center for Community Inclusion, UAP
5717 Corbett Hall, Room 100
University of Maine
Orono, ME 04469-5717
(207) 581-1084

MARYLAND

CLIENT ASSISTANCE PROGRAM

Client Assistance Program
Department of Education
Division of Rehabilitation Services
2301 Argonne Drive
Baltimore, MD 21218
(410) 554-9358 or (800) 638-6243

GOVERNOR'S OFFICE FOR INDIVIDUALS WITH DISABILITIES

Governor's Office for Individuals with Disabilities
One Market Center, Box 10
300 West Lexington Street
Baltimore, MD 21201-3435
(410) 333-3098 (V/TTY)
e-mail: ojd@clark.net

OFFICE OF STATE COORDINATOR OF VOCATIONAL EDUCATION FOR STUDENTS WITH DISABILITIES

Division of Career Technology and Adult Education
200 West Baltimore Street
Baltimore, MD 21201
(410) 767-0531

PARENT-TO-PARENT

Family Support Network/Maryland Infants and Toddlers Program
Department of Education
Division of Special Education
200 West Baltimore Street, Fourth Floor
Baltimore, MD 21201
(800) 535-0182

PARENT TRAINING AND INFORMATION PROJECT

Parents Place of Maryland, Inc.
801 Cromwell Park Drive, Suite 103
Glen Burnie, MD 21061
(410) 768-9100
http://www.ppmd.org

PROGRAMS FOR CHILDREN WITH DISABILITIES: AGES THREE THROUGH FIVE

Program Development and Assistance Branch
Division of Special Education
200 West Baltimore Street
Baltimore, MD 21201
(410) 767-0237

PROGRAMS FOR CHILDREN WITH SPECIAL HEALTH-CARE NEEDS

Department of Health & Mental Hygiene
Children's Medical Services - Unit 50
201 West Preston Street
Baltimore, MD 21201
(410) 225-5580

PROGRAMS FOR INFANTS AND TODDLERS WITH DISABILITIES: AGES BIRTH THROUGH TWO

Department of Education
Division of Special Education
200 West Baltimore Street, Fourth Floor
Baltimore, MD 21201
(410) 767-0261 or (410) 767-0342
(800) 535-0182 (in MD only)

PROTECTION AND ADVOCACY AGENCY

Maryland Disability Law Center
1800 N. Charles, Suite 204
Baltimore, MD 21201
(410) 234-2791

STATE DEPARTMENT OF EDUCATION: SPECIAL EDUCATION

Department of Education, Division of Special Education
200 West Baltimore Street
Baltimore, MD 21201-2595
(410) 767-0238

STATE DEVELOPMENTAL DISABILITIES PLANNING COUNCIL

Maryland Developmental Disabilities Council
300 West Lexington Street, Box 10
Baltimore, MD 21201-2323
(410) 333-3688

STATE EDUCATION AGENCY RURAL REPRESENTATIVE

Program Administration and Support
Division of Special Education/Department of Education
200 West Baltimore Street, Fourth Floor
Baltimore, MD 21201
(410) 767-0249

STATE MENTAL HEALTH AGENCY

Mental Hygiene Administration
Department of Health and Mental Hygiene
201 West Preston Street, Room 416A
Baltimore, MD 21201
(410) 767-6860

STATE MENTAL HEALTH REPRESENTATIVE FOR CHILDREN AND YOUTH

Division of Child and Adolescent Services
Department of Health and Mental Hygiene
201 West Preston Street
Baltimore, MD 21201
(410) 767-6649

STATE MENTAL RETARDATION PROGRAM

Developmental Disabilities Administration
Department of Health and Mental Hygiene
201 West Preston Street
O'Connor Building, Fourth Floor

Baltimore, MD 21201
(410) 767-5600

STATE VOCATIONAL REHABILITATION AGENCY

Division of Rehabilitation Services
Department of Education, Maryland Rehabilitation Center
2301 Argonne Drive
Baltimore, MD 21218-1696
(410) 554-9385

TECHNOLOGY-RELATED ASSISTANCE

Maryland Technology Assistance Program
Office for Individuals with Disabilities
2301 Argonne Drive, Rm T-17
Baltimore, MD 21218
(410) 333-4975 (V/TTY) or (800) TECH-TAP
http://www.mdtap.org

UNIVERSITY-AFFILIATED PROGRAM

The Kennedy Krieger Institute
707 North Broadway
Baltimore, MD 21205-1890
(410) 550-9483; (410) 550-8446; (800) 873-3377

MASSACHUSETTS

CLIENT ASSISTANCE PROGRAM

Client Assistance Program
Massachusetts Office on Disability
One Ashburton Place, Room 1305
Boston, MA 02108
(617) 727-7440 or (800) 322-2020 (in MA)

OFFICE OF STATE COORDINATOR OF VOCATIONAL EDUCATION FOR STUDENTS WITH DISABILITIES

School to Employment
Department of Education
350 Main Street
Malden, MA 02148-5023
(617) 388-3300

PARENT-TO-PARENT

Families Ties
c/o Massachusetts Dept. of Public Health
250 Washington Street
Boston, MA 02108
(617) 624-5070

Greater Boston Association for Retarded Citizens
1505 Commonwealth Avenue
Boston, MA 02135
(617) 783-3900

Massachusetts Families Organizing for Change
P.O. Box 50
Raynham, MA 02768
(800) 406-3632

PARENT TRAINING AND INFORMATION PROJECT

Federation for Children with Special Needs
1135 Tremont Street, Suite 420
Boston, MA 02120
(617) 236-7210 (V/TTY) or (800) 331-0688 (in MA)
http://www.fcsn.org

PROGRAMS FOR CHILDREN WITH DISABILITIES: AGES THREE THROUGH FIVE

Early Learning Services
Department of Education
350 Main Street
Malden, MA 02148-5023
(617) 388-3300

PROGRAMS FOR CHILDREN WITH SPECIAL HEALTH-CARE NEEDS

Division for Children with Special Health Care Needs
Department of Public Health
250 Washington Street, Fourth Floor
Boston, MA 02108-4619
(617) 624-5070

PROGRAMS FOR INFANTS AND TODDLERS WITH DISABILITIES: AGES BIRTH THROUGH TWO

Early Intervention Services
Department of Public Health
250 Washington Street, Fourth Floor
Boston, MA 02108
(617) 624-5070

PROTECTION AND ADVOCACY AGENCY

Disability Law Center, Inc.
11 Beacon Street, Suite 925
Boston, MA 02108
(617) 723-8455

STATE DEPARTMENT OF EDUCATION: SPECIAL EDUCATION

Educational Improvement Group
Department of Education
350 Main Street
Malden, MA 02148-5023
(617) 388-3300

STATE DEVELOPMENTAL DISABILITIES PLANNING COUNCIL

Massachusetts Developmental Disabilities Council
174 Portland Street, Fifth Floor
Boston, MA 02114
(617) 727-6374, ext. 100 or (617) 727-1885 (TTY)

STATE MENTAL HEALTH AGENCY

Department of Mental Health
25 Staniford Street
Boston, MA 02114
(617) 727-5600

STATE MENTAL HEALTH REPRESENTATIVE FOR CHILDREN AND YOUTH

Child-Adolescent Services
Department of Mental Health
25 Staniford Street

Boston, MA 02114
(617) 727-5600

STATE MENTAL RETARDATION PROGRAM

Department of Mental Retardation
160 North Washington Street
Boston, MA 02114
(617) 727-5608

STATE VOCATIONAL REHABILITATION AGENCY

Massachusetts Rehabilitation Commission
Fort Point Place
27-43 Wormwood Street
Boston, MA 02210-1606
(617) 727-2172

TECHNOLOGY-RELATED ASSISTANCE

Massachusetts Assistive Technology Partnership
MATP Center; Children's Hospital
1295 Boylston Street, Suite 310
Boston, MA 02215
(800) 848-8867 (V/TTY, in MA); (617) 355-7820;
    (617) 355-7301 (TTY)

UNIVERSITY-AFFILIATED PROGRAMS

Eunice Shriver Center UAP
200 Trapello Road
Waltham, MA 02154
(617) 642-0238

Institute for Community Inclusion UAP
Children's Hospital
300 Longwood Avenue
Boston, MA 02115
(617) 355-6506 or (617) 355-6956 (TTY)

MICHIGAN

CLIENT ASSISTANCE PROGRAM

State of Michigan, Michigan Jobs Commission
Michigan Rehabilitation Services, Client Assistance
    Program
P.O. Box 30008

Lansing, MI 48909
(517) 373-8193

OFFICE OF STATE COORDINATOR OF VOCATIONAL EDUCATION FOR STUDENTS WITH DISABILITIES

Special Populations, Programs, and Services
Vocational, Technical Education Service/Dept. of
    Education
P.O. Box 30009
Lansing, MI 48909
(517) 373-6866

PARENT-TO-PARENT

Parent Participation Program
1200 Sixth St., Third Floor, South Tower, Suite 316
Detroit, MI 48226
(313) 256-2186 or (800) 359-3722 (parent
    hotline)

PARENT TRAINING AND INFORMATION PROJECTS

Citizens Alliance to Uphold Special Education (CAUSE)
3303 West Saginaw Street, Suite F1
Lansing, MI 48917-2303
(517) 886-9167 or (800) 221-9105 (in MI)

Parents Training Parents Project/ Parents are Experts
23077 Greenfield Road, Suite 205
Southfield, MI 48075-3744
(248) 557-5070 (V/TTY)

PROGRAMS FOR CHILDREN AND YOUTH WHO ARE DEAF OR HARD OF HEARING

Division on Deafness
Michigan Family Independence Agency
350 North Washington Square, Box 30659
Lansing, MI 48909
(517) 334-7363 (V/TTY)

PROGRAMS FOR CHILDREN WITH DISABILITIES: AGES THREE THROUGH FIVE

Office of Special Education Services
Department of Education

P.O. Box 30008
Lansing, MI 48909
(517) 373-8215

PROGRAMS FOR CHILDREN WITH SPECIAL HEALTH-CARE NEEDS

Children's Special Health Care Services
Bureau of Child and Family Services
Department of Community Health
3423 North Logan, Martin Luther King Boulevard
P.O. Box 30195
Lansing, MI 48909
(517) 335-8969

PROGRAMS FOR INFANTS AND TODDLERS WITH DISABILITIES: AGES BIRTH THROUGH TWO

Comprehensive Program in Health and Early Childhood
Department of Education
P.O. Box 30008
Lansing, MI 48909
(517) 373-6335

PROTECTION AND ADVOCACY AGENCY

Michigan Protection and Advocacy Service
4095 Legacy Parkway, Suite 500
Lansing, MI 48911-4263
(517) 487-1755 or (800) 288-5923
http://www.mpas.org

STATE AGENCY FOR THE VISUALLY IMPAIRED

Commission for the Blind
Family Independence Agency
201 North Washington Square
P.O. Box 30015
Lansing, MI 48909
(517) 373-2062

STATE DEPARTMENT OF EDUCATION: SPECIAL EDUCATION

Office of Special Education Services
Department of Education
P.O. Box 30008
Lansing, MI 48909-7508
(517) 373-9433

STATE DEVELOPMENTAL DISABILITIES PLANNING COUNCIL

Michigan Developmental Disabilities Council
Lewis Cass Building, Sixth Floor
Lansing, MI 48913
(517) 334-6123

STATE MENTAL HEALTH AGENCY

Department of Community Health
Lewis Cass Building
320 South Walnut Boulevard
Lansing, MI 48913
(517) 373-3500

STATE MENTAL HEALTH REPRESENTATIVE FOR CHILDREN AND YOUTH

Office of Children's Services
Department of Community Health
Lewis Cass Building, Sixth Floor
Lansing, MI 48913
(517) 373-1839

STATE MENTAL RETARDATION PROGRAM

Bureau of Community Residential Services
Department of Community Health
Lewis Cass Building, Sixth Floor
Lansing, MI 48913
(517) 373-8209

STATE VOCATIONAL REHABILITATION AGENCY

Michigan Jobs Commission
Michigan Rehabilitation Services
P.O. Box 30010
Lansing, MI 48909
(517) 373-3391

TECHNOLOGY-RELATED ASSISTANCE

Tech 2000: Michigan's Assistive Technology Project
3815 W. St. Joseph Highway
Lansing, MI 48913-3623
(517) 334-6502 or (517) 334-6499 (TTY)

UNIVERSITY-AFFILIATED PROGRAM

Developmental Disabilities Institute, Wayne State University
326 Justice Building
6001 Cass Avenue
Detroit, MI 48202
(313) 577-2654

MINNESOTA

CLIENT ASSISTANCE PROGRAM

Legal Aid Society of Minneapolis
430 First Avenue, N., Suite 300
Minneapolis, MN 55401-1780
(612) 332-1441

OFFICE OF STATE COORDINATOR OF VOCATIONAL EDUCATION FOR STUDENTS WITH DISABILITIES

Secondary Vocational Education
Capitol Square Building, 550 Cedar Street
St. Paul, MN 55101
(612) 296-1085

PARENT-TO-PARENT

Arc Duluth/Pilot Parents
201 Ordean Building
Duluth, MN 55802
(218) 726-4725

PARENT TRAINING AND INFORMATION PROJECT

PACER Center, Inc.
8161 Normandale Boulevard
Minneapolis, MN 55417-1098
(952) 838-9000; (952) 838-0190 (TTY);
    (800) 537-2237 (in MN)
http://www.pacer.org

PROGRAMS FOR CHILDREN AND YOUTH WHO ARE DEAF OR HARD OF HEARING

Minnesota Commission Serving Deaf and Hard of Hearing People
Human Services Building
444 Lafayette Road

St. Paul, MN 55155-3814
(612) 297-7305 (V/TTY)

PROGRAMS FOR CHILDREN WITH DISABILITIES: AGES THREE THROUGH FIVE

Community Collaboration Team
Minnesota Department of Children, Families and Learning
986 Capitol Square Building
550 Cedar Street
St. Paul, MN 55101
(612) 296-5007

PROGRAMS FOR CHILDREN WITH SPECIAL HEALTH-CARE NEEDS

Minnesota Children with Special Health Needs
Department of Health
717 Delaware Street, S.E.
Minneapolis, MN 55440
(612) 623-5150 or (800) 728-5420

PROGRAMS FOR INFANTS AND TODDLERS WITH DISABILITIES: AGES BIRTH THROUGH TWO

Interagency Early Intervention Project for Young Children with Disabilities and Their Families
Minnesota Department of Children, Families and Learning
Capitol Square Building, Room 927
550 Cedar Street
St. Paul, MN 55101
(612) 296-7032

PROTECTION AND ADVOCACY AGENCY

Minnesota Disability Law Center
430 First Avenue N., Suite 300
Minneapolis, MN 55401-1780
(612) 332-1441

STATE AGENCY FOR THE VISUALLY IMPAIRED

State Services for the Blind and Visually Handicapped
Department of Jobs and Training

2200 University Avenue W., #240
St. Paul, MN 55114
(612) 642-0500

STATE DEPARTMENT OF EDUCATION:
SPECIAL EDUCATION

Minnesota Department of Children, Families and Learning
Office of Special Education
811 Capitol Square Building, 550 Cedar Street
St. Paul, MN 55101
(612) 296-1793

STATE DEVELOPMENTAL DISABILITIES
PLANNING COUNCIL

Governor's Council on Developmental Disabilities
300 Centennial Office Building
658 Cedar Street
St. Paul, MN 55155
(612) 296-4018

STATE DEVELOPMENTAL DISABILITIES
PROGRAM

Division for Persons with Developmental Disabilities
Department of Human Services
444 Lafayette Road
St. Paul, MN 55155-3825
(612) 296-2160

STATE EDUCATION AGENCY LOW
INCIDENCE REPRESENTATIVE

Department of Education
Capitol Square Building, Room 819
St. Paul, MN 5510l
(612) 296-5174

STATE MENTAL HEALTH AGENCY

Department of Human Services
Health and Continuing Care Strategies
Human Services Building
444 Lafayette Road
St. Paul, MN 55155-3852
(612) 296-2710

STATE MENTAL HEALTH
REPRESENTATIVE FOR CHILDREN
AND YOUTH

Children's Mental Health Section
Department of Human Services
Human Services Building
444 Lafayette Road
St. Paul, MN 55155-3828
(612) 297-3510

STATE VOCATIONAL
REHABILITATION AGENCY

Rehabilitation Services Branch
Department of Economic Security
390 North Robert Street, First Floor
St. Paul, MN 55101
(612) 296-1822

TECHNOLOGY-RELATED
ASSISTANCE

Minnesota Star Program
300 Centennial Building
658 Cedar Street
St. Paul, MN 55155
(800) 657-3862 (V); (612) 296-2771 (V);
   (800) 657-3895 (TTY); (612) 296-9478 (TTY)

UNIVERSITY-AFFILIATED PROGRAM

Institute on Community Integration (UAP)
University of Minnesota
102 Pattee Hall
150 Pillsbury Drive SE
Minneapolis, MN 55455
(612) 624-6300

MISSISSIPPI

CLIENT ASSISTANCE PROGRAM

Client Assistance Program, Easter Seals Society
3226 North State Street
Jackson, MS 39216
(601) 982-7051

OFFICE OF STATE COORDINATOR OF VOCATIONAL EDUCATION FOR STUDENTS WITH DISABILITIES

Special Vocational Services for the Handicapped
Office of Vocational and Technical Education
Department of Education
P.O. Box 771
Jackson, MS 39205-0771
(601) 359-3465

PARENT TRAINING AND INFORMATION PROJECTS

Parent Partners
3111 N. State Street
Jackson, MS 39216
(601) 366-5707 or (800) 366-5707 (in MS)

Project Empower
1427 S. Main, Suite Eight
Greenville, MS 38701
(601) 332-4852 or (800) 337-4852

PROGRAMS FOR CHILDREN WITH DISABILITIES: AGES THREE THROUGH FIVE

Office of Special Education, Department of Education
P.O. Box 771
Jackson, MS 39205-0771
(601) 359-3498

PROGRAMS FOR CHILDREN WITH SPECIAL HEALTH-CARE NEEDS

Children's Medical Program, Department of Health
P.O. Box 1700
Jackson, MS 39215
(601) 987-3965 or (800) 844-0898 (National/WATS)

PROGRAMS FOR INFANTS AND TODDLERS WITH DISABILITIES: AGES BIRTH THROUGH TWO

First Steps Early Intervention System
MS State Department of Health (MSDH)

P.O. Box 1700
2423 North State Street, Room 105A
Jackson, MS 39215-1700
(601) 960-7622 or (800) 451-3903

PROTECTION AND ADVOCACY AGENCY

5330 Executive Place, Suite A
Jackson, MS 39206
(601) 981-8207 or (800) 772-4057

STATE DEPARTMENT OF EDUCATION: SPECIAL EDUCATION

Office of Special Education, Department of Education
P.O. Box 771
Jackson, MS 39205-0771
(601) 359-3490

STATE DEVELOPMENTAL DISABILITIES PLANNING COUNCIL

Developmental Disabilities Planning Council
1101 Robert E. Lee Building, 239 N. Lamar Street
Jackson, MS 39201
(601) 359-1288

STATE MENTAL HEALTH AGENCY

Department of Mental Health
1101 Robert E. Lee Building, 239 North Lamar Street
Jackson, MS 39201
(601) 359-1288

STATE MENTAL HEALTH REPRESENTATIVE FOR CHILDREN AND YOUTH

Division of Children and Youth Services
Department of Mental Health
1101 Robert E. Lee Building, 239 North Lamar Street
Jackson, MS 39201
(601) 359-1288

STATE MENTAL RETARDATION PROGRAM

Bureau of Mental Retardation
Department of Mental Health
1101 Robert E. Lee Building, 239 North Lamar Street
Jackson, MS 39201
(601) 359-1288

STATE VOCATIONAL REHABILITATION AGENCY

Mississippi Office of Vocational Rehabilitation
Department of Rehabilitation Services
P.O. Box 1698
Jackson, MS 39215-1698
(601) 853-5230

TECHNOLOGY-RELATED ASSISTANCE

Mississippi Project Start
P.O. Box 1698
Jackson, MS 39215-1698
(601) 853-5171 (V/TTY)

UNIVERSITY-AFFILIATED PROGRAM

Mississippi University Affiliated Program
University of Southern Mississippi
P.O. Box 5163
Hattiesburg, MS 39406-5163
(601) 266-5163

MISSOURI

OFFICE OF STATE COORDINATOR OF VOCATIONAL EDUCATION FOR STUDENTS WITH DISABILITIES

Vocational Special Needs
Department of Elementary and Secondary Education
P.O. Box 480
Jefferson City, MO 65102
(573) 751-3500

PARENT TRAINING AND INFORMATION PROJECTS

Missouri Parents Act (MPACT)
1901 Wind River Drive
Jefferson City, MO 65101
(573) 635-1189 or (573) 635-7802

Missouri Parents Act (MPACT)
3100 Main Street, Suite 303
Kansas City, MO 64111
(816) 531-7070 or (816) 931-2992 (TTY)

Missouri Parents Act (MPACT)
2100 South Brentwood, Suite G
Springfield, MO 63108
(417) 882-7434 or (800) 743-7634 (in MO)

Missouri Parents Act (MPACT)
4144 Lindell Boulevard, Suite 405
St. Louis, MO 63108
(314) 531-5922 or (800) 995-3160 (in MO)

PROGRAMS FOR CHILDREN AND YOUTH WHO ARE DEAF OR HARD OF HEARING

Missouri Commission for the Deaf
915 Leslie Boulevard, Suite E
Jefferson City, MO 65101
(573) 526-5205 (V/TTY) or (800) 796-6499 (V/TTY)

PROGRAMS FOR CHILDREN WITH DISABILITIES: AGES THREE THROUGH FIVE

Department of Elementary and Secondary Education
P.O. Box 480
Jefferson City, MO 65102
(573) 751-0187

PROGRAMS FOR CHILDREN WITH SPECIAL HEALTH-CARE NEEDS

Bureau of Special Health Care Needs/ Department of Health
P.O. Box 570, 1730 East Elm
Jefferson City, MO 65102
(573) 751-6246

PROGRAMS FOR INFANTS AND TODDLERS WITH DISABILITIES: AGES BIRTH THROUGH TWO

Section of Early Childhood Special Education
Department of Elementary and Secondary Education
P.O. Box 480
Jefferson City, MO 65102
(573) 751-0187

PROTECTION AND ADVOCACY AGENCY

Missouri Protection and Advocacy Services
925 South Country Club Drive, Unit B-1
Jefferson City, MO 65109
(573) 893-3333 or (800) 392-8667 (in MO)

STATE AGENCY FOR THE VISUALLY IMPAIRED

Rehabilitation Service for the Blind
Division of Family Services/Department of Social
    Services
619 East Capital Avenue
Jefferson City, MO 65101
(573) 751-4249

STATE DEPARTMENT OF EDUCATION: SPECIAL EDUCATION

Division of Special Education
Department of Elementary and Secondary Education
P.O. Box 480
Jefferson City, MO 65102
(573) 751-2965

STATE DEVELOPMENTAL DISABILITIES PLANNING COUNCIL

**Missouri Planning Council for Developmental
    Disabilities**
Division of MR/Developmental Disabilities,
    Department of Mental Health
1706 East Elm, P.O. Box 687
Jefferson City, MO 65102
(573) 751-8611 or (800) 500-7878 (in MO)

STATE EDUCATION AGENCY RURAL REPRESENTATIVE

Department of Education
Department of Elementary and Secondary Education
P.O. Box 480
Jefferson City, MO 65102
(573) 751-4426

STATE MENTAL HEALTH AGENCY

Department of Mental Health
1706 East Elm, P.O. Box 687
Jefferson City, MO 65102
(573) 751-3070

STATE MENTAL HEALTH REPRESENTATIVE FOR CHILDREN AND YOUTH

**Children and Youth Services Department of
    Mental Health**
1706 East Elm, P.O. Box 687
Jefferson City, MO 65102
(573) 751-9482

STATE MENTAL RETARDATION PROGRAM

**Division of Mental Health and Mental
    Retardation**
1706 East Elm, P.O. Box 687
Jefferson City, MO 65102
(573) 751-4054

STATE VOCATIONAL REHABILITATION AGENCY

Division of Vocational Rehabilitation
Department of Education
3024 W. Trauma Boulevard
Jefferson City, MO 65109-0525
(573) 751-3251

TECHNOLOGY-RELATED ASSISTANCE

Missouri Assistive Technology Project
4731 South Cochise, Suite 114
Independence, MO 64055-6975
(800) 647-8557 or (816) 373-5193

UNIVERSITY-AFFILIATED PROGRAM

Institute for Human Development
University of MO at Kansas City
2220 Holmes Street, Third Floor
Kansas City, MO 64108
(816) 235-1770

MONTANA

OFFICE OF STATE COORDINATOR OF VOCATIONAL EDUCATION FOR STUDENTS WITH DISABILITIES

K-12 Vocational Education
Office of Public Instruction
P.O. Box 202501

Helena, MT 59620-2501
(406) 444-9019

PARENT TRAINING/INFORMATION PROJECTS

Parents, Let's Unite For Kids (PLUK)

MSU/B-SPED, Room 183
1500 North 30th Street
Billings, MT 59101-0298
(406) 657-2055 or (800) 222-7585 (MT only)

PROGRAMS FOR CHILDREN WITH DISABILITIES: AGES THREE THROUGH FIVE

Office of Public Instruction

P.O. Box 202501
Helena, MT 59620-2501
(406) 444-4425

PROGRAMS FOR CHILDREN WITH SPECIAL HEALTH CARE NEEDS

Special Health Services

Family and Community Health Bureau
Department of Public Health and Human
    Services
Cogswell Building, P.O. Box 200901
Helena, MT 59620-0901
(406) 444-3622

PROGRAMS FOR INFANTS AND TODDLERS WITH DISABILITIES: AGES BIRTH THROUGH TWO

Developmental Disabilities Program

Department of Public Health and Human Services
P.O. Box 4210
Helena, MT 59604
(406) 444-2995

PROTECTION AND ADVOCACY AGENCY

Montana Advocacy Program

P.O. Box 1681, 400 North Park, Second Floor
Helena, MT 59624
(406) 449-2344 or (800) 245-4743 (V/TTY, in MT)
http://www.mtadv.org

STATE DEPARTMENT OF EDUCATION: SPECIAL EDUCATION

Special Education Division

Office of Public Instruction
P.O. Box 202501
Helena, MT 59620-2501
(406) 444-4429

STATE DEVELOPMENTAL DISABILITIES PLANNING COUNCIL

Developmental Disabilities Planning and Advisory Council

P.O. Box 526
Helena, MT 59624
(406) 444-1334 or (800) 337-9942 (in MT)

STATE DEVELOPMENTAL DISABILITIES PROGRAMS

Disability Services Division

Department of Public Health and Human Services
111 Sanders Street, Room 307
P.O. Box 4210
Helena, MT 59604
(406) 444-2590

STATE EDUCATION AGENCY RURAL REPRESENTATIVE

Office of Public Instruction

P.O. Box 202501
Helena, MT 59620-2501
(406) 444-5541

STATE MENTAL HEALTH AGENCY

Addictive and Mental Disorders Division

Department of Public Health and Human Services
Cogswell Building - C118
1400 Broadway, P.O. Box 202951
Helena, MT 59620-2951
(406) 444-3969

STATE MENTAL HEALTH REPRESENTATIVE FOR CHILDREN AND YOUTH

Addictive and Mental Disorders Division

Department of Public Health and Human Services
Cogswell Building - C118

1400 Broadway, P.O. Box 202951
Helena, MT 59620-2951
(406) 444-1290

STATE VOCATIONAL REHABILITATION AGENCY

Disability Services Division
Department of Public Health and Human Services
111 Sanders Street, Room 307
P.O. Box 4210
Helena, MT 59604-4210
(406) 444-2590

TECHNOLOGY-RELATED ASSISTANCE

MonTECH
The University of Montana, MUARID, MonTECH
634 Eddy Avenue
Missoula, MT 59812
(406) 243-5676 or (800) 732-0323 (V/TTY)

UNIVERSITY-AFFILIATED PROGRAM

Montana University Affiliated Rural
Institute on Disabilities Program
The University of Montana
52 Corbin Hall
Missoula, MT 59812
(406) 243-5467 (V/TTY)
http://ruralinstitute.umt.edu

NEBRASKA

CLIENT ASSISTANCE PROGRAM

Division of Vocational Rehabilitation Services
Department of Education
301 Centennial Mall South
Lincoln, NE 68509
(402) 471-3656 or (800) 742-7594 (in NE)

OFFICE OF STATE COORDINATOR OF VOCATIONAL EDUCATION FOR STUDENTS WITH DISABILITIES

Student Personnel Services
Career Guidance and Counseling
Vocational Special Needs/Nebraska Dept. of Educ.

P.O. Box 94987
301 Centennial Mall South
Lincoln, NE 68509
(402) 471-4811

PARENT-TO-PARENT

Pilot Parents
3610 Dodge Street, Suite 101
Omaha, NE 68131
(402) 346-5220

PARENT TRAINING AND INFORMATION PROJECTS

Nebraska Parent's Information and Training Center
3135 N. 93rd St.
Omaha, NE 68134
(402) 346-0525 (V/TTY) or (800) 284-8520 (V/TTY, in NE)
info@pti-nebraska.org
http://www.pti-nebraska.org

PROGRAMS FOR CHILDREN AND YOUTH WHO ARE DEAF OR HARD OF HEARING

Nebraska Commission for the Hearing Impaired
4600 Valley Road, Suite 420
Lincoln, NE 68510
(402) 471-3593 (V/TTY) or (800) 545-6244 (V, in NE)

PROGRAMS FOR CHILDREN WITH DISABILITIES: AGES THREE THROUGH FIVE

Special Populations Office
Department of Education
P.O. Box 94987
Lincoln, NE 68509
(402) 471-4319

PROGRAMS FOR CHILDREN WITH SPECIAL HEALTH-CARE NEEDS

Nebraska Health and Human Services
Department of Social Services
Special Services for Children and Adults
P.O. Box 95044

Lincoln, NE 68509-5044
(402) 471-9345

PROGRAMS FOR INFANTS AND TODDLERS WITH DISABILITIES: AGES BIRTH THROUGH TWO

Special Populations Office
State Department of Education
P.O. Box 94987
Lincoln, NE 68509
(402) 471-2463

PROTECTION AND ADVOCACY AGENCY

Nebraska Advocacy Services, Inc.
522 Lincoln Center Building
215 Centennial Mall South
Lincoln, NE 68508
(402) 474-3183 or (800) 422-6691

STATE AGENCY FOR THE VISUALLY IMPAIRED

Division of Rehabilitation Services for the Visually
Impaired/Department of Health and Human Services
4600 Valley Road, Suite 100
Lincoln, NE 68510
(402) 471-2891

STATE DEPARTMENT OF EDUCATION: SPECIAL EDUCATION

Special Populations, Department of Education
P.O. Box 94987
Lincoln, NE 68509-4987
(402) 471-2471 (V/TTY) or (402) 471-0117
http://www.nde.state.ne.us/SPED/sped.html

STATE DEVELOPMENTAL DISABILITIES PLANNING COUNCIL

Developmental Disabilities Planning Council/HHS
P.O. Box 95044
301 Centennial Mall South
Lincoln, NE 68509
(402) 471-2330

STATE DEVELOPMENTAL DISABILITIES PROGRAMS

Developmental Disabilities System
Department of Health and Human Services
P.O. Box 94728
Lincoln, NE 68509-4728
(402) 479-5110

STATE EDUCATION AGENCY RURAL REPRESENTATIVE

Department of Education
301 Centennial Mall South
P.O. Box 94987
Lincoln, NE 68509-4987
(402) 471-2783

STATE MENTAL HEALTH AGENCY

Department of Health and Human Services
P.O. Box 94728
Lincoln, NE 68509-4728
(402) 471-2851, ext. 5507

STATE MENTAL HEALTH REPRESENTATIVE FOR CHILDREN AND YOUTH

Office of Community Mental Health
Department of Health and Human Services
P.O. Box 94728
Lincoln, NE 68509-4728
(402) 479-5512

STATE VOCATIONAL REHABILITATION AGENCY

Division of Rehabilitation Services
Department of Education
P.O. Box 94987
301 Centennial Mall South, Sixth Floor
Lincoln, NE 68509
(402) 471-3649

TECHNOLOGY-RELATED ASSISTANCE

Nebraska Assistive Technology Project
301 Centennial Mall South
P.O. Box 94987
Lincoln, NE 68509-4987

(402) 471-0734 (V/TTY)
http://www.nde.state.ne.us/ATP/TECHome.html

UNIVERSITY-AFFILIATED PROGRAM

Meyer Rehabilitation Institute
University of Nebraska Medical Center
600 South 42nd Street
Omaha, NE 68198-5450
(402) 559-6400

NEVADA

CLIENT ASSISTANCE PROGRAM

State of Nevada, Client Assistance Program
1755 E. Plumb Lane, #109
Reno, NV 89502
(702) 688-1440 or (800) 633-9879

OFFICE OF STATE COORDINATOR OF VOCATIONAL EDUCATION FOR STUDENTS WITH DISABILITIES

Occupational and Continuing Education Branch
Department of Education
700 E. Fifth Street, Suite 111
Carson City, NV 89701-5096
(702) 687-9190

PARENT-TO-PARENT

Nevada Parent Network
Research and Educational Planning Center, College of Education, MS 285
University of Nevada, Reno
Reno, NV 89557-0082
(702) 784-4921 or (800) 216-7988
http://repc.unr.edu

PARENT TRAINING AND INFORMATION PROJECT

Nevada PEP
2355 Red Rock Street, Suite 106
Las Vegas, NV 89146
(702) 388-8899 or
    (800) 216-5188
http://www.nvpep.org

PROGRAMS FOR CHILDREN WITH DISABILITIES: AGES THREE THROUGH FIVE

Educational Equity, Department of Education
700 E. Fifth Street, Suite 113
Carson City, NV 89701-5096
(702) 687-9142

PROGRAMS FOR CHILDREN WITH SPECIAL HEALTH-CARE NEEDS

Bureau of Family Health Services, Division of Health
Dept. of Human Resources
505 East King Street, Room 200
Carson City, NV 89701-4792
(702) 687-4885

PROGRAMS FOR INFANTS AND TODDLERS WITH DISABILITIES: AGES BIRTH THROUGH TWO

Early Childhood Services
Department of Human Resources
3987 S. McCarran Boulevard
Reno, NV 89502
(702) 688-2284

PROTECTION AND ADVOCACY AGENCY

Travis Wall, Director
Nevada Disability Advocacy and Law Center
401 S. Third Street, Suite 403
Las Vegas, NV 89101
(702) 383-8150; (702) 383-7097 (TTY);
    (800) 992-5715 (in NV)

STATE DEPARTMENT OF EDUCATION: SPECIAL EDUCATION

Educational Equity, Department of Education
700 E. Fifth Street, Suite 113
Carson City, NV 89701-5096
(702) 687-9142

STATE DEVELOPMENTAL DISABILITIES PLANNING COUNCIL

Office of Community Based Services
711 South Stewart Street
Carson City, NV 89701
(702) 687-4452

STATE MENTAL HEALTH AGENCY

Division of Mental Hygiene and Mental Retardation
Department of Human Resources
Kinkead Building, Suite 602
505 East King Street
Carson City, NV 89701-3790
(702) 687-5943

STATE MENTAL HEALTH REPRESENTATIVE FOR CHILDREN AND YOUTH

Division of Child/Family Services
711 East Fifth Street
Carson City, NV 89701
(702) 687-5982

STATE MENTAL RETARDATION PROGRAM

Division of Mental Hygiene and Mental Retardation
Department of Human Resources
Kinkead Building, Suite 602
505 East King Street
Carson City, NV 89701-3790
(702) 687-5943

STATE VOCATIONAL REHABILITATION AGENCY

Rehabilitation Division, Dept. of Employment, Training, and Rehabilitation
505 East King Street, Room 502
Carson City, NV 89710
(702) 687-4440

TECHNOLOGY-RELATED ASSISTANCE

Nevada Assistive Technology Collaborative
Rehabilitation Division
Office of Community Based Services
711 South Stewart Street
Carson City, NV 89710
(702) 687-4452 or (702) 687-3388 (TTY)

Nevada Special Education Technology Assistance Project
P.O. Box 603
Carson City, NV 89702
(702) 885-6268

UNIVERSITY-AFFILIATED PROGRAM

University Affiliated Program
Research and Education Planning Center
College of Education/MS285
University of Nevada, Reno
Reno, NV 89557
(702) 784-4921 (V/TTY) or (800) 216-7988

NEW HAMPSHIRE

CLIENT ASSISTANCE PROGRAM

Governor's Commission on Disability
Client Assistance Program
57 Regional Drive
Concord, NH 03301-8506
(603) 271-2773 or (800) 852-3405 (in NH)

PARENT-TO-PARENT

P.O. Box 622
Hanover, NH 03755
(603) 448-6393 or (800) 698-5465 (in NH and VT)

PROGRAMS FOR CHILDREN WITH DISABILITIES: AGES THREE THROUGH FIVE

Bureau of Early Learning, Dept. of Education
101 Pleasant Street
Concord, NH 03301-3860
(603) 271-2178

PROGRAMS FOR CHILDREN WITH SPECIAL HEALTH-CARE NEEDS

Bureau of Special Medical Services
Office of Health Management
Six Hazen Drive
Concord, NH 03301-6527
(603) 271-4596

PROGRAMS FOR INFANTS AND TODDLERS WITH DISABILITIES: AGES BIRTH THROUGH TWO

New Hampshire Early Support and Services
Division of Developmental Services
105 Pleasant Street
Concord, NH 03301-3860
(603) 271-5144

PROTECTION AND ADVOCACY AGENCY

Disabilities Rights Center, Inc.
P.O. Box 3660
Concord, NH 03302-3660
(603) 228-0432 or (800) 834-1721

STATE DEPARTMENT OF EDUCATION: SPECIAL EDUCATION

New Hampshire Department of Education
101 Pleasant Street
Concord, NH 03301-3860
(603) 271-3842

STATE DEVELOPMENTAL DISABILITIES PLANNING COUNCIL

New Hampshire Developmental Disabilities Council, The Concord Center
10 Ferry Street, Unit 315
Concord, NH 03301-5004
(603) 271-3236

STATE EDUCATION AGENCY RURAL REPRESENTATIVE

Bureau for Early Learning
Department of Education
101 Pleasant Street
Concord, NH 03301-3860
(603) 271-3730

STATE MENTAL HEALTH AGENCY

Division of Behavioral Health
Department of Health and Human Services
105 Pleasant Street
Concord, NH 03301
(603) 271-5167

STATE MENTAL HEALTH REPRESENTATIVE FOR CHILDREN AND YOUTH

Division of Behavioral Health
State Office Park South, 105 Pleasant Street
Concord, NH 03301
(603) 271-5095

STATE MENTAL RETARDATION PROGRAM

Division of Developmental Services
105 Pleasant Street
Concord, NH 03301
(603) 271-5013

STATE VOCATIONAL REHABILITATION AGENCY

Division of Adult Learning and Rehabilitation
New Hampshire Department of Education
78 Regional Drive, Building Two
Concord, NH 03301
(603) 271-3471

TECHNOLOGY-RELATED ASSISTANCE

New Hampshire Technology Partnership Project
Institute on Disability/UAP
University of New Hampshire
#14, 10 Ferry Street
The Concord Center
Concord, NH 03301
(603) 224-0630 (V/TTY)

UNIVERSITY-AFFILIATED PROGRAM

Institute on Disability/UAP
University of New Hampshire
Seven Leavitt Lane, Suite 101
Durham, NH 03824-3522
(603) 862-4320 (V/TTY)
http://iod.unh.edu

VOCATIONAL EDUCATION FOR STUDENTS WITH DISABILITIES

Educational Consultant
New Hampshire Department of Education
101 Pleasant Street
Concord, NH 03301-3860
(603) 271-2454

NEW JERSEY

OFFICE OF STATE COORDINATOR OF VOCATIONAL EDUCATION FOR STUDENTS WITH DISABILITIES

Department of Human Services
Office of School-to-Career and College Initiatives
New Jersey Department of Education
P.O. Box 710

Trenton, NJ 08625
(609) 292-2121

PARENT-TO-PARENT

New Jersey Self-Help Clearinghouse
Northwest Covenant Medical Center
25 Pocono Road
Denville, NJ 07834-2995
(201) 625-9053 or (800) 367-6274 (in NJ)

New Jersey Statewide Parent-to-Parent
35 Halsey Street
Newark, NJ 07102
(973) 642-8100 or (800) 372-6510

PARENT TRAINING AND INFORMATION PROJECT

Statewide Parent Advocacy Network (SPAN)
35 Halsey Street
Newark, NJ 07102
(973) 642-8100 or (973) 642-8080
http://www.spannj.org

PROGRAMS FOR CHILDREN AND YOUTH WHO ARE DEAF OR HARD OF HEARING

Division of the Deaf and Hard of Hearing
New Jersey Department of Human Services
P.O. Box 074
Trenton, NJ 08625-0074
(609) 984-7281 (V/TTY) or (800) 792-8339
(V/TTY, in NJ)

PROGRAMS FOR CHILDREN WITH DISABILITIES: AGES THREE THROUGH FIVE

Office of Special Education Programs/ Department of Education
P.O. Box 500
Trenton, NJ 08625-0500
(609) 292-4692

PROGRAMS FOR CHILDREN WITH SPECIAL HEALTH-CARE NEEDS

New Jersey Department of Health and Senior Services
Special Child and Adult Health Services
50 E. State Street

P.O. Box 364
Trenton, NJ 08625
(609) 984-0755

PROGRAMS FOR INFANTS AND TODDLERS WITH DISABILITIES: AGES BIRTH THROUGH TWO

New Jersey Department of Health and Senior Services
P.O. Box 364
Trenton, NJ 08625
(609) 777-7734

PROTECTION AND ADVOCACY AGENCY

New Jersey Protection and Advocacy, Inc.
210 South Broad Street, Third Floor
Trenton, NJ 08608
(609) 292-9742; (609) 633-7106 (TTY);
(800) 922-7233 (in NJ)

STATE AGENCY FOR THE VISUALLY IMPAIRED

Commission for the Blind and Visually Impaired
Department of Human Services
P.O. Box 47017
153 Halsey Street
Newark, NJ 07101
(201) 648-2324
e-mail: NJCBVI@Edu.GTE.net

STATE DEPARTMENT OF EDUCATION: SPECIAL EDUCATION

Office of Special Education Program, Dept. of Education
100 Riverview Plaza
P.O. Box 500
Trenton, NJ 08625-0500
(609) 292-0147

STATE DEVELOPMENTAL DISABILITIES PLANNING COUNCIL

New Jersey Developmental Disabilities Council
20 West State Street
P.O. Box 700

Trenton, NJ 08625
(609) 292-3745

STATE EDUCATION AGENCY RURAL REPRESENTATIVE

Special Education
High Point Regional High School
299 Pigeon Hill Road
Sussex, NJ 07461
(201) 875-3102

STATE MENTAL HEALTH AGENCY

Division of Mental Health Services/ Dept. of Human Services
50 East State Street, Capitol Center
P.O. Box 727
Trenton, NJ 08625
(609) 777-0702

STATE MENTAL HEALTH REPRESENTATIVE FOR CHILDREN AND YOUTH

Office of Children's Services
Division of Mental Health Services
Capitol Center
P.O. Box 727
Trenton, NJ 08625
(609) 777-0707

STATE MENTAL RETARDATION PROGRAM

Division of Developmental Disabilities
Department of Human Services
50 East State Street
P.O. Box 726
Trenton, NJ 08625
(609) 292-7260

STATE VOCATIONAL REHABILITATION AGENCY

New Jersey Dept. of Labor, Div. of Vocational Rehabilitation Services
P.O. Box 398
Trenton, NJ 08625-0398
(609) 292-5987 or
    (609) 292-2919 (TTY)

TECHNOLOGY-RELATED ASSISTANCE

New Jersey Technology Assistive Resource Program
135 East State Street
Trenton, NJ 08625
(609) 292-7498 or (800) 382-7765 (TTY)

UNIVERSITY-AFFILIATED PROGRAM

The University Affiliated Program of New Jersey
University of Medicine and Dentistry of New Jersey
Robert Wood Johnson Medical School
Brookwood II
45 Knightsbridge Road
P.O. Box 6810
Piscataway, NJ 08855-6810
(732) 235-4447 or (732) 235-4407 (TTY)

NEW MEXICO

OFFICE OF STATE COORDINATOR OF VOCATIONAL EDUCATION FOR STUDENTS WITH DISABILITIES

Adult Basic Education, State Dept. of Education
Education Building, 300 Don Gaspar
Santa Fe, NM 87501-2786
(505) 827-6655

PARENT-TO-PARENT

Parents Reaching Out (P.R.O.)
1000 A Main Street, NW
Los Lunas, NM 87031
(505) 865-3700 or (800) 524-5176 (in NM)

PARENT TRAINING AND INFORMATION PROJECTS

Education for Parents of Indian Children with Special Needs/(EPICS) Project
P.O. Box 788
Bernalillo, NM 87004
(505) 867-3396 or (800) 765-7320 (V/TTY)

Parents Reaching Out (P.R.O.), Project Adobe
1000 A Main Street, NW

Los Lunas, NM 87031
(505) 865-3700 or (800) 524-5176 (in NM)

STEP*HI PARENT/INFANT PROGRAM

New Mexico School for the Deaf
Early Childhood Programs
1060 Cerrillos Road
Santa Fe, NM 87503
(505) 827-6789 (V/TTY)

PROGRAMS FOR CHILDREN AND YOUTH WHO ARE DEAF OR HARD OF HEARING

New Mexico Commission for the Deaf and Hard of Hearing
1435 St. Francis Drive
Santa Fe, NM 87501
(505) 827-7584 (V/TTY); (505) 827-7588 (TTY);
    (800) 489-8536 (V/TTY, in NM);
    (800) 873-8897 (V/TTY, News Line in NM)

PROGRAMS FOR CHILDREN WITH DISABILITIES: AGES THREE THROUGH FIVE

Early Childhood Consultant
Special Education Unit, Department of Education
300 Don Gasper Avenue
Santa Fe, NM 87501-2786
(505) 827-6788

PROGRAMS FOR CHILDREN WITH SPECIAL HEALTH-CARE NEEDS

Department of Health
Public Health Division, Children's Medical Services
P.O. Box 22110
Santa Fe, NM 87502
(505) 827-2548

Family Health Bureau, Dept. of Health
1190 Saint Francis Drive
Santa Fe, NM 87502
(505) 827-2350

PROGRAMS FOR INFANTS AND TODDLERS WITH DISABILITIES: AGES BIRTH THROUGH TWO

Department of Health
Development Disabilities Division
1190 St. Francis Drive

P.O. Box 26110
Santa Fe, NM 87502-6110
(505) 827-2573

PROTECTION AND ADVOCACY AGENCY

Protection and Advocacy System, Inc.
1720 Louisiana Boulevard, N.E., Suite 204
Albuquerque, NM 87110
(505) 256-3100 or (800) 432-4682 (in NM)

STATE AGENCY FOR THE VISUALLY IMPAIRED

Commission for the Blind
PERA Building, Room 553
Santa Fe, NM 87503
(505) 827-4479

STATE DEPARTMENT OF EDUCATION: SPECIAL EDUCATION

Special Education, Department of Education - Education Building
300 Don Gaspar Avenue
Santa Fe, NM 87501-2786
(505) 827-6541

STATE DEVELOPMENTAL DISABILITIES PLANNING COUNCIL

New Mexico Developmental Disabilities Planning Council
435 Saint Michael's Drive, Building D
Santa Fe, NM 87505
(505) 827-7590
(505) 827-7589 (fax)

STATE EDUCATION AGENCY RURAL REPRESENTATIVE

Department of Education, Special Education
300 Don Gaspar, Education Building
Santa Fe, NM 87501-2786
(505) 827-6541

STATE MENTAL HEALTH AGENCY

Division of Mental Health, Department of Health
1190 St. Francis Drive, Room 3078N
Santa Fe, NM 87502
(505) 827-2651

STATE MENTAL HEALTH REPRESENTATIVE FOR CHILDREN AND YOUTH

Children, Youth and Families Department
Prevention and Intervention Division
P.O. Box 5160
Santa Fe, NM 87502-5160
(505) 827-5888

STATE MENTAL RETARDATION PROGRAM

Long-Term Services, Dept. of Health
1190 Saint Francis Drive, P.O. Box 26110
Santa Fe, NM 87502-6110
(505) 827-2574

STATE VOCATIONAL REHABILITATION AGENCY

Div. of Vocational Rehabilitation, Dept. of Education
435 St. Michaels Drive, Building D
Santa Fe, NM 87505
(505) 827-3511

TECHNOLOGY-RELATED ASSISTANCE

New Mexico Technology Assistance Program
435 St. Michael's Drive, Building D
Santa Fe, NM 87505
(800) 866-ABLE (V); (505) 954-8539;
   (800) 659-4915 (TTY)

UNIVERSITY-AFFILIATED PROGRAM

University of New Mexico
Health Sciences Center
Center for Developmental Disabilities
School of Medicine
Albuquerque, NM 87131-5020
(505) 272-3000

NEW YORK

CLIENT ASSISTANCE PROGRAM

New York Committee on Quality of Care
99 Washington Avenue, Suite 1002
Albany, NY 12210
(518) 473-7378

PARENT-TO-PARENT

Family Support Project for the Developmentally Disabled
North Central Bronx Hospital
3424 Kossuth Avenue, Room 15A10
Bronx, NY 10467
(718) 519-4797

Parent to Parent of New York State
P.O. Box 1296
Tupper Lake, NY 12986
(800) 305-8817 or (518) 359-3006
http://www.parenttoparentnys.org

PARENT TRAINING AND INFORMATION PROJECT

Advocates for Children of New York (New York City)
151 W. 30th Street, Fifth Floor
New York, NY 10001
(212) 947-9779
http://www.advocatesforchildren.org

Parent Network Center
250 Delaware Avenue, Suite Three
Buffalo, NY 14202
(716) 853-1570; (800) 724-7408 (in NY);
   (716) 853-1573 (TTY)

Resources for Children with Special Needs, Inc.
200 Park Avenue South, Suite 816
New York, NY 10003
(212) 667-4650
e-mail: resourcesnyc@prodigy.net

Sinergia/Metropolitan Parent Center
15 West 65th Street, Sixth Floor
New York, NY 10023
(212) 496-1300
e-mail: intake@sinergiany.org
http://www.sinergiany.org

PROGRAMS FOR CHILDREN AND YOUTH WHO ARE DEAF OR HARD OF HEARING

Office of Vocational and Educational Services for Individuals with Disabilities
State Education Department
One Commerce Plaza, Room 1603
Albany, NY 12234
(518) 474-5652 (V/TTY) or (800) 222-5627 (V/TTY)

PROGRAMS FOR CHILDREN WITH DISABILITIES: AGES THREE THROUGH FIVE

State Education Department
Special Education Services
One Commerce Plaza, Room 1607
Albany, NY 12234
(518) 473-6108

PROGRAMS FOR CHILDREN WITH SPECIAL HEALTH-CARE NEEDS

Bureau of Child and Adolescent Health, Dept. of Health
Tower Building, Room 208
Albany, NY 12237-0618
(518) 474-2084

PROGRAMS FOR INFANTS AND TODDLERS WITH DISABILITIES: AGES BIRTH THROUGH TWO

Early Intervention Program
Bureau of Child and Adolescent Health
Corning Tower, Room 208
Albany, NY 12237
(518) 473-7016

PROTECTION AND ADVOCACY AGENCY

New York Commission on Quality of Care
99 Washington Avenue, Suite 1002
Albany, NY 12210
(518) 473-7378

STATE AGENCY FOR THE VISUALLY IMPAIRED

Commission for the Blind and Visually Handicapped
Department of Social Services
40 North Pearl Street
Albany, NY 12243
(518) 473-1801

STATE DEPARTMENT OF EDUCATION: SPECIAL EDUCATION

Office of Vocational and Educational Services for Individuals with Disabilities
One Commerce Plaza, Room 1606
Albany, NY 12234
(518) 474-2714

STATE DEVELOPMENTAL DISABILITIES PLANNING COUNCIL

NYS Developmental Disabilities Planning Council
155 Washington Avenue, Second Floor
Albany, NY 12210
(518) 432-8233

STATE EDUCATION AGENCY RURAL REPRESENTATIVE

Department of Education
Bureau of School District Reorganization Unit
Education Building Annex, Room 876
Albany, NY 12234
(518) 474-3936

STATE MENTAL HEALTH AGENCY

Office of Mental Health
44 Holland Avenue
Albany, NY 12229
(518) 474-4403

STATE MENTAL HEALTH REPRESENTATIVE FOR CHILDREN AND YOUTH

Office of Children and Families
Office of Mental Health
44 Holland Avenue
Albany, NY 12229
(518) 473-6902

STATE MENTAL RETARDATION PROGRAM

New York State Office of Mental Retardation and Developmental Disabilities
44 Holland Avenue
Albany, NY 12229
(518) 473-1997

STATE VOCATIONAL REHABILITATION AGENCY

Office of Vocational and Educational Services for Individuals with Disabilities
Department of Education

One Commerce Plaza, Room 1606
Albany, NY 12234
(518) 474-2714

TECHNOLOGY-RELATED ASSISTANCE

New York State TRAID Project
New York State Commission on Quality of Care
    and Advocacy for Persons with Disabilities
One Empire State Plaza, Suite 1001
Albany, NY 12223-1150
(518) 474-2825 (V); (800) 522-4369 (V/TTY/
    Spanish, in NY); (518) 473-4231 (TTY)
http://www.oapwd.org

UNIVERSITY-AFFILIATED PROGRAM

**Developmental Disabilities Center/St. Lukes
    - Roosevelt Hospital Center**
1000 10th Avenue
New York, NY 10019
(212) 523-6230

Strong Center for Developmental Disorders
University of Rochester Medical Center
601 Elmwood Avenue, Box 671
Rochester, NY 14642
(716) 275-2986

**University Affiliated Program/
    Rose F. Kennedy Center**
Albert Einstein Coll. of Medicine/Yeshiva University
1410 Pelham Parkway South
Bronx, NY 10461
(718) 430-4228

WIHD/University Affiliated Program
Westchester County Medical Center
Valhalla, NY 10595
(914) 285-8204

NORTH CAROLINA

CLIENT ASSISTANCE PROGRAM

Client Assistance Program
P.O. Box 26053
Raleigh, NC 27611
(919) 733-6300 (V/TTY)

OFFICE OF STATE COORDINATOR OF VOCATIONAL EDUCATION FOR STUDENTS WITH DISABILITIES

Workforce Development Education
Department of Public Instruction
301 N. Wilmington Street
Raleigh, NC 27601-2825
(919) 715-1644

PARENT-TO-PARENT

**Family Support Network of North Carolina/
    Central Directory of Resources**
CB #7340
University of North Carolina at Chapel Hill
Chapel Hill, NC 27599-7340
(919) 966-2841 or (800) 852-0042
http://www.fnnc.org

PARENT TRAINING AND INFORMATION PROJECT

**ECAC, Inc. (Exceptional Children's
    Assistance Center)**
P.O. Box 16
Davidson, NC 28036
(704) 892-1321(V/TTY) or (800) 962-6817 (in NC)

PROGRAMS FOR CHILDREN AND YOUTH WHO ARE DEAF OR HARD OF HEARING

**Division of Services for the Deaf and Hard of
    Hearing**
Department of Human Resources
319 Chapanoke Road, Suite 108
Raleigh, NC 27603
(919) 773-2963 or (919) 773-2966 (TTY)

PROGRAMS FOR CHILDREN WITH SPECIAL HEALTH-CARE NEEDS

**Children and Youth Section, Dept. of
    Environment, Health, and Natural
    Resources, Maternal and Child Health
    Division**
P.O. Box 29597
1330 St. Mary's Street
Raleigh, NC 27626-0597
(919) 733-7437

PROGRAMS FOR INFANTS AND TODDLERS WITH DISABILITIES: AGES BIRTH THROUGH TWO

Developmental Disabilities Services Section
Division of Mental Health, Developmental
  Disabilities and Substance Abuse Services
Department of Human Resources
325 North Salisbury Street
Raleigh, NC 27603
(919) 733-3654

PROTECTION AND ADVOCACY AGENCY

Governor's Advocacy Council for Persons with Disabilities
Bryan Building
2113 Cameron Street, Suite 218
Raleigh, NC 27605
(919) 733-9250

STATE AGENCY FOR THE VISUALLY IMPAIRED

Division of Services for the Blind/ Dept. of Human Resources
309 Ashe Avenue
Raleigh, NC 27606
(919) 733-9822

STATE DEPARTMENT OF EDUCATION: SPECIAL EDUCATION

Exceptional Children Division
Department of Public Instruction
301 N. Wilmington Street, Education Building, #570
Raleigh, NC 27601-2825,
(919) 715-1565

STATE DEVELOPMENTAL DISABILITIES PLANNING COUNCIL

North Carolina Council on Developmental Disabilities
1508 Western Boulevard
Raleigh, NC 27606
(919) 733-6566

STATE DEVELOPMENTAL DISABILITIES PROGRAM

Developmental Disability Services Section
Division of Mental Health, Developmental Disabilities and Substance Abuse Services

Department of Human Resources
325 North Salisbury Street
Raleigh, NC 27603
(919) 733-3654

STATE MENTAL HEALTH AGENCY

Division of Mental Health, Developmental Disabilities and Substance Abuse Services
Department of Human Resources
325 North Salisbury Street
Raleigh, NC 27603
(919) 733-7011

STATE MENTAL HEALTH REPRESENTATIVE FOR CHILDREN AND YOUTH

Child and Family Services Section
Division of Mental Health, Developmental Disabilities and Substance Abuse Services
Department of Human Resources
325 North Salisbury Street
Raleigh, NC 27603
(919) 733-0598

STATE VOCATIONAL REHABILITATION AGENCY

Division of Vocational Rehabilitation Services
Department of Human Resources
P.O. Box 26053
Raleigh, NC 27611
(919) 733-3364 or (919) 733-5924 (TTY)

TECHNOLOGY-RELATED ASSISTANCE

North Carolina Assistive Technology Project
Department of Human Resources
Division of Vocational Rehabilitation Services
1110 Navaho Drive, Suite 101
Raleigh, NC 27609-7322
(919) 850-2787 (V/TTY) or (800) 852-0042

UNIVERSITY-AFFILIATED PROGRAM

Clinical Center for the Study of Development and Learning
CB# 7255
University of North Carolina
Chapel Hill, NC 27599-7255
(919) 966-5171

NORTH DAKOTA

CLIENT ASSISTANCE PROGRAM

Client Assistance Program
Office of Vocational Rehabilitation
Department of Human Services
600 S. Second Street, Suite 1B
Bismarck, ND 58504-5729
(701) 328-8947 or (800) 207-6122

OFFICE OF STATE COORDINATOR OF VOCATIONAL EDUCATION FOR STUDENTS WITH DISABILITIES

Supervisor of Special Needs
State Board for Vocational Education
15th Floor, Capitol Tower
600 East Boulevard
Bismarck, ND 58505-0610
(701) 328-3178

PARENT TRAINING AND INFORMATION PROJECTS

Native American Family Network System/ Pathfinder Family Center
1600 Second Avenue, S.W.
Suite 18
Arrowhead Shopping Center
Minot, ND 58701-3459
(701) 837-7510 or (888) 763-7277
http://www.pathfinder.minot.com/index2.html

PROGRAMS FOR CHILDREN WITH DISABILITIES: AGES THREE THROUGH FIVE

Special Education Division, Dept. of Public Instruction
600 E. Boulevard Avenue
Bismarck, ND 58505-0440
(701) 328-2277

PROGRAMS FOR CHILDREN WITH SPECIAL HEALTH-CARE NEEDS

Children's Special Health Services
Department of Human Services
State Capitol, 600 East Boulevard Avenue
Bismarck, ND 58505-0269
(701) 328-2436 or (800) 755-2714 (in ND)

PROGRAMS FOR INFANTS AND TODDLERS WITH DISABILITIES: AGES BIRTH THROUGH TWO

Developmental Disabilities Unit
North Dakota Department of Human Services
600 S. Second Street, Suite 1A
Bismarck, ND 58504-5729
(701) 328-8930 or (800) 755-8529 (in ND)

PROTECTION AND ADVOCACY AGENCY

Protection and Advocacy Project
400 East Broadway, Suite 409
Bismarck, ND 58501-4071
(701) 328-3295; (800) 472-2670 (in ND);
    (800) 642-6694; (800) 366-6888 (TDD)
http://www.ndpanda.org

STATE DEPARTMENT OF EDUCATION: SPECIAL EDUCATION

Special Education, Department of Public Instruction
600 East Boulevard Avenue
Bismarck, ND 58505-0440
(701) 328-2277

STATE DEVELOPMENTAL DISABILITIES PLANNING COUNCIL

North Dakota Developmental Disabilities Council
Department of Human Services
600 S. Second Street, Suite 1B
Bismarck, ND 58504-5729
(701) 328-8953

STATE EDUCATION AGENCY RURAL REPRESENTATIVE

Programs Administrator
Department of Public Instruction
State Capitol
600 East Boulevard Avenue
Bismarck, ND 58505-0440
(701) 328-4525

STATE MENTAL HEALTH AGENCY

Division of Mental Health and Substance Abuse Services
Department of Human Services

600 S. Second Street, Suite 1D
Bismarck, ND 58504-5729
(701) 328-8940 or (800) 755-2719 (in ND)

STATE MENTAL RETARDATION PROGRAM

Developmental Disabilities Unit
North Dakota Department of Human Services
600 S. Second Street, Suite 1A
Bismarck, ND 58504-5729
(701) 328-8930 or (800) 755-8529 (in ND)

STATE VOCATIONAL REHABILITATION AGENCY

Vocational Rehabilitation
600 S. Second Street, Suite 1B
Bismarck, ND 58504-5729
(701) 328-8950; (701) 328-8968 (TTY); (800) 755-2745 (in ND)

TECHNOLOGY-RELATED ASSISTANCE

North Dakota Interagency Project for Assistive Technology
P.O. Box 743
Cavalier, ND 58220
(701) 265-4807 (V/TTY) or (800) 265-4728 (V/TTY)
http://www.ndipat.org

OHIO

CLIENT ASSISTANCE PROGRAM

Ohio Client Assistance Program
Governor's Office of Advocacy for People with Disabilities
35 E. Chestnut Street, Fifth Floor
Columbus, OH 43215-2541
(614) 466-9956 (V/TTY) or (800) 228-5405

OFFICE OF STATE COORDINATOR OF VOCATIONAL EDUCATION FOR STUDENTS WITH DISABILITIES

Division of Special Education
Ohio Department of Education
933 High Street
Worthington, OH 43085
(614) 466-2650

PARENT-TO-PARENT

Ohio Coalition for the Education of Children with Disabilities
165 W. Center Street, Suite 302
Bank One Building
Marion, OH 43302-3741
(800) 374-2806

PARENT TRAINING AND INFORMATION PROJECTS

Child Advocacy Center
1821 Summit Road, #303
Cincinnati, OH 45237
(513) 821-2400 (V/TTY)

Ohio Coalition for the Education of Children with Disabilities
Bank One Building
165 West Center Street, Suite 302
Marion, OH 43302-3741
(614) 382-5452 or (800) 374-2806 (V/TTY)

PROGRAMS FOR CHILDREN WITH DISABILITIES: AGES THREE THROUGH FIVE

Division of Early Childhood Education
Ohio Department of Education
65 South Front Street, Room 309
Columbus, OH 43215-4183 or (614) 466-0224

PROGRAMS FOR CHILDREN WITH SPECIAL HEALTH-CARE NEEDS

Bureau for Children with Medical Handicaps
Ohio Department of Health
P.O. Box 1603
Columbus, OH 43216-1603
(614) 466-1700

PROGRAMS FOR INFANTS AND TODDLERS WITH DISABILITIES: AGES BIRTH THROUGH TWO

Ohio Department of Health
P.O. Box 118
246 North High Street, Fifth Floor
Columbus, OH 43266-0118
(614) 644-8389

PROTECTION AND ADVOCACY AGENCY

Ohio Legal Rights Service
8 East Long Street, Fifth Floor
Columbus, OH 43215
(614) 466-7264; (614) 728-2553 (TTY);
    (800) 282-9181 (in OH)

STATE DEPARTMENT OF EDUCATION:
SPECIAL EDUCATION

**Division of Special Education, Ohio
    Department of Education**
933 High Street
Worthington, OH 43085-4017
(614) 466-2650

STATE DEVELOPMENTAL DISABILITIES
PLANNING COUNCIL

**Ohio Developmental Disabilities Planning
    Council**
Eight East Long Street
Atlas Building, 12th Floor
Columbus, OH 43215
(614) 466-5205

STATE EDUCATION AGENCY RURAL
REPRESENTATIVE

**Division of Special Education, Ohio
    Department of Education**
933 High Street
Worthington, OH 43085
(614) 466-2650

STATE MENTAL HEALTH AGENCY

Ohio Department of Mental Health
30 East Broad Street, Room 1180
Columbus, OH 43215
(614) 466-2337/4217

STATE MENTAL HEALTH
REPRESENTATIVE FOR CHILDREN
AND YOUTH

Office of Children's Services
Department of Mental Health
30 East Broad Street, Eighth Floor
Columbus, OH 43215
(614) 466-1984

STATE MENTAL RETARDATION PROGRAM

**Ohio Department of Mental Retardation
    and Developmental Disabilities**
30 East Broad Street, Room 1280
Columbus, OH 43224
(614) 466-5214

STATE VOCATIONAL
REHABILITATION AGENCY

Rehabilitation Services Commission
400 East Campus View Boulevard
Columbus, OH 43235-4604
(614) 438-1210 (V/TTY)

TECHNOLOGY-RELATED ASSISTANCE

Ohio Train
Ohio Supercomputer Center
1224 Kinnear Road
Columbus, OH 43212
(614) 292-2426 (V/TTY) or (800) 784-3425
    (V/TTY, in OH)
(614) 292-3162 (TTY)

UNIVERSITY-AFFILIATED PROGRAM

The Nisonger Center
Ohio State University
1581 Dodd Drive
Columbus, OH 43210-1296
(614) 292-8365

**University Affiliated Cincinnati Center
    for Developmental Disorders**
Pavilion Building
3333 Burnet Avenue
Cincinnati, OH 45229-3039
(513) 636-4688

OKLAHOMA

CLIENT ASSISTANCE PROGRAM

Oklahoma Client Assistance Program
Office of Handicapped Concerns
2712 Villa Prom Street
Oklahoma City, OK 73107-2423
(405) 521-3756 or (800) 522-8224 (in OK)

OKLAHOMA DEPARTMENT OF VOCATIONAL AND TECHNICAL EDUCATION

Department of Vocational Technical Education

1500 West Seventh Avenue
Stillwater, OK 74074
(405) 377-2000, ext. 138; (405) 743-5138;
(800) 522-5810

PARENT TRAINING AND INFORMATION PROJECT

Parents Reaching Out in OK (PRO-Oklahoma)

1917 South Harvard Drive
Oklahoma City, OK 73128
(405) 681-9710 or (800) 759-4142 (V/TTY)
http://www.iser.com

PROGRAMS FOR CHILDREN WITH DISABILITIES: AGES THREE THROUGH FIVE

Special Education Section, Department of Education

2500 North Lincoln Boulevard, Room 411
Oklahoma City, OK 73105
(405) 521-3351

PROGRAMS FOR CHILDREN WITH SPECIAL HEALTH CARE NEEDS

Family Support Services

Department of Human Services
P.O. Box 25352
Oklahoma City, OK 73125
(405) 521-3076

PROGRAMS FOR INFANTS AND TODDLERS WITH DISABILITIES: AGES BIRTH THROUGH TWO

Early Intervention

Special Education Section, Department of Education
2500 North Lincoln Boulevard, Room 411
Oklahoma City, OK 73105-4599
(405) 521-3351

PROTECTION AND ADVOCACY AGENCY

Oklahoma Disability Law Center, Inc.

2828 E. 51st Street, Suite 302
Tulsa, OK 74105
(918) 743-6220 (V/TTY) or (800) 226-5883
(V/TTY, in OK)

2915 Classen Boulevard
300 Cameron Building
Oklahoma City, OK 73106
(405) 525-7755 (V/TTY) or (800) 880-7755
(V/TTY, in OK)

STATE DEPARTMENT OF EDUCATION: SPECIAL EDUCATION

Special Education Services, Department of Education

2500 N. Lincoln Boulevard
Oklahoma City, OK 73105-4599
(405) 521-3351

STATE DEVELOPMENTAL DISABILITIES PLANNING COUNCIL

Oklahoma Developmental Disabilities Council

3033 N. Walnut, Suite 105E
P.O. Box 25352
Oklahoma City, OK 73125
(405) 528-4984 or (800) 836-4470
e-mail:OPCDD@aol.com

STATE MENTAL HEALTH AGENCY

Department of Mental Health and Substance Abuse Services

P.O. Box 53277
Oklahoma City, OK 73152-3277
(405) 522-3877

STATE MENTAL HEALTH REPRESENTATIVE FOR CHILDREN AND YOUTH

Department of Mental Health and Substance Abuse Services

P.O. Box 53277
Oklahoma City, OK 73152
(405) 522-3839

STATE MENTAL RETARDATION PROGRAM

Developmental Disabilities Services
Department of Human Services
P.O. Box 25352
Oklahoma City, OK 73125
(405) 521-3571

STATE VOCATIONAL REHABILITATION AGENCY

Department of Rehabilitation Services
3535 NW 58th, Suite 500
Oklahoma City, OK 73112
(405) 951-3400

TECHNOLOGY-RELATED ASSISTANCE

Oklahoma ABLE Tech
Oklahoma State University
Wellness Center
1514 W. Hall of Fame
Stillwater, OK 74078-2026
(405) 744-9864; (800) 257-1705 (V/TTY);
     (888) 885-5588 (ABLE Tech Info-line)
http://www.okabletech.okstate.edu

UNIVERSITY-AFFILIATED PROGRAM

UAP of Oklahoma
University of Oklahoma Health Sciences Center
P.O. Box 26901, ROB 316
Oklahoma City, OK 73190-3042
(405) 271-2688

OREGON

CLIENT ASSISTANCE PROGRAM

Oregon Disabilities Commission
1257 Ferry Street SE
Salem, OR 97310
(503) 378-3599 or (503) 378-3142 (TTY)

OFFICE OF STATE COORDINATOR OF VOCATIONAL EDUCATION FOR STUDENTS WITH DISABILITIES

Disadvantaged and Handicapped
Oregon Department of Education
255 Capitol Street, N.E.

Salem, OR 97310-0203
(503) 378-3584

PARENT TRAINING AND INFORMATION PROJECT

Oregon COPE Project (Coalition in OR for Parent Education)
999 Locust Street, N.E.
Salem, OR 97303
(503) 581-8156 (V/TTY) or (888) 505-COPE
     (V/TTY)
http://community.open.org

PROGRAMS FOR CHILDREN AND YOUTH WHO ARE DEAF OR HARD OF HEARING

Deaf and Hearing Impaired Access Program
Oregon Disabilities Commission
1257 Ferry Street, SE
Salem, OR 97310
(503) 378-3142 (V/TTY); (800) 358-3117 (V/TTY, in OR); (800) 521-9615 (V/TTY, in OR)

PROGRAMS FOR CHILDREN WITH DISABILITIES: AGES THREE THROUGH FIVE

Office of Special Education, Department of Education
255 Capitol Street, N.E.
Salem, OR 97310-0203
(503) 378-3598, ext. 639
http://www.ode.state.or.us

PROGRAMS FOR CHILDREN WITH SPECIAL HEALTH-CARE NEEDS

Child Development and Rehabilitation Center
Oregon Health Sciences University
P.O. Box 574
Portland, OR 97207
(503) 494-8362

PROGRAMS FOR INFANTS AND TODDLERS WITH DISABILITIES: AGES BIRTH THROUGH TWO

Office of Special Education
Department of Education

255 Capitol Street, N.E.
Salem, OR 97310-0203
(503) 378-3598, ext. 637
http://www.ode.state.or.us

PROTECTION AND ADVOCACY AGENCY

Oregon Advocacy Center
620 SW Fifth Avenue, Fifth Floor
Portland, OR 97204-1428
(503) 243-2081 or (503) 323-9161 (TTY)
http://www.oradvocacy.org

REGIONAL ADA ASSISTIVE TECHNOLOGY AGENCY

Washington State Govenor's Committee on Disability Issue and Employment
P.O. Box 9046, MS 6000
Olympia, WA 98507-9046
(360) 438-4116 (V/TTY)
http://access.wa.gov

STATE AGENCY FOR THE VISUALLY IMPAIRED

Oregon Commission for the Blind
535 SE 12th Avenue
Portland, OR 97214
(503) 731-3221
e-mail: charles.young@state.or.us
http://www.cfb.state.or.us

STATE DEPARTMENT OF EDUCATION: SPECIAL EDUCATION

Office of Special Education
Department of Education
255 Capitol Street, NE
Salem, OR 97310-0203
(503) 378-3598, ext. 639
http://www.ode.state.or.us

STATE DEVELOPMENTAL DISABILITIES PLANNING COUNCIL

Oregon Developmental Disabilities Council
540 24th Place, NE
Salem, OR 97301-4517
(503) 945-9941 or (800) 292-4154 (in OR)
http://www.ocdd.org

STATE MENTAL HEALTH AGENCY

Mental Health and Developmental Disabilities Services Division
Department of Human Resources
2575 Bittern Street, NE
Salem, OR 97310-0520
(503) 945-9499

STATE MENTAL HEALTH REPRESENTATIVE FOR CHILDREN AND YOUTH

Office of Mental Health Services
Mental Health and Developmental Disabilities
   Services Division
2575 Bittern Street, NE
Salem, OR 97310-0520
(503) 945-9718

STATE MENTAL RETARDATION PROGRAM

Office of Developmental Disabilities Services
Mental Health and Developmental Disability
   Services Division
Department of Human Resources
2575 Bittern Street, NW
Salem, OR 97310
(503) 945-9774

STATE VOCATIONAL REHABILITATION AGENCY

Vocational Rehabilitation Division, Dept. of Human Resources
500 Summer Street, NE
Salem, OR 97310-1018
(503) 945-5880

TECHNOLOGY-RELATED ASSISTANCE

Oregon Technology Access for Life Needs Project
1257 Ferry Street, SE
Salem, OR 97310
(503) 361-1201 or (800) 677-7512 (V/TTY)

UNIVERSITY-AFFILIATED PROGRAM

Center on Human Development—Clinical Services
College of Education

5252 University of Oregon-Eugene
Eugene, OR 97403-1265
(541) 346-3591
http://www.uoregon.edu

Child Development and Rehabilitation Center
Oregon Health Sciences University
3181 SW Sam Jackson Park Road
Portland, OR 97239
(503) 494-8311
http://www.ohsu.edu/outreach/cdrc

PENNSYLVANIA

CLIENT ASSISTANCE PROGRAM

Center for Disability Law and Policy
1617 JFK Boulevard, Suite 800
Philadelphia, PA 19103
(215) 557-7112 (V/TTY)

OFFICE OF STATE COORDINATOR OF VOCATIONAL EDUCATION FOR STUDENTS WITH DISABILITIES

Special Populations Section, Department of Education
Bureau of Vocational-Technical Education
333 Market Street, Sixth Floor
Harrisburg, PA 17126-0333
(717) 787-5293

PARENT TRAINING AND INFORMATION PROJECTS

Parent Education Network
2107 Industrial Highway
York, PA 17402
(717) 845-9722; (800) 522-5827 (V/TTY, in PA);
    (800) 441-5028 (Spanish)
http://www.parentednet.org

Parents Union for Public Schools
311 South Juniper Street, Suite 200
Philadelphia, PA 19107
(215) 546-1166

PROGRAMS FOR CHILDREN AND YOUTH WHO ARE DEAF OR HARD OF HEARING

Office for the Deaf and Hard of Hearing
1110 Labor and Industry Building

Seventh and Forster Streets
Harrisburg, PA 17120-0019
(717) 783-4912 (V/TTY) or (800) 233-3008 (V/TTY, in PA)

PROGRAMS FOR CHILDREN WITH DISABILITIES: AGES THREE THROUGH FIVE

Division of Early Intervention
Bureau of Special Education, Department of Education
333 Market Street, Seventh Floor
Harrisburg, PA 17126-0333
(717) 783-6879

PROGRAMS FOR CHILDREN WITH SPECIAL HEALTH-CARE NEEDS

Division of Special Health Care Programs
Department of Health, Room 724
P.O. Box 90
Harrisburg, PA 17108
(717) 783-5436

PROGRAMS FOR INFANTS AND TODDLERS WITH DISABILITIES: AGES BIRTH THROUGH TWO

Children's Services Division
Office of Mental Retardation, Department of Public Welfare
P.O. Box 2675
Harrisburg, PA 17105-2675
(717) 783-8302

PROTECTION AND ADVOCACY AGENCY

Pennsylvania Protection and Advocacy, Inc.
1414 N. Cameron Street
Suite C
Harrisburg, PA 17103
(717) 236-8110 or (800) 692-7443 (V/TTY, in PA)

STATE AGENCY FOR THE VISUALLY IMPAIRED

Blindness and Visual Services, Dept. of Public Welfare
P.O. Box 2675
Harrisburg, PA 17105
(717) 787-6176 or (800) 622-2842 (in PA)

STATE DEPARTMENT OF EDUCATION: SPECIAL EDUCATION

Bureau of Special Education, Department of Education
333 Market Street, Seventh Floor
Harrisburg, PA 17126-0333
(717) 783-2311

STATE DEVELOPMENTAL DISABILITIES PLANNING COUNCIL

Developmental Disabilities Planning Council
568 Forum Building, Commonwealth Avenue
Harrisburg, PA 17120
(717) 787-6057

STATE EDUCATION AGENCY RURAL REPRESENTATIVE

Advisory Service, Department of Education
333 Market Street, 6th Floor
Harrisburg, PA 17126
(717) 787-8022

STATE MENTAL HEALTH AGENCY

Office of Mental Health, Department of Public Welfare
Health and Welfare Building, Room 502
P.O. Box 2675
Harrisburg, PA 17105-2675
(717) 787-6443

STATE MENTAL HEALTH REPRESENTATIVE FOR CHILDREN AND YOUTH

Bureau of Children's Services
Office of Mental Health Department of Public
   Welfare
P.O. Box 2675
Harrisburg, PA 17105
(717) 772-2351

STATE MENTAL RETARDATION PROGRAM

Department of Public Welfare
Health and Welfare Building, Room 512
P.O. Box 2675
Harrisburg, PA 17105-2675
(717) 787-3700

STATE VOCATIONAL REHABILITATION AGENCY

Office of Vocational Rehabilitation, Department of Labor and Industry
1300 Labor and Industry Building, Seventh and
   Forster Streets
Harrisburg, PA 17120
(717) 787-5244

TECHNOLOGY-RELATED ASSISTANCE

Pennsylvania's Initiative on Assistive Technology
Institute on Disability/UAP
1301 Cecil B. Moore Avenue
Ritter Hall Annex 423
Philadelphia, PA 19122
(215) 204-1356 (V/TTY); (800) 204-PIAT (V);
   (800) 750-PIAT (TTY)

UNIVERSITY AFFILIATED PROGRAM

Institute on Disabilities UAP
Temple University, Ritter Annex, Room 423
1301 Cecil B. Moore Avenue
Philadelphia, PA 19122
(215) 204-1356 (V/TTY)
http://www.disabilities.temple.edu

RHODE ISLAND

OFFICE OF STATE COORDINATOR OF VOCATIONAL EDUCATION FOR STUDENTS WITH DISABILITIES

State Department of Education
Office of Special Needs Center
Shepard Building
255 Westminster Street
Providence, RI 02903-3400
(401) 277-4600, ext. 2216

PARENT TRAINING AND INFORMATION PROJECT

Rhode Island Parent Info Network (RIPIN)
500 Prospect Street
Pawtucket, RI 02860
(401) 727-4144 or (800) 464-3399 (in RI)

PROGRAMS FOR CHILDREN AND YOUTH WHO ARE DEAF OR HARD OF HEARING

Commission on the Deaf and Hard of Hearing
One Capitol Hill, Ground Level
Providence, RI 02908-5850
(401) 222-1204 (V) or (401) 222-1205 (TTY)
e-mail: cdhh@cdhh.ri.gov
http://www.cdhh.ri.gov/cdhh/committee.php

PROGRAMS FOR CHILDREN WITH DISABILITIES: AGES THREE THROUGH FIVE

Special Education Program Services Unit
Shepard Building
255 Westminster Street
Providence, RI 02903-3400
(401) 277-4600, ext. 2135

PROGRAMS FOR CHILDREN WITH SPECIAL HEALTH-CARE NEEDS

Office for Children with Special Health Care Needs
Department of Health
Three Capitol Hill
Providence, RI 02908
(401) 277-2313 or (401) 277-2312

PROGRAMS FOR INFANTS AND TODDLERS WITH DISABILITIES: AGES BIRTH THROUGH TWO

Division of Family Health
State Department of Health
Three Capitol Hill, Rm. 302
Providence, RI 02908-5097
(401) 277-2313 or (401) 277-2312

PROTECTION AND ADVOCACY AGENCY

Rhode Island Disability Law Center
151 Broadway
Providence, RI 02903
(401) 831-3150; (401) 831-5335 (TTY);
    (800) 733-5332 (in RI)

STATE AGENCY FOR THE VISUALLY IMPAIRED

Services for the Blind and Visually Impaired, Department of Human Services
40 Fountain Street
Providence, RI 02903
(401) 277-2300 or (800) 752-8088, ext. 2300
http://www.ors.state.ri.us

STATE DEPARTMENT OF EDUCATION: SPECIAL EDUCATION

Office of Special Needs
Department of Education, Shepard Building
255 Westminster Street, Room 400
Providence, RI 02903-3400
(401) 277-4600, ext. 2301

STATE DEVELOPMENTAL DISABILITIES PLANNING COUNCIL

Rhode Island Developmental Disabilities Council
600 New London Avenue
Cranston, RI 02920
(401) 464-3191 (V/TTY)

STATE EDUCATION AGENCY RURAL REPRESENTATIVE

Office of Special Needs
Department of Education, Shepard Building
255 Westminster Street, Room 400
Providence, RI 02903-3400
(401) 277-3505

STATE MENTAL HEALTH AGENCY

Department of Mental Health, Retardation, and Hospitals
600 New London Avenue
Cranston, RI 02920
(401) 464-3201

STATE MENTAL HEALTH REPRESENTATIVE FOR CHILDREN AND YOUTH

Children's Mental Health and Education
Department of Children, Youth, and Families
610 Mt. Pleasant Avenue, Building Seven
Providence, RI 02908
(401) 457-4514

STATE MENTAL RETARDATION PROGRAM

Division of Developmental Disabilities
Department of Mental Health, Retardation and
    Hospitals

Aime J. Forand Building
600 New London Avenue
Cranston, RI 02920
(401) 464-3234

STATE VOCATIONAL REHABILITATION AGENCY

Office of Rehabilitation Services
Department of Human Services
40 Fountain Street
Providence, RI 02903
(401) 421-7005, ext. 301
http://www.ors.state.ri.us

TECHNOLOGY-RELATED ASSISTANCE

Rhode Island Assistive Technology Access Partnership
Office of Rehabilitation Services
40 Fountain Street
Providence, RI 02903-1898
(800) 752-8088, ext. 2608 (in RI);
    (401) 421-7005; (401) 421-7016 (TTY)
http://www.atap.state.ri.us

UNIVERSITY-AFFILIATED PROGRAM

UAP of Rhode Island
Institute for Developmental Disabilities at Rhode
    Island College
600 Mount Pleasant Avenue
Providence, RI 02908
(401) 456-8072 or (401) 456-8150 (TTY)

SOUTH CAROLINA

CLIENT ASSISTANCE PROGRAM

Office of Governor; Division of Ombudsman and Citizen Services
Edgar Brown Building, Room 308
1205 Pendelton Street
Columbia, SC 29201
(803) 734-0285 or (800) 868-0040 (in SC)

OFFICE OF STATE COORDINATOR OF VOCATIONAL EDUCATION FOR STUDENTS WITH DISABILITIES

Office of Occupational Education
Rutledge Building, Ninth Floor, 924

Columbia, SC 29201
(803) 734-8486

PROGRAMS FOR CHILDREN WITH DISABILITIES: AGES THREE THROUGH FIVE

Office of Programs for Exceptional Children
1429 Senate Street, Eighth Floor
Columbia, SC 29201
(803) 734-8811

PROGRAMS FOR CHILDREN WITH SPECIAL HEALTH-CARE NEEDS

Division of Children's Rehabilitative Services
Department of Health and Environmental Control
1751 Calhoun Street, Box 101106
Columbia, SC 29211
(803) 737-4072

PROGRAMS FOR INFANTS AND TODDLERS WITH DISABILITIES: AGES BIRTH THROUGH TWO

Department of Health and Environmental Control/Baby Net
Robert Mills Complex, Box 101106
Columbia, SC 29211
(803) 737-4046

PROTECTION AND ADVOCACY AGENCY

Protection and Advocacy for People with Disabilities
3710 Landmark Drive, Suite 208
Columbia, SC 29204
(803) 782-0639; (800) 922-5225 (in SC);
    (800) 531-9781 (Spanish)

STATE DEPARTMENT OF EDUCATION: SPECIAL EDUCATION

State Department of Education
Office of Programs for Exceptional Children
1429 Senate Street, Room 808
Columbia, SC 29201
(803) 734-8806

STATE DEVELOPMENTAL DISABILITIES PLANNING COUNCIL

South Carolina Developmental Disabilities Council
Edgar Brown Building

1205 Pendleton Street, Room 372
Columbia, SC 29201
(803) 734-0465

STATE DISABILITIES AND SPECIAL NEEDS

Department of Disabilities and Special Needs
3440 Harden Street Extension
P.O. Box 4706
Columbia, SC 29240
(803) 737-6444
http://www.state.sc.us/ddsn

STATE EDUCATION AGENCY RURAL REPRESENTATIVE

Family Connection of South Carolina, Inc.
2712 Middleburg Drive, Suite 103B
Columbia, SC 29204
(803) 252-0914 (in Columbia); (864) 455-6213
    (in Greenville); (800) 578-8750

ORTHOPEDICALLY HANDICAPPED, DEPARTMENT OF EDUCATION

Office of Technical Assistance
1429 Senate Street, 506 Rutledge Building
Columbia, SC 29201-3730
(803) 734-8223

SOUTH CAROLINA SERVICES INFORMATION SYSTEM

Center for Developmental Disabilities
University of South Carolina School of Medicine
Columbia, SC 29208
(803) 935-5231 (Admin. number);
    (803) 935-5300 (Columbia area);
    (800) 922-1107

STATE MENTAL HEALTH AGENCY

Department of Mental Health
Box 485
Columbia, SC 29202
(803) 734-7780

STATE MENTAL HEALTH REPRESENTATIVE FOR CHILDREN AND YOUTH

Division of Children, Adolescents and Their Families
Department of Mental Health

2414 Bull Street, Room 304
Columbia, SC 29201
(803) 734-7859

STATE SCHOOL FOR THE DEAF AND THE BLIND

South Carolina School for the Deaf and the Blind
355 Cedar Springs Road
Spartanburg, SC 29302-4699
(864) 585-7711

STATE VOCATIONAL REHABILITATION AGENCY

Vocational Rehabilitation Department
1410 Boston Avenue, P.O. Box 15
West Columbia, SC 29171-0015
(803) 896-6504

TECHNOLOGY-RELATED ASSISTANCE

South Carolina Assistive Technology Project
USC School of Medicine
Center for Developmental Disabilities
Columbia, SC 29208
(803) 935-5263

UNIVERSITY-AFFILIATED PROGRAM

UAP of South Carolina
USC School of Medicine
Center for Developmental Disabilities
Columbia, SC 29208
(803) 935-5231

THE VISUALLY IMPAIRED

Donald Gist, Commissioner
Commission for the Blind
1430 Confederate Avenue
Columbia, SC 29201
(803) 734-7520

SOUTH DAKOTA

PARENT-TO-PARENT

Parent to Parent, Inc.
2501 West 26th Street
Sioux Falls, SD 57105

(605) 334-3119 or (800) 658-5411 (in SD)

PARENT TRAINING AND INFORMATION PROJECT

South Dakota Parent Connection
3701 W. 49th Street, Suite 102
Sioux Falls, SD 57106
(605) 361-3171 or (800) 640-4553 (in SD)
http://www.sdparent.org

PROGRAMS FOR CHILDREN AND YOUTH WHO ARE DEAF OR HARD OF HEARING

Communication Services for the Deaf
102 N. Krohn Place
Sioux Falls, SD 57103
(605) 367-5760 (V/TTY) or (800) 640-6410
   (V/TTY, in SD)

PROGRAMS FOR CHILDREN WITH DISABILITIES: AGES THREE THROUGH FIVE

Office of Special Education
700 Governor's Drive
Pierre, SD 57501-2291
(605) 773-3678

PROGRAMS FOR CHILDREN WITH SPECIAL HEALTH-CARE NEEDS

Children's Special Health Services
Health Medical Services and Laboratory
Department of Health
615 E. Fourth Street
Pierre, SD 57501
(605) 773-3737

PROGRAMS FOR INFANTS AND TODDLERS WITH DISABILITIES: AGES BIRTH THROUGH TWO

Education Program Assistant Manager
Office of Special Education
700 Governor's Drive
Pierre, SD 57501-2291
(605) 773-3678

PROTECTION AND ADVOCACY AGENCY

Mental Health Advocacy Program
South Dakota Advocacy Services
221 S. Central Avenue
Pierre, SD 57501
(605) 224-8294 or (800) 658-4782 (in SD)

STATE AGENCY FOR THE VISUALLY IMPAIRED

Service to the Blind and Visually Impaired
East Highway 34
c/o 500 E. Capitol
Pierre, SD 57501
(605) 773-4644

STATE DEPARTMENT OF EDUCATION: SPECIAL EDUCATION

Office of Special Education
700 Governor's Drive
Pierre, SD 57501-2291
(605) 773-3678

STATE DEVELOPMENTAL DISABILITIES PLANNING COUNCIL

South Dakota Governor's Planning Council on Developmental Disabilities
Hillsview Plaza, E. Hwy 34
c/o 500 East Capitol
Pierre, SD 57501-5070
(605) 773-6415

STATE DEVELOPMENTAL DISABILITIES PROGRAM

Division of Developmental Disabilities
Hillsview Plaza, East Highway 34
c/o 500 East Capitol
Pierre, SD 57501
(605) 773-3438
http://www.state.sd.us

STATE DEVELOPMENTAL DISABILITIES REPRESENTATIVE FOR CHILDREN AND YOUTH

Department of Human Services
Hillsview Plaza, East Highway 34
c/o 500 East Capitol

Pierre, SD 57501
(605) 773-3438

STATE MENTAL HEALTH AGENCY

Division of Mental Health
South Dakota Human Services Center
3515 Broadway Avenue
P.O. Box 76
Yankton, SD 57078
(605) 668-3102

STATE MENTAL HEALTH REPRESENTATIVE FOR CHILDREN AND YOUTH

Division of Mental Health
3515 Broadway Avenue
P.O. Box 76
Yankton, SD 57078
(605) 668-3548

STATE RESPITE CARE PROGRAM

Department of Human Services
Hillsview Plaza, East Highway 34
c/o 500 East Capitol
Pierre, SD 57501
(605) 773-3438
http://www.state.sd.us/dhs/dd/respite

STATE VOCATIONAL REHABILITATION AGENCY

Division of Rehabilitation Services
Hillsview Plaza, E. Highway 34
c/o 500 East Capitol
Pierre, SD 57501-5070
(605) 773-3195
http://www.state.sd.us/dhs/drs

TECHNOLOGY-RELATED ASSISTANCE

DakotaLink
1925 Plaza Boulevard
Rapid City, SD 57702
(605) 394-1876 (V/TTY) or (800) 645-0673 (V/TTY)

UNIVERSITY-AFFILIATED PROGRAM

South Dakota University Affiliated Program
Health Science Center

1400 West 22nd Street
Sioux Falls, SD 57105
(605) 357-1439 or (800) 658-3080 (V/TTY)

TENNESSEE

OFFICE OF STATE COORDINATOR OF VOCATIONAL EDUCATION FOR STUDENTS WITH DISABILITIES

Division of Vocational Education
Andrew Johnson Tower, Fourth Floor
710 James Robertson Parkway
Nashville, TN 37243-0383
(615) 532-2800

PARENT-TO-PARENT

Parents Encouraging Parents (PEP) Program
Cordell Hull Building, Fifth Floor
426 Fifth Avenue North
Nashville, TN 37247-4850
(615) 741-8530

PARENT TRAINING AND INFORMATION PROJECT

Support and Training for Exceptional Parents (STEP)
712 Professional Plaza
Greeneville, TN 37745
(423) 639-0125; (800) 280-7837 (in TN);
    (423) 639-2464 (TTY)
e-mail: information@tnstep.org
http://www.tnstep.org

PROGRAMS FOR CHILDREN AND YOUTH WHO ARE DEAF OR HARD OF HEARING

Tennessee Council for the Hearing Impaired
400 Deaderick Street, 11th Floor
Nashville, TN 37248-6300
(615) 313-4913 (V/TTY) or (615) 313-5695
    (24-hour answering machine)

PROGRAMS FOR CHILDREN WITH SPECIAL HEALTH-CARE NEEDS

Children's Special Services
Department of Health
Cordell Hull Building, Fifth Floor

425 Fifth Avenue North
Nashville, TN 37247-4701
(615) 741-8530

PROGRAMS FOR INFANTS AND TODDLERS WITH DISABILITIES: AGES BIRTH THROUGH TWO

Contact STATE DEPARTMENT OF EDUCATION: SPECIAL EDUCATION
Andrew Johnson Tower, Fifth floor
710 James Robertson Parkway
Nashville, TN 37243
(615) 741-2851

PROTECTION AND ADVOCACY AGENCY

Tennessee Protection and Advocacy, Inc.
P.O. Box 121257
Nashville, TN 37212
(615) 298-1080 or (800) 342-1660 (in TN)

STATE DEPARTMENT FOR CHILDREN AND YOUTH IN STATE CUSTODY

Tennessee Department of Children's Services
Seventh Floor, Cordell Hull Building
436 Sixth Avenue North
Nashville, TN 37243-1290
(615) 741-9699

STATE DEPARTMENT OF EDUCATION: SPECIAL EDUCATION

Division of Special Education
Department of Education
Andrew Johnson Tower, Fifth Floor
710 James Robertson Parkway
Nashville, TN 37243-0380
(615) 741-2851

STATE DEVELOPMENTAL DISABILITIES PLANNING COUNCIL

Tennessee Developmental Disabilities Council
Andrew Johnson Tower, 10th Floor
710 James Robertson Parkway
Nashville, TN 37243-0675
(615) 532-6615

STATE EDUCATION AGENCY RURAL REPRESENTATIVE

Department of Education, Division of Special Education
Andrew Johnson Tower, Fifth Floor
710 James Robertson Parkway
Nashville, TN 37243-0380
(615) 741-2851

STATE MENTAL HEALTH AGENCY

Department of Mental Health and Mental Retardation
Andrew Johnson Tower, 11th Floor
710 James Robertson Parkway
Nashville, TN 37243-0675
(615) 532-6500

STATE MENTAL HEALTH REPRESENTATIVE FOR CHILDREN AND YOUTH

Office of Children and Adolescent Services
Department of Mental Health and Mental Retardation
Andrew Johnson Tower, 10th Floor
710 James Robertson Parkway
Nashville, TN 37243-0675
(615) 532-6767

STATE MENTAL RETARDATION PROGRAM

Division of Mental Retardation
Department of Mental Health and Mental Retardation
Andrew Johnson Tower, 11th Floor
710 James Robertson Parkway
Nashville, TN 37243-0675
(615) 532-6530

STATE VOCATIONAL REHABILITATION AGENCY

Division of Rehabilitation Services
Department of Human Services
400 Deaderick Street, 15th Floor
Nashville, TN 37248-0060
(615) 313-4714

TECHNOLOGY-RELATED ASSISTANCE

Tennessee Technology Access Project
710 James Robertson Parkway
Andrew Johnson Tower, 10th Floor
Nashville, TN 37243-0675
(615) 532-6558; (615) 741-4566 (TTY);
    (800) 732-5059 (in TN)

UNIVERSITY-AFFILIATED PROGRAM

Boling Center for Developmental Disabilities—UAT
The University of Tennessee, Memphis
711 Jefferson Avenue
Memphis, TN 38105
(901) 448-6512
http://www.utmem.edu/bcdd

TEXAS

CLIENT ASSISTANCE PROGRAM

Client Assistant Program
Advocacy, Inc.
7800 Shoal Creek Boulevard, Suite 171-E
Austin, TX 78757
(512) 454-4816
http://www.advocacyinc.org

PARENT TRAINING AND INFORMATION PROJECTS

Grassroots Consortium
6202 Belmark
P.O. Box 61628
Houston, TX 77208-1628
(713) 643-9576

Partners Resource Network, Inc.
1090 Longfellow Drive, Suite B
Beaumont, TX 77706-4819
(409) 898-4684 or (800) 866-4726 (in TX)
http://www.partnerstx.org

Project PODER
1017 N. Main Avenue, Suite 207
San Antonio, TX 78212
(210) 222-2637 or (800) 682-9747 (in TX)

PROGRAMS FOR CHILDREN AND YOUTH WHO ARE DEAF OR HARD OF HEARING

Texas Commission for the Deaf and Hard of Hearing
P.O. Box 12904
Austin, TX 78711-2904
(512) 451-8494 (V/TTY)

PROGRAMS FOR CHILDREN WITH DISABILITIES: AGES THREE THROUGH FIVE

Special Education Programs
Texas Education Agency
1701 North Congress Avenue
Austin, TX 78701-1494
(512) 463-9414

PROGRAMS FOR CHILDREN WITH SPECIAL HEALTH-CARE NEEDS

CSHCN Planning and Policy Development
Bureau of Children's Health
Texas Department of Health
1100 West 49th Street
Austin, TX 78756-3179
(512) 458-7355

PROGRAMS FOR INFANTS AND TODDLERS WITH DISABILITIES: AGES BIRTH THROUGH TWO

Early Childhood Intervention Program
4900 N. Lamar Boulevard
Austin, TX 78751-2399
(512) 424-6754 or (800) 250-2246 (Information and referral)

PROTECTION AND ADVOCACY AGENCY

Advocacy, Inc.
7800 Shoal Creek Boulevard, Suite 171-E
Austin, TX 78757
(512) 454-4816 or (800) 252-9108 (in TX)

STATE AGENCY FOR THE BLIND AND VISUALLY IMPAIRED

Texas Commission for the Blind
P.O. Box 12866

Austin, TX 78711
(512) 459-2500

STATE DEPARTMENT OF EDUCATION
CAREER AND TECHNOLOGY EDUCATION

Texas Education Agency
1701 North Congress Avenue
Austin, TX 78701
(512) 463-9446 or (512) 475-3575

STATE DEPARTMENT OF EDUCATION:
SPECIAL EDUCATION

Texas Education Agency
Division of Special Education
1701 North Congress Avenue
Austin, TX 78701-1494
(512) 463-9414

STATE DEVELOPMENTAL DISABILITIES
PLANNING COUNCIL

**Texas Planning Council for Developmental
   Disabilities**
4900 North Lamar Boulevard
Austin, TX 78751-2399
(512) 424-4080; (800) 262-0334;
   (512) 424-4099 (TTY)

STATE EDUCATION AGENCY RURAL
REPRESENTATIVE

Special Education
Texas Education Agency
1701 North Congress Avenue
Austin, TX 78701-1494
(512) 463-9414

STATE MENTAL HEALTH AGENCY

**Texas Department of Mental Health and
   Mental Retardation**
P.O. Box 12668, Capitol Station
Austin, TX 78711-2668
(512) 206-4588

STATE MENTAL HEALTH
REPRESENTATIVE FOR CHILDREN
AND YOUTH

Children's Services
Texas Department of Mental Health and Mental
   Retardation

P.O. Box 12668
Austin, TX 78711-2668
(512) 206-4722

STATE VOCATIONAL
REHABILITATION AGENCY

Texas Rehabilitation Commission
4900 North Lamar, Room 7102
Austin, TX 78751-2399
(512) 424-4001

TECHNOLOGY-RELATED ASSISTANCE

Texas Assistive Technology Partnership
Texas UAP for Developmental Disabilities
University of Texas at Austin
SZB 252/D5100
Austin, TX 78712
(512) 471-7621 or (512) 471-1844 (TTY)
(800) 828-7839

UNIVERSITY-AFFILIATED PROGRAM

Texas UAP for Developmental Disabilities
University of Texas at Austin
SZB 252/D5100
Austin, TX 78712-1290
(512) 471-7621; (800) 828-7839;
   (512) 471-1844 (TTY)

UTAH

OFFICE OF STATE COORDINATOR
OF VOCATIONAL EDUCATION
FOR STUDENTS WITH DISABILITIES

Transition and Applied Technology
Services for At Risk Students (SARS)
State Office of Education
250 East 500 South
Salt Lake City, UT 84111
(801) 538-7700

PARENT-TO-PARENT

Hope—A Parent to Parent Network
2290 East 4500 South, Suite 110
Salt Lake City, UT 84117
(801) 272-0493 or (800) 468-1160 (in UT)

PARENT TRAINING AND INFORMATION PROJECT

Utah Parent Center
2290 East 4500 South, Suite 110
Salt Lake City, UT 84117
(801) 272-1051 (V/TTY) or (800) 468-1160 (in UT)
http://www.utahparentcenter.org

PROGRAMS FOR CHILDREN AND YOUTH WHO ARE DEAF OR HARD OF HEARING

Utah Community Center for the Deaf
Utah State Office of Rehabilitation
5709 South 1500 West
Salt Lake City, UT 84123
(801) 263-4860 (V/TTY) or (800) 860-4860
    (V/TTY, in UT)
http://www.deafservices.utah.gov

PROGRAMS FOR CHILDREN WITH SPECIAL HEALTH-CARE NEEDS

Utah Department of Health
Community and Family Health Services
Children with Special Health Care Needs
44 North Medical Drive
Box 144650 BHCS
Salt Lake City, UT 84114-4650
(801) 584-8240

PROGRAMS FOR CHILDREN WITH DISABILITIES: AGES THREE THROUGH FIVE

Special Education Services Unit, State Office of Education
250 East Fifth South
Salt Lake City, UT 84111
(801) 538-7708

PROGRAMS FOR INFANTS AND TODDLERS WITH DISABILITIES: AGES BIRTH THROUGH TWO

Utah Dept. of Health
Community and Family Health Services
Children with Special Health Care Needs—BWEIP
Box 144720
Salt Lake City, UT 84114-4720
(801) 584-8226 or (801) 584-8496

PROTECTION AND ADVOCACY AGENCY

Disability Law Center
455 East 400 South, Suite 410
Salt Lake City, UT 84111
(801) 363-1347 or (800) 662-9080 (V/TTY, in UT)

STATE AGENCY FOR THE VISUALLY IMPAIRED

Division of Services for the Blind and Visually Impaired
309 East 100 South
Salt Lake City, UT 84111
(801) 323-4343
http://www.usor.utah.gov/dsbvi.htm

STATE DEPARTMENT OF EDUCATION: SPECIAL EDUCATION

At Risk and Special Education Services
State Office of Education
250 East 500 South
Salt Lake City, UT 84111-3204
(801) 538-7706

STATE DEVELOPMENTAL DISABILITIES PLANNING COUNCIL

Utah Governor's Council for People with Disabilities
555 East 300 South, #201
Salt Lake City, UT 84102
(801) 533-4128

STATE EDUCATION AGENCY RURAL REPRESENTATIVE

Rural Education, Utah State Office of Education
250 East 500 South
Salt Lake City, UT 84111
(801) 538-7892

STATE MENTAL HEALTH AGENCY

Division of Mental Health, Department of Human Services
120 North 200 West, Fourth Floor
Salt Lake City, UT 84103
(801) 538-4270

STATE MENTAL HEALTH REPRESENTATIVE FOR CHILDREN AND YOUTH

Division of Mental Health, Department of Social Services
120 North 200 West, Fourth Floor
P.O. Box 45500
Salt Lake City, UT 84145-0500
(801) 538-4270

STATE MENTAL RETARDATION PROGRAM

Division of Services for People with Disabilities
Department of Human Services
120 North 200 West, #411
Salt Lake City, UT 84103
(801) 538-4200 or (800) 837-6811
http://www.dspd.utah.gov

STATE VOCATIONAL REHABILITATION AGENCY

Utah State Office of Rehabilitation
250 East 500 South
Salt Lake City, UT 84111
(801) 538-7530 (V/TTY)
http://www.usor.state.ut.us/ucat/index.htm

TECHNOLOGY-RELATED ASSISTANCE

Utah Assistive Technology Program
Center for Persons with Disabilities
6855 Old Main Hill
Logan, UT 84322-6855
(800) 524-5152
http://www.uatpat.org

UNIVERSITY-AFFILIATED PROGRAM

Center for Persons with Disabilities
Utah State University
6800 Old Main Hill
Logan, UT 84322-6800
(435) 797-1981 or (866) 284-2821
http://www.cpd.usu.edu

VERMONT

CLIENT ASSISTANCE PROGRAM

Client Assistance Program
264 North Winooski Avenue
P.O. Box 1367
Burlington, VT 05402-1367
(802) 863-2881 or (800) 747-5022 (V/TTY)

OFFICE OF STATE COORDINATOR OF VOCATIONAL EDUCATION FOR STUDENTS WITH DISABILITIES

Vocational Education for Disadvantaged and Handicapped Programs
Department of Education
120 State Street
Montpelier, VT 05620
(802) 828-3101

PARENT-TO-PARENT

Parent-to-Parent Program of Vermont
600 Blair Park Road, Suite 240
Williston, VT 05495-7549
(800) 800-4005 or (802) 764-5290
http://www.partoparvt.org

PARENT TRAINING AND INFORMATION PROJECT

Vermont Parent Information Center
600 Blair Park Road, Suite 301
Williston, VT 05495-7589
(802) 876-5315 or (800) 639-7170 (in VT)
http://www.vtpic.com

PROGRAMS FOR CHILDREN WITH DISABILITIES: AGES THREE THROUGH FIVE

Special Education Unit, Department of Education
120 State Street
Montpelier, VT 05620-2501
(802) 828-3130

PROGRAMS FOR CHILDREN WITH SPECIAL HEALTH-CARE NEEDS

Division for Children with Special Health Needs
Department of Health
108 Cherry Street, P.O. Box 70
Burlington, VT 05402
(802) 863-7338 or (800) 660-4427

PROGRAMS FOR INFANTS AND TODDLERS WITH DISABILITIES: AGES BIRTH THROUGH TWO

Family, Infant and Toddlers Project
108 Cherry Street
P.O. Box 70
Burlington, VT 05402
(802) 651-1786 or (800) 660-4427 (V/TTY)

PROTECTION AND ADVOCACY AGENCY

Disability Law Project
264 North Winooski Avenue
P.O. Box 1367
Burlington, VT 05402-1367
(802) 863-2881 (V/TTY) or (800) 889-2047

Vermont Protection and Advocacy, Inc.
21 E. State Street, #101
Montpelier, VT 05602
(802) 229-1355 or (800) 834-7890 (in VT)

STATE AGENCY FOR THE VISUALLY IMPAIRED

Division for the Blind and Visually Impaired
Dept. of Aging and Disabilities, Agency of Human Services
Osgood Building
103 South Main Street
Waterbury, VT 05671-2304
(802) 241-2210 or (888) 405-5005
http://www.dad.state.vt.us/dbvi

STATE DEPARTMENT OF EDUCATION: SPECIAL EDUCATION

Family and Educational Support Team
120 State Street, State Office Building
Montpelier, VT 05620-2501
(802) 828-3130

STATE DEVELOPMENTAL DISABILITIES PLANNING COUNCIL

Vermont Developmental Disabilities Council
103 South Main Street
Waterbury, VT 05671-0206
(802) 241-2612 (TTY)

STATE EDUCATION AGENCY RURAL REPRESENTATIVE

Department of Education, Special Education Unit
120 State Street
Montpelier, VT 05602
(802) 828-3130 or (802) 229-4126

STATE MENTAL HEALTH AGENCY

Department of Developmental and Mental Health Services
Agency of Human Services
103 South Main Street, Weeks Building
Waterbury, VT 05671-1601
(802) 241-2610
http://www.dail.state.vt.us/DSwebsite

STATE MENTAL HEALTH REPRESENTATIVE FOR CHILDREN AND YOUTH

Division of Mental Health
103 South Main Street, Weeks Building
Waterbury, VT 05671-1601
(802) 241-2650
http://www.dail.state.vt.us/DSwebsite

STATE MENTAL RETARDATION PROGRAM

Division of Developmental Services
Department of Developmental and Mental Health Services
103 South Main Street, Weeks Building
Waterbury, VT 05671-1601
(802) 241-2614

STATE VOCATIONAL REHABILITATION AGENCY

Vocational Rehabilitation Division
Dept. of Aging and Disabilities, Agency of Human Services
103 South Main Street
Waterbury, VT 05671-2303
(802) 241-2186
http://www.dad.state.vt.us

TECHNOLOGY-RELATED ASSISTANCE

Vermont Assistive Technology Project
103 South Main Street, Weeks Building

Waterbury, VT 05671-2305
(802) 241-2620 (V/TTY)

VIRGINIA

CLIENT ASSISTANCE PROGRAM

Contact PROTECTION AND ADVOCACY AGENCY

OFFICE OF STATE COORDINATOR OF VOCATIONAL EDUCATION FOR STUDENTS WITH DISABILITIES

Office of Vocational and Adult Education Services
Department of Education
P.O. Box 2120
Richmond, VA 23218-2120
(804) 225-2847

PARENT RESOURCE CENTERS

Office of Special Education Services
Virginia Department of Education
P.O. Box 2120
Richmond, VA 23218-2120
(800) 422-2083 or (804) 371-7420

PARENT-TO-PARENT

Parent to Parent of Virginia
Family and Children's Service
1518 Willow Lawn Drive
Richmond, VA 23230
(804) 282-4255

PARENT TRAINING AND INFORMATION PROJECT

Parent Educational Advocacy Training Center (PEATC)
6320 Augusta Drive #1200
Springfield, VA 22150
(703) 691-7826 or (800) 869-6782
http://www.peatc.org

PROGRAMS FOR CHILDREN AND YOUTH WHO ARE DEAF OR HARD OF HEARING

Ratcliffe Building, Suite 203
1602 Rolling Hills Drive

Richmond, VA 23229-5012
(804) 662-9502 (V/TTY) or (800) 552-7917 (V/TTY)

PROGRAMS FOR CHILDREN WITH SPECIAL HEALTH CARE NEEDS

Division of Child and Adolescent Health
Virginia Department of Health
P.O. Box 2448
Richmond, VA 23218
(804) 786-7367
http://www.vdh.state.va.us

PROGRAMS FOR CHILDREN WITH DISABILITIES: AGES THREE THROUGH FIVE

Office of Special Education Services, Department of Education
P.O. Box 2120
Richmond, VA 23218-2120
(804) 225-2675

PROGRAMS FOR INFANTS AND TODDLERS WITH DISABILITIES: AGES BIRTH THROUGH TWO

Children/Family Services
Office of Mental Retardation Services
Department of Mental Health, Mental Retardation
and Substance Abuse Services
P.O. Box 1797
Richmond, VA 23214
(804) 786-0992

PROTECTION AND ADVOCACY AGENCY

Department for Rights of Virginians with Disabilities
Ninth Street Office Building, Ninth Floor
202 North Ninth Street
Richmond, VA 23219
(804) 225-2042 (Voice/TTY) or (800) 552-3962
(in VA)

STATE AGENCY FOR THE VISUALLY IMPAIRED

Department for the Blind and Visually Handicapped
397 Azalea Avenue
Richmond, VA 23227

(804) 371-3140

http://www.vdbvi.org

STATE DEPARTMENT OF EDUCATION: SPECIAL EDUCATION

Division of Special Education and Student Services

Department of Education

P.O. Box 2120

Richmond, VA 23218-2120

(804) 225-2402

STATE DEVELOPMENTAL DISABILITIES PLANNING COUNCIL

Virginia Board for People with Disabilities

Ninth Street Office Building

202 North Ninth Street, Ninth Floor

Richmond, VA 23219

(804) 786-0016 (V/TTY) or (800) 846-4464 (in VA)

STATE HEALTH DEPARTMENT: CHILD AND ADOLESCENT HEALTH

Division of Child and Adolescent Health

Virginia Department of Health

P.O. Box 2448

Richmond, VA 23218

(804) 786-7367

http://www.vdh.state.va.us

STATE MENTAL HEALTH AGENCY

Department of Mental Health, Mental Retardation and Substance Abuse Services

P.O. Box 1797

Richmond, VA 23218

(804) 786-3921

STATE MENTAL HEALTH REPRESENTATIVE FOR CHILDREN AND YOUTH

Department of Mental Health

Mental Retardation and Substance Abuse Services

P.O. Box 1797

Richmond, VA 23218

(804) 371-2185

STATE MENTAL RETARDATION PROGRAM

Office of Mental Retardation Services

Department of Mental Health, Mental Retardation and Substance Abuse

P.O. Box 1797

Richmond, VA 23219

(804) 786-1746

STATE VOCATIONAL REHABILITATION AGENCY

Virginia Department of Rehabilitative Services

P.O. Box K300

8004 Franklin Farm Drive

Richmond, VA 23288-0300

(804) 662-7000

TECHNOLOGY-RELATED ASSISTANCE

Virginia Assistive Technology System

8004 Franklin Farms Drive

P.O. Box K300

Richmond, VA 23288-0300

(804) 662-9990 or (800) 435-8490 (in VA only)

UNIVERSITY-AFFILIATED PROGRAM

Virginia Institute for Developmental Disabilities

Virginia Commonwealth University

301 West Franklin Street, Box 843020

Richmond, VA 23284-3020

(804) 828-3876 (V/TTY)

WASHINGTON

CLIENT ASSISTANCE PROGRAM

Client Assistance Program

P.O. Box 22510

Seattle, WA 98122

(206) 721-5999 or (800) 544-2121 (in WA)

OFFICE OF STATE COORDINATOR OF VOCATIONAL EDUCATION FOR STUDENTS WITH DISABILITIES

Special Needs and OCR

P.O. Box 47200

Olympia, WA 98504-7200
(360) 753-0555

PARENT-TO-PARENT

Parent-to-Parent Support Programs
10550 Lake City Way N.E., Suite A
Seattle, WA 98125-7752
(206) 364-3814 or (800) 821-5927 (in WA, OR, and ID)

PARENT TRAINING AND INFORMATION PROJECTS

Parents Are Vital in Education (PAVE)
6316 South 12th Street
Tacoma, WA 98465
(253) 565-2266 (V/TTY) or (800) 572-7368 (in WA)

PAVE/STOMP

6316 South 12th Street
Tacoma, WA 98465
(253) 565-2266 (V/TTY) or (800) 572-7368

PROGRAMS FOR CHILDREN AND YOUTH WHO ARE DEAF OR HARD OF HEARING

Office of Deaf and Hard of Hearing Services
Department of Social and Health Services
P.O. Box 45300
Olympia, WA 98504-5300
(360) 902-8000 (V/TTY); (360) 753-0699 (TTY);
(800) 422-7930 (Voice message only);
(800) 422-7941 (TTY message only)

PROGRAMS FOR CHILDREN WITH DISABILITIES: AGES THREE THROUGH FIVE

Office of Superintendent of Public Instruction
P.O. Box 47200
Olympia, WA 98504-7200
(360) 753-0317

PROGRAMS FOR CHILDREN WITH SPECIAL HEALTH-CARE NEEDS

Community and Family Health
Department of Health
P.O. Box 47830

Olympia, WA 98504-7830
(360) 753-7021

PROGRAMS FOR INFANTS AND TODDLERS WITH DISABILITIES: AGES BIRTH THROUGH TWO

Infant Toddler Early Intervention Program
Department of Social and Health Services
P.O. Box 45201
Olympia, WA 98504-5201
(360) 902-8490 (Voice) or (360) 902-7864 (TTY)
http://www1.dshs.wa.gov/iteip

PROTECTION AND ADVOCACY AGENCY

Washington Protection and Advocacy System
1401 East Jefferson, Suite 506
Seattle, WA 98122
(206) 324-1521

STATE AGENCY FOR THE VISUALLY IMPAIRED

Dept. of Services for the Blind
1400 South Evergreen Drive, SW, Suite 100
P.O. Box 40933
Olympia, WA 98504-0933
(360) 586-1224 or (800) 552-7103
http://www.wa.gov/dsb

STATE DEPARTMENT OF EDUCATION: SPECIAL EDUCATION

Special Education Section
Superintendent of Public Instruction
P.O. Box 47200
Olympia, WA 98504-7200
(360) 753-6733

STATE DEVELOPMENTAL DISABILITIES PLANNING COUNCIL

Developmental Disabilities Council
P.O. Box 48314
Olympia, WA 98504-8314
(360) 753-3908

STATE DEVELOPMENTAL DISABILITIES PROGRAM

Division of Developmental Disabilities
Department of Social and Health Services

P.O. Box 45310
Olympia, WA 98504-5310
(360) 902-8484

STATE MENTAL HEALTH AGENCY

Mental Health Division
Department of Social and Health Services
P.O. Box 45320
Olympia, WA 98504-5320
(360) 902-0790

STATE MENTAL HEALTH REPRESENTATIVE FOR CHILDREN AND YOUTH

Community Services, Mental Health Division
Department of Social and Health Services
P.O. Box 45320
Olympia, WA 98504-5320
(360) 902-8070

STATE VOCATIONAL REHABILITATION AGENCY

Division of Vocational Rehabilitation
Department of Social and Health Services
P.O. Box 45340
Olympia, WA 98504-5340
(360) 438-8008

TECHNOLOGY-RELATED ASSISTANCE

Washington Assistive Technology Alliance
ATRC/University of Washington
P.O. Box 357920
Seattle, WA 98195-7920
(260) 685-6836 (V/TTY)

UNIVERSITY-AFFILIATED PROGRAM

Center on Human Development and Disability
Box 357920, University of Washington
Seattle, WA 98195-7920
(206) 543-2832

WASHINGTON, D.C.

CLIENT ASSISTANCE PROGRAM

Client Assistance Program
300 I Street, NE, Suite 202

Washington, DC 20002
(202) 547-0198 (V) or (202) 547-2657 (TTY)

D.C. PUBLIC SCHOOLS SPECIAL EDUCATION BRANCH

Giddings School
315 G Street, SE
Washington, DC 20003
(202) 724-2477

D.C. VOCATIONAL REHABILITATION AGENCY

Rehabilitation Services Administration
Department of Human Services
800 Ninth Street, SW
Washington, DC 20024

OFFICE OF STATE COORDINATOR OF VOCATIONAL EDUCATION FOR STUDENTS WITH DISABILITIES

Vocational Transition Services Unit
Walker Jones Elementary School
First and K Street, NW
Washington, DC 20001
(202) 724-3878

PROGRAMS FOR CHILDREN WITH SPECIAL HEALTH-CARE NEEDS

Health Services for Children with Special Needs Clinic
D.C. General Hospital, Building 10
19th and Massachusetts Avenue, S.E.
Washington, DC 20003
(202) 675-5214

PROGRAMS FOR INFANTS AND TODDLERS WITH DISABILITIES: AGES BIRTH THROUGH TWO

D.C. Early Intervention Program
609 H Street, NE, Fifth Floor
Washington, DC 20002
(202) 727-5930

PROTECTION AND ADVOCACY AGENCY

University Legal Services: Protection and Advocacy
300 I Street, NE, Suite 202

Washington, DC 20002
(202) 547-0198 or (202) 547-2657 (TTY)

STATE DEVELOPMENTAL DISABILITIES PLANNING COUNCIL

D.C. Developmental Disabilities State Planning Council
2700 Martin Luther King Jr. Avenue, SE
Department of Human Services/801 East Building
Washington, DC 20032
(202) 279-6086

STATE MENTAL HEALTH AGENCY

Commission on Mental Health Services
Department of Human Services/Building A, Room 105
2700 Martin Luther King Jr. Avenue, SE
Washington, DC 20032
(202) 373-7166

STATE MENTAL HEALTH REPRESENTATIVE FOR CHILDREN AND YOUTH

D.C. Commission on Mental Health Services
Child Youth Services Administration
2700 Martin Luther King Avenue, SE
St. Elizabeth's Hospital, #L Building
Washington, DC 20032
(202) 373-7225

STATE MENTAL RETARDATION PROGRAM

Mental Retardation/Developmental Disabilities Administration
Commission on Social Services
Department of Human Services
429 O Street, N.W., #202
Washington, DC 20001
(202) 673-7678

UNIVERSITY-AFFILIATED PROGRAM

Georgetown University Child Development Center
3307 M Street, NW, Suite 401
Washington, DC 20007
(202) 687-8635

WEST VIRGINIA

CLIENT ASSISTANCE PROGRAM

Client Assistance Program
West Virginia Advocates
1207 Quarrier Street, Fourth Floor
Charleston, WV 25301

OFFICE OF STATE COORDINATOR OF VOCATIONAL EDUCATION FOR STUDENTS WITH DISABILITIES

Special Populations Services
Division of Technical and Adult Education Services
West Virginia Department of Education
1900 Kanawha Boulevard East
Building Six, Room 230
Charleston, WV 25305-0330
(304) 558-2349

PARENT TEACHER ASSOCIATION (PTA)

West Virginia Congress of Parents and Teachers
P.O. Box 3557
Parkersville, WV 26103-3557
(304) 420-9576 or (304) 229-8407

PARENT-TO-PARENT

Common Bonds: A Regional Parent-to-Parent
P.O. Box 3698 @ DTC
Charleston, WV 25336
(304) 768-3901 or (800) 282-3901 (in WV)

Parent-Educator Resource Center
116 East King Street
Martinsburg, WV 25401
(304) 263-5717

PARENT TRAINING AND INFORMATION PROJECT

West Virginia Parent Training and Information Project (WVPTI)
371 Broaddus Avenue
Clarksburg, WV 26301
(304) 624-1436 (V/TTY) or (800) 281-1436 (in WV)

PROGRAMS FOR CHILDREN AND YOUTH WHO ARE DEAF OR HARD OF HEARING

West Virginia Commission for the Deaf and Hard of Hearing
4190 Washington Street West
Charleston, WV 25313
(304) 558-2175 (V/TTY)

PROGRAMS FOR CHILDREN WITH DISABILITIES: AGES THREE THROUGH FIVE

Preschool Disabilities
Office of Special Education
1900 Kanawha Boulevard East
Building Six, Room 304
Charleston, WV 25305
(304) 558-2696

PROGRAMS FOR CHILDREN WITH SPECIAL HEALTH-CARE NEEDS

Children's Specialty Care
Office of Maternal and Child Health
Department of Health and Human Services
1116 Quarrier Street
Charleston, WV 25301
(304) 558-3071

PROGRAMS FOR INFANTS AND TODDLERS WITH DISABILITIES: AGES BIRTH THROUGH TWO

West Virginia Birth to Three
Office of Maternal and Child Health
Bureau of Public Health
1116 Quarrier Street
Charleston, WV 25301
(304) 558-3071

PROTECTION AND ADVOCACY AGENCY

West Virginia Advocates
Litton Building, Fourth Floor
1207 Quarrier Street
Charleston, WV 25301
(304) 346-0847 (V/TTY) or (800) 950-5250
    (in WV)

STATE DEPARTMENT OF EDUCATION: SPECIAL EDUCATION

Office of Special Education
Department of Education
1900 Kanawha Boulevard East
Building Six, Room B-304
Charleston, WV 25305
(304) 558-2696

STATE DEVELOPMENTAL DISABILITIES PLANNING COUNCIL

Developmental Disabilities Planning Council
110 Stockton Street
Charleston, WV 25312
(304) 558-0416 or (304) 558-2376 (TTY)

STATE MENTAL HEALTH AGENCY

Office of Behavioral Health
Department of Health and Human Resources
State Capitol Complex, Building Six, Room B-717
1900 Kanawha Boulevard, East
Charleston, WV 25305
(304) 558-0627

STATE MENTAL HEALTH REPRESENTATIVE FOR CHILDREN AND YOUTH

Division of Children's Mental Health Services
Office of Behavioral Health Services
Department of Health and Human Resources
Capitol Complex, Building Six, Room B-717
Charleston, WV 25305
(304) 558-0627

STATE MENTAL RETARDATION PROGRAM

Division of Developmental Disabilities
Office of Behavioral Health Services
Department of Health and Human Resources
Capitol Complex, Building Six, Room 727
Charleston, WV 25305
(304) 558-0627

STATE VOCATIONAL REHABILITATION AGENCY

Division of Rehabilitation Services
State Board of Rehabilitation

State Capitol Complex
P.O. Box 50890
Charleston, WV 25305-0890
(304) 766-4601
http://www.wvdrs.wvnet.edu

TECHNOLOGY-RELATED ASSISTANCE

West Virginia Assistive Technology System
West Virginia Division of Rehabilitation Services
P.O. Box 50890
State Capitol Complex
Charleston, WV 25305-0890
(304) 766-4694 or (304) 293-4692 (TTY)
(800) 642-8207

UNIVERSITY-AFFILIATED PROGRAM

West Virginia University
University Affiliated Center for
Developmental Disabilities (UACDD)
Research and Office Park
955 Hartman Run Road
Morgantown, WV 26505
(304) 293-4692

WISCONSIN

CLIENT ASSISTANCE PROGRAM

Client Assistance Program
One West Wilson Street, Room 558
Madison, WI 53707-7850
(608) 266-5378

OFFICE OF STATE COORDINATOR OF VOCATIONAL EDUCATION FOR STUDENTS WITH DISABILITIES

Division for Learning Support: Equity and Advocacy
Department of Public Instruction
P.O. Box 7841
Madison, WI 53707-7841
(608) 266-3701 or (800) 441-4563

PARENT-TO-PARENT

Mothers United for Moral Support, Inc.
150 Custer Court
Green Bay, WI 54301-1243
(920) 336-5333

Parent Projects, Waisman Center UAP
1500 Highland Avenue
Madison, WI 53705-2280
(608) 265-2063
http://www.waisman.wisc.edu/birthto3

PARENT TRAINING AND INFORMATION PROJECT

Parent Education Project of Wisconsin, Inc.
2192 South 60th Street
West Allis, WI 53219
(414) 328-5520; (414) 328-5525 (TTY);
    (800) 231-8382 (in WI)

PROGRAMS FOR CHILDREN AND YOUTH WHO ARE DEAF OR HARD OF HEARING

Office for the Deaf and Hard of Hearing
Department of Health and Family Services
2917 International Lane
P.O. Box 7852
Madison, WI 53707-7852
(608) 243-5625 or (608) 243-5626 (TTY)

PROGRAMS FOR CHILDREN WITH DISABILITIES: AGES THREE THROUGH FIVE

Early Childhood: Exceptional Educational Needs Programs
Division for Learning Support: Equity and Advocacy
Department of Public Instruction
P.O. Box 7841
Madison, WI 53707
(608) 267-9625; (608) 267-9172;
    (800) 441-4563

PROGRAMS FOR CHILDREN WITH SPECIAL HEALTH-CARE NEEDS

CSHCN Program
1414 East Washington Avenue, Room 167
Madison, WI 53703
(608) 266-3886 or (800) 441-4576

PROGRAMS FOR INFANTS AND TODDLERS WITH DISABILITIES: AGES BIRTH THROUGH TWO

Division of Supported Living
Department of Health and Family Services
P.O. Box 7851, Room 418

Madison, WI 53707
(608) 266-8276

WISCONSIN PERSONNEL DEVELOPMENT PROJECT

231 Waisman Center
1500 Highland Avenue
Madison, WI 53705
(608) 263-5022
http://www.waisman.wisc.edu/earlyint

PROTECTION AND ADVOCACY AGENCY

Lynn Breedlove, Executive Director
Wisconsin Coalition for Advocacy
16 North Carroll Street, Suite 400
Madison, WI 53703
(608) 267-0214 or (800) 928-8778 (in WI)

STATE CHILDREN'S SERVICES

Division of Child and Family Services
Department of Health and Social Services
P.O. Box 7850
Madison, WI 53707
(608) 267-3905

STATE DEPARTMENT OF EDUCATION: SPECIAL EDUCATION

Division for Learning Support: Equity and Advocacy
125 South Webster Street, P.O. Box 7841
Madison, WI 53707-7841
(608) 266-1649 or (800) 441-4563
http://www.dpi.state.wi.us/dpi/dlsea/een

STATE DEVELOPMENTAL DISABILITIES PLANNING COUNCIL

Wisconsin Council on Developmental Disabilities
722 Williamson Street, Second Floor
P.O. Box 7851
Madison, WI 53707-7851
(608) 266-7826

STATE DEVELOPMENTAL DISABILITIES PROGRAM

Bureau of Developmental Disabilities Services
Department of Health and Family Services

P.O. Box 7851
Madison, WI 53707
(608) 266-0805

STATE EDUCATION AGENCY RURAL REPRESENTATIVE

Department of Public Instruction
125 South Webster Street
P.O. Box 7841
Madison, WI 53707
(608) 266-9401

STATE MENTAL HEALTH AGENCY

Bureau of Community Mental Health
Department of Health and Family Services
P.O. Box 7851
Madison, WI 53707
(608) 267-7792

STATE MENTAL HEALTH COUNCIL

Bureau of Community Mental Health
Department of HFS
P.O. Box 7851
Madison, WI 53707
(608) 267-9282

STATE MENTAL HEALTH REPRESENTATIVE FOR CHILDREN AND YOUTH DHFS-DSL-BCMH

Bureau of Community Mental Health
One West Wilson Street, Room 543
P.O. Box 7851
Madison, WI 53707-7851
(608) 267-7792

STATE VOCATIONAL REHABILITATION AGENCY

Vocational Rehabilitation
Department of Workforce Development
2917 International Lane, Suite 300
P.O. Box 7852
Madison, WI 53707-7852
(608) 243-5603

TECHNOLOGY-RELATED ASSISTANCE

Wistech
Division of Supportive Living

P.O. Box 7852
2917 International Lane
Madison, WI 53707-7852
(608) 243-5675 or (608) 243-5601 (TTY)

UNIVERSITY AFFILIATED PROGRAM

Waisman Center UAP
University of Wisconsin-Madison
1500 Highland Avenue
Madison, WI 53705-2280
(608) 263-5940

WYOMING

CLIENT ASSISTANCE PROGRAM

Client Assistance Program
Wyoming Protection and Advocacy System, Inc.
320 West 25th Street, Second Floor
Cheyenne, WY 82001
(307) 632-3496
http://wypanda.vcn.com

OFFICE OF STATE COORDINATOR OF VOCATIONAL EDUCATION FOR STUDENTS WITH DISABILITIES

Department of Education, Special Programs Unit
Hathaway Building, Second Floor
2300 Capitol Avenue
Cheyenne, WY 82002-0050
(307) 777-7417

PARENT-TO-PARENT

Division of Public Health, Department of Health
Children's Health Services
Fourth Floor, Hathaway Building
Cheyenne, WY 82002
(307) 777-3637 or (800) 438-5795

Governor's Planning Council on Developmental Disabilities
122 West 25th Street
Herschler Building, First Floor/West
Cheyenne, WY 82002
(307) 777-7230 or (800) 438-5791 (in WY)

PARENT TRAINING AND INFORMATION PROJECT

Parent Information Center
Five N. Lobban
Buffalo, WY 82834
(307) 684-2277 or (800) 660-9742 (in WY)

PROGRAMS FOR CHILDREN WITH DISABILITIES: AGES THREE THROUGH FIVE

Department of Health, Division of Developmental Disabilities
Herschler Building, First Floor West
122 West 25th Street
Cheyenne, WY 82002
(307) 777-5246

PROGRAMS FOR CHILDREN WITH SPECIAL HEALTH-CARE NEEDS

Division of Public Health
Department of Health
Fourth Floor, Hathaway Building
Cheyenne, WY 82002
(307) 777-7941

PROGRAMS FOR INFANTS AND TODDLERS WITH DISABILITIES: AGES BIRTH THROUGH TWO

Division of Developmental Disabilities
Department of Health
Herschler Building, First Floor West
122 West 25th Street
Cheyenne, WY 82002
(307) 777-6972 (V/TTY)

PROTECTION AND ADVOCACY AGENCY

Wyoming Protection and Advocacy System
320 West 25th Street, Second Floor
Cheyenne, WY 82001
(307) 632-3496
http://wypanda.vcn.com

STATE DEPARTMENT OF EDUCATION: SPECIAL EDUCATION

Department of Education, Special Programs Unit
Hathaway Building, Second Floor
2300 Capitol Avenue

Cheyenne, WY 82002
(307) 777-7417
http://www.k12.wy.us

STATE DEVELOPMENTAL DISABILITIES PLANNING COUNCIL

Governor's Planning Council on Developmental Disabilities

122 West 25th Street
Herschler Building, First W
Cheyenne, WY 82002
(307) 777-7230 (TTY) or (800) 442-4333 (in WY)

STATE EDUCATION AGENCY RURAL REPRESENTATIVE

Social Studies/Facilities Consultant

Department of Education
Hathaway Building, Second Floor
Cheyenne, WY 82002
(307) 777-6198

STATE MENTAL HEALTH AGENCY

Division of Behavioral Health-Community Programs

Department of Health
447 Hathaway Building
2300 Capitol Avenue
Cheyenne, WY 82002-0480
(307) 777-7094

STATE MENTAL HEALTH REPRESENTATIVE FOR CHILDREN AND YOUTH

Mental Health Program

Division of Behavioral Health-Community
Programs

450 Hathaway Building, Fourth Floor
Cheyenne, WY 82002
(307) 777-6495

STATE MENTAL RETARDATION PROGRAM

Division of Developmental Disabilities

Department of Health
Herschler Building, First Floor West
122 West 25th Street
Cheyenne, WY 82002
(307) 777-7115

STATE VOCATIONAL REHABILITATION AGENCY

Division of Vocational Rehabilitation

Department of Employment
1100 Herschler Building
Cheyenne, WY 82002
(307) 777-7389

UNIVERSITY-AFFILIATED PROGRAM

Wyoming Institute for Disabilities

Department 4298
1000 E. University Avenue
Laramie, WY 82071-4298
(307) 766-2761 (V) or (307) 766-2720 (TTY)
http://wind.uwyo.edu/wind/default.asp

APPENDIX V
COLLABORATIVE PROGRAMS
OF EXCELLENCE IN AUTISM (CPEA)

Readers interested in taking part in one of the following CPEA studies or who want more information about one of the sites should contact the nearest network site. Individuals may participate in as many studies as possible but only one study of genetics. The success of this research depends on family participation.

Boston University

Helen Tager-Flusberg, Ph.D.
Laboratory of Developmental Cognitive
    Neuroscience
Department of Anatomy and Neurobiology, Boston University School of Medicine
715 Albany Street, L-814
Boston, MA 02118-2526
(617) 414-1312
e-mail: htagerf@bu.edu

This site conducts studies of social-communicative abilities in autism, language delays and problems in autism, and brain pathology underlying social-communicative and language impairments in autism, using structural and functional magnetic resonance imaging.

University of California, Davis

Sally Rogers, Ph.D.
U.C. Davis M.I.N.D. Institute
2825 50th Street
Sacramento, CA 95817
(888) 883-0961 or (916) 703-0268
e-mail: sjrogers@ucdavis.edu

This site conducts studies of imitation and motor function in autism, measurement, predictors, course, causes, and external validity of regression in autism, and a longitudinal study of the developmental course of autism.

University of California, Los Angeles

Marian Sigman, Ph.D.
UCLA Center for Autism Research and Treatment
    (CART)
760 Westwood Plaza
Los Angeles, CA 92868
(310) 825-0180
e-mail: info@autism.ucla.edu
http://www.autism.ucla.edu

This site conducts studies of how social, communication, and language deficits in autism start and develop, follow-up and extension of certain treatments for autism, phenotype and genotype in inversion and duplication of chromosome 15, and neuroimaging and deficits in social communication in autism.

University of Pittsburgh

Nancy Minshew, M.D.
University of Pittsburgh Autism Research Program
Webster Hall, Suite 300
3811 O'Hara Street
Pittsburgh, PA 15213
(866) 647-3436
e-mail: autismrecruiter@msx.upmc.edu
http://www.pitt.edu/~nminshew

This site conducts studies of organizing information into concepts in persons with high-functioning autism and Asperger's syndrome, visual perception and visual processing in persons with high-functioning autism and Asperger's syndrome, sensory, motor, and executive problems in persons with high-functioning autism and Asperger's syndrome, and functional brain imaging of language and cognition in persons with high-functioning autism and Asperger's syndrome. This research is done in conjunction with Carnegie Mellon University and the University of Illinois, Chicago.

University of Rochester Medical Center
Patricia Rodier, Ph.D.
University of Rochester Medical Center
610 Elmwood Avenue
Box 603
Rochester, NY 14642
(716) 275-2582
e-mail: Patricia_Rodier@mrmc.rochester.edu

This site conducts studies of animal models and mechanisms of injury in autism, behaviors that distinguish autism from other disorders, and mutations in genes involved in early development and influences on gene function. This research is done in conjunction with the University of Rochester Medical Center's Departments of Pediatrics and Neurology, the Hospital for Sick Children (Toronto), Cornell Medical College, and the U.S. Environmental Protection Agency.

University of Utah
William McMahon, M.D.
Utah Autism Research Project
421 Wakara Way
Suite 143
Salt Lake City, UT 84108
(801) 585-9098
http://utahautismresearchprogram.genetics.utah.edu

This site conducts studies of genetics and genetic susceptibility of autism, brain development, and serotonin function and immune system functioning in autism.

University of Washington
Geraldine Dawson, Ph.D.
Autism Research Program Project
Autism Center at the Center for Human Development and Disability
Box 357920
University of Washington
Seattle, WA 98195
800-994-9701
e-mail: cbrock@u.washington.edu
http://depts.washington.edu/uwautism/research/participation.html

This site conducts studies of the relationships between the brain and behavior in autism, language problems characteristic of autism, early diagnosis of autism and resulting outcomes, neuroimaging studies of autism, and the genetics of autism.

Yale University
Fred Volkmar, M.D.
Yale Child Study Center
230 South Frontage Road
New Haven, CT 06520-7900
(203) 785-5930
http://info.med.yale.edu/chldstdy

This site conducts studies of genetics of persons with autism; the genetics of persons with autism and Asperger's syndrome, their families, and family members with related disorders; changes to the nervous system in autism; behavior problems, epilepsy, and puberty in adolescents with autism; and regression studies that seek to define the phenomena, predict outcomes, and evaluate medical factors that may play a role, such as vaccines, seizures, and prenatal conditions. This research is done in conjunction with the University of Michigan, the University of Chicago, and Harvard University.

APPENDIX VI
CLINICAL TRIALS IN AUTISTIC DISORDER

Clinical trials are a kind of research study that compares a specific treatment currently recognized as the best available (called the "standard of care") with a new treatment that the study's researchers believe is even safer or more effective. If clinical trials prove a new treatment to be more effective than current therapies, then it may become the new standard of care.

Until 1997, clinical trials generally included only adults because of the risks, but in the past few years the U.S. Food and Drug Administration (FDA) has recognized the importance of including children in research—especially in assessing the safety of medications in young people. Today, the FDA encourages pharmaceutical manufacturers to conduct research with children, and many more trials involving children are under way.

However, children are a particularly vulnerable group, and for that reason research on children must comply with strict federal regulations. Many studies conducted on adults cannot be approved for children. Researchers who wish to enroll children in a clinical trial must make sure that the child's parents or guardians provide informed consent. They also must make sure that the child has indicated a willingness to enter the study if they are age seven or above.

The Institutional Review Board (IRB) alone can approve studies in children if the trial poses only a minor increase in risk—or that may directly benefit the children in the trial. For studies that pose more than minor risk, the federal government and a panel of experts must approve the study. The American Academy of Pediatrics also has guidelines for research involving children.

Some patients agree to participate in clinical trials because this is a way to obtain high-quality, free care with constant monitoring. If patients are in a study and do not receive the new treatment being tested, they will still receive the best standard treatment, which may be as good as or better than the new approach. If a new treatment approach is proven to work, patients taking this treatment in the clinical trial may be among the first to benefit.

On the other hand, there is no way to be sure whether the new treatment will work. New treatments being studied are not always better than (or even as good as) standard care, and they may have side effects that doctors do not expect or that are worse than those of standard treatment. Moreover, not everyone benefits from a new treatment. In addition, participants in randomized trials will not be able to choose the approach they receive. Health insurance and managed care providers may not cover all patient care costs in a study, and participants may need to make more visits and undergo more procedures than they would if they were not in the clinical trial.

Phases of Clinical Trials

Clinical trials move through phases, from one (I) to three (III), before the final outcome leads to a potential new treatment.

Phase I These small trials are the first step in testing new treatments in patients, and are designed to determine how the treatment should be given and at what dose. Because less is known about the possible risks and benefits in Phase I trials, these studies usually include only a small number of patients who would not be helped by other known treatments.

Phase II In this phase, researchers next examine possible side effects and how well the treatment works (for example, whether brain lesions fade away or whether trembling lessens). Although larger than Phase I trials, still only a small number of patients enter Phase II trials because the usefulness and the side effects of the new treatments are still unknown.

Phase III Phase III trials compare the results of people taking the new treatment with results of people taking standard treatment to see which group has better survival rates and fewer side effects. Patients are randomly divided into each treatment group: one receiving the new treatment, and the other receiving the current standard of care treatment. Sometimes patients do not know which group they are in.

Usually studies move into Phase III testing only after a treatment has shown promise in Phases I and II. Phase III trials may include many hundreds of people around the country.

Safety

Clinical trials are tightly regulated and closely monitored by the federal government to make sure each phase of the study is as safe as possible. All clinical trials must follow a detailed plan (the "protocol") written by the researchers and approved by the IRB at each institution. This board, which includes at least five doctors, consumers, statistical experts, health professionals, and clergy, reviews the protocol to try to be sure that the research will not expose patients to extreme or unethical risks. The IRB must approve all clinical trials before they start and re-approve them at least once every year. The IRB also evaluates the merits of a trial and makes sure that the clinical trial poses no unnecessary or inappropriate risks.

Informed consent In addition, each patient (and parents of minor patients) must receive all the facts about a study before deciding whether to take part, including details about treatments, tests, possible benefits, and risks—a process called "informed consent." The informed consent document is a written description of what will happen in the study. In some clinical trials, the informed consent document may be several pages. Patients must receive this written explanation about the content of clinical research and ethical responsibilities of researchers.

Each patient must sign an informed consent form that highlights key facts. The informed consent process continues throughout the study. (For instance, if new risks of the treatment are discovered during a trial, the patients will be told of any new findings and must sign a new consent form to stay in the study.) Signing a consent form does not mean patients are required to stay in the study; patients can withdraw at any time.

Because clinical trials are not all the same, some informed consent documents may not include all the same sections. Informed consent documents generally include the following sections:

Introduction: The informed consent document usually begins with a general overview of the patient's rights as a study participant.

Purpose: This brief statement describes why the clinical trial is being done, and should discuss any experimental medications patients will be taking that are not yet approved.

Subject selection: This section describes the selection criteria for the study, and how many participants will be enrolled.

Procedure: All of the tests and procedures that patients will undergo (including hospitalizations, clinic visits, questionnaires, and lab tests) are discussed in this section.

Risks: This section lists all the potential risks and the likelihood of their occurrence, such as side effects or complications from medications or procedures.

Benefits: This section highlights the benefits patients can expect. However, trials testing new drugs will not include a benefits section, since researchers do not yet know what the benefits will be.

Alternatives: Here patients can read about options if they choose not to participate in the study, including standard therapies for specific medical conditions.

Participation and withdrawal: This vital section reminds patients of their right to quit a clinical trial at any time. It also may include a list of reasons why a researcher may remove a participant from a trial.

Cost or payment: Here patients will find a list of potential expenses, along with any compensation.

Injuries: This section outlines who is responsible for paying for the participant's treatment of research-related injuries. Federal guidelines require this section to be included in all informed consent documents, even for clinical trials that pose minor risk.

Confidentiality: This section describes how researchers make sure information from the trial remains confidential.

Preclinical studies: Before the human studies begin, scientists must have completed preclinical studies that show that a new treatment is safe and effective in laboratory and animal tests. Scientists also must use a strict protocol—an outline prepared before the beginning of a study that describes exactly what will take place during the trial.

Deciding Whether to Participate

A patient has no guarantee how the trial will turn out, and the treatment may cause discomfort, inconvenience, and expense. Each patient (or the parents of a patient) must decide whether joining a clinical trial is worthwhile, based on the possible benefits and risks. Patients should evaluate the details of a clinical trial carefully before making any decision. Before signing on to a clinical trial, patients should consider a number of issues, including:

- the nature of the study
- adverse effects
- how much time the study would take, including number and length of time of clinic visits
- expenses, including travel, parking, and meals
- possible tests and type of treatment
- whether enrolling in the study will be of benefit, or provide satisfaction from helping others
- private information the scientists may need to know and how they plan to protect patient privacy
- where to call if the patient has questions

Study Participant Rights

Patients who participate in medical studies have a number of rights guaranteed by the government. Patients have the right

- to join a research study, but they must never be pressured or coerced to join a study
- to join a clinical trial if eligibility criteria are met. They cannot be excluded on the basis of age, sex, race, or any other characteristic (unless this is explicitly stated in the approved protocol).

- to know about any alternatives
- to leave a research study at any point, and not be pressured or coerced to stay in a study. Patients cannot lose access to regular medical care if they leave a study.
- to full and complete information about what the study means ("informed consent")
- to ask questions about the study, both before it begins and as it continues

Genetics and Autism

Clinical trials may collect genetic information in an effort to clarify the relationship between heredity and autism. There are several important issues to consider before joining a genetic study.

Because entire families can be affected by a participant's genetic information, family members may have strong feelings about discovering or avoiding the results of genetic tests. Most genes tested in clinical trials do not cause disease in everyone who has them, but having certain genes does raise a person's chance of getting the disease. Finding out that a person carries a particular gene that might cause a disease could make that person uncomfortable, or trigger a strong emotional response. Participants should ask whether the clinical trial covers the costs of counseling before the trial starts.

The Process

Once a participant has read the informed consent and decided to join a trial, the first part of the study begins. Typically, a study researcher asks questions about the participant's medical history and conducts an examination. The patient will be assigned to receive a drug or a placebo (a drug that looks the same but does not contain active medication). In a double blind study, neither the participant nor the researcher knows which drug the patient is taking. (However, in an emergency, information about what drug you are taking can be obtained quickly from the study sponsor.)

Depending on the study, at each visit, the study researcher may perform a physical exam, take a medical history, review any symptoms, administer a urine pregnancy test (for women of childbearing potential), or take blood. Usually, participants will complete a questionnaire about possible side effects for each visit. In addition, some studies require a researcher to contact participants by phone to assess compliance.

If Patients Are Harmed

By law, researchers must advise participants who will pay for treatment if the subjects are injured in a research study. This information is included in the informed consent document. Clinical trial sponsors may deal with research-related injuries in different ways, reimbursing all medical expenses from all research-related injuries, reimbursing just medical expenses that are not covered by medical insurance, or paying back some or all medical expenses—but only after they have been reviewed.

ONGOING AUTISM CLINICAL TRIALS

Citalopram for Children with Autism and Repetitive Behavior
Study ID Number 1U54 MH066398-01 A1

The primary aim of this study is to determine the efficacy in improving global functioning, as well as the tolerability and safety of citalopram, a selective serotonin reuptake inhibitor (SSRI), as compared to placebo in the treatment of children with a diagnosis of an autism spectrum disorder (ASD) or pervasive developmental disorder (PDD).

The study is sponsored by the National Institute of Mental Health (NIMH), the National Institute of Neurological Disorders and Stroke (NINDS), the National Institute of Child Health and Human Development (NICHD), the National Institute on Deafness and Other Communication Disorders (NIDCD), and the National Institute of Environmental Health Sciences (NIEHS).

Children between the ages of five and 17 years of age are eligible for this study. In addition, children must be diagnosed with autistic disorder, Asperger's disorder, or PDD-NOS, and able to walk. They must demonstrate a mental age above 18 months as determined by the Vineland Adaptive Behavior Scales. In addition, they must not have taken fluoxetine for at least one month, other SSRIs and neuroleptics for two weeks, or stimulants for five days prior to baseline ratings. Finally, they must be able

to take medication and agree to keep appointments for study contacts and tests.

Studies will be held at the UCLA Neuropsychiatric Institute; Yale University; the Dartmouth-Hitchcock Medical Center in Lebanon, NH; the Mount Sinai School of Medicine in New York; the North Shore–Long Island Jewish Hospital in Great Neck; and the University of North Carolina at Chapel Hill.

Improving Attention Skills of Children with Autism
Study ID Number R21MH64927

This study is designed to teach caregivers how to initiate and maintain episodes of joint engagement with their children. Participants will be randomized to either the intervention group or to a wait list control group.

Children with autism have problems sustaining a shared interest in social interaction and using specific joint attention skills, such as pointing and showing. The importance of joint attention is underscored by data suggesting these skills are important to later language skills. Targeting joint attention deficits in developmentally young children using familiar caregivers may result in better child language outcomes.

Each caregiver and child in the intervention group will participate in 24 one-hour sessions, three times a week for two months. In these sessions, caregivers will be taught 10 different modules for teaching joint attention skills to their children. Outcome measures will include language and joint attention skills in the child and caregiver adherence to the intervention protocols. Children and caregivers will be assessed at baseline, during the eight-week intervention, and 10 weeks after the end of the intervention. Participants assigned to the wait list group will begin the intervention at week 12.

To be eligible for the study, boys or girls must be between 12 and 36 months of age, and must be diagnosed with autism based on the Autism Diagnostic Interview Revised (ADI-R) and Autism Diagnostic Observation Schedule (ADOS) criteria Exclusion Criteria. In addition, they may not have seizures or medical or psychiatric diagnoses other than autism that could contribute to developmental delay (such as genetic syndromes).

The study is sponsored by the National Institute of Child Health and Human Development (NICHD) and the National Institute of Mental Health (NIMH). The study will take place at the University of California at Los Angeles.

Valproate Response in Aggressive Autistic Adolescents
Study ID Numbers P30HD02528; K08MH01516

This study will examine the effect of valproate, a medication used to treat seizures and bipolar disorder, on aggressive behavior in children and adolescents with autism.

Some people with autism become very aggressive and can hurt others or themselves. This study will test the hypothesis that aggressive autistic adolescents will show a significantly greater response to valproate maintained at blood levels of 75–100 mcg/ml than to placebo. The study will also assess the safety of valproate in autistic adolescents.

This represents the first double-blind study of valproate in mentally retarded/developmentally delayed populations. Participants in this study will undergo DSM-IV evaluation, the Autism Diagnostic Interview-Revised and Autism Diagnostic Observation Schedule, and baseline blood tests.

After baseline screening, all participants will be given a placebo for one week. Participants will then be randomized to receive either valproate or placebo for eight weeks. Dosage adjustment according to blood levels drawn at the end of weeks two and four will be arranged with parents by a child psychiatrist without breaking the blind.

The Aberrant Behavior Checklist-Community (ABC-C) irritability subscale will be the primary measure; the Overt Aggression Scale (OAS), ABC-C hyperactivity subscale, Clinical Global Impressions (CGI) problem severity, Self-Injurious Behavior Questionnaire (SIB-Q), and a valproate side effects checklist will be secondary measures.

The study is open to those ages six through 21 years. Both males and females are accepted; participants must have been diagnosed with autism and must live in the Kansas City, Kansas, area.

Children may not participate if they take psychoactive maintenance medication, have a degenerative central nervous system disorder, have unstable medical illness, or have had seizures in the six months prior to study entry. In addition, they must not have a history of valproate sensitivity or previous liver disease, a history of ovarian cysts, or a low platelet count or raised liver transaminases.

The study is sponsored by the National Institute of Child Health and Human Development (NICHD) and the National Institute of Mental Health (NIMH). It takes place at the Outpatient MR/Autism Clinic at the University of Kansas in Kansas City.

Risperidone and Behavioral Therapy in Treatment of Children and Adolescents with Autistic Disorder
Study ID Numbers U10 MH66764; U10 MH66766; U10 MH66768

The purpose of this study is to compare the safety and effectiveness of medication treatment alone to medication treatment in combination with a structured parent management training program for children with pervasive developmental disorders (PDDs).

PDD can be a profoundly disabling condition across social, emotional, and academic domains, and safe and effective treatments for PDD are needed.

Participants are randomly assigned to receive either risperidone plus parent management training or risperidone alone for 24 weeks. Participants who show deterioration after the fourth week will be offered an alternative medication treatment (aripiprazole). These participants will remain in their original treatment group (either med alone or med plus parent management training). After six months of treatment, participants who respond to their treatment will be gradually discontinued from their medication to see if the response can be sustained without continued medication treatment. Adaptive and behavioral outcomes are assessed during the study and at a year follow-up visit.

Children must be between the ages of four and 13 (both boys and girls), and have a diagnosis either of autistic disorder, Asperger's disorder, or pervasive developmental disorder–not otherwise specified (PDD-NOS). Children must weigh more than 30 pounds and have an IQ at or above 35, or a mental age of at least 18 months.

Children cannot participate if they have a psychotic disorder, a history of intolerance or nonresponse to risperidone, a history of neuroleptic malignant syndrome, or if they are pregnant.

The study, which is sponsored by the National Institute of Mental Health (NIMH), will be administered in Connecticut at Yale University; in Indiana at Indiana University at Indianapolis; in Ohio at Ohio State University at Columbus.

Drug Treatment for Autism (Donepezil HCl)
Study ID Number NIMH-65941-01

The purpose of this study is to examine the safety and effectiveness of donepezil HCl (Aricept) in children and adolescents with autism spectrum disorder (ASD). These children often have problems with communication and social interaction, along with repetitive and stereotyped patterns of behavior. While most research has attempted to treat the behavioral deficits commonly associated with ASD, few studies have tried to improve the core features of this disorder.

A recent study found that donepezil HCl helped to improve speech production, attention span, and ability to express emotions in a group of children with autism. This study will provide an opportunity to conduct further testing of the effects of donepezil HCl on the cognitive deficits presumed to underlie the core features of ASD.

The first week of the study begins with a baseline assessment. Participants are then randomly assigned to either donepezil HCl or placebo. Participants will start with either a 5 mg/day dose of donepezil HCl or placebo followed by a cognitive assessment after four weeks on this dose; they will then have their dose increased to 10 mg/day. Another cognitive assessment will be given after one month on this dose.

Boys and girls are eligible for this study if they are between ages eight and 17 and have been diagnosed with either ASD or Asperger's disorder. They must have an IQ of 75 or above and have baseline assessment tests within the acceptable range.

Children may not participate if they have bipolar disorder, schizophrenia, schizoaffective disorder, psychotic disorder, a seizure disorder requiring anticonvulsant medications, congenital rubella, cytomegalovirus, or tuberous sclerosis. In addition, they will not be eligible if they take certain medications prescribed for behavior management or medications known to interact with donepezil HCl. Also prevented from participating will be children with significant medical illness, endocrinopathies, cardiovascular disease, or severe chronic malnutrition, and pregnant or sexually active girls not using a reliable method of contraception.

Sponsored by the National Institute of Mental Health (NIMH), the study is administered at the Western Psychiatric Institute and Clinic in Pittsburgh, Pennsylvania.

Early Characteristics of Autism
Sponsored by National Institute of Mental Health (NIMH)
Study ID Numbers 1U54 MH066399-01A1; U54 MH066399

The purpose of this study is to identify factors that distinguish children with autism from children with developmental delay and those with normal development. This study will also assess the effectiveness of a therapy program designed to help children with autism.

By understanding the social, linguistic, psychological, and physiological differences that distinguish autistic children, developmentally delayed children, and children with typical development, researchers may be able to recognize autism early in life so that children with autism can be helped as early as possible and their long-term outcome can be improved. Children in this study will be enrolled for two years. They will undergo a magnetic resonance imaging (MRI) scan and will complete various activities to determine brain functioning. In addition, children with autism will take part in intensive behavioral therapy at least four hours every day for the entire six months. Communication and social behavior scales, an early development interview, and observations of parent/child interaction will be used to assess participants.

This study, which is sponsored by the National Institute of Mental Health, is administered at the University of Washington, Seattle.

Diet and Behavior in Young Children with Autism
Study ID Number 1U54 MH066397-01A1

The purpose of this study is to determine whether a gluten- and casein-free diet has specific benefits for children with autism.

Studies suggest that a gluten- and casein-free diet may have a therapeutic effect on children with autism. This study will examine the effects of such a diet in autistic boys and girls from 30 months through four-and-a-half years of age. Children in this study will be randomly assigned to follow either a gluten- and casein-free diet or a standard diet for 16 weeks. All participants will receive a supplement regimen, and educational and behavioral services will be provided. Standard autism evaluation methods, weekly diet and sleep diaries, and laboratory tests will be used to assess participants. A follow-up assessment will be completed 30 weeks after the start of the study.

Children with autism spectrum disorder or pervasive developmental disorder are eligible to participate. In addition, participants must participate in applied behavioral analysis classes for at least four months, with at least 20 hours a week of service, at least one of which must be in the home. Participations also must score above 30 on the Mullen Early Learning scale, and be able to maintain a gluten- and casein-free diet during the study.

This study takes place at the University of Rochester Medical Center, in Rochester, New York.

GLOSSARY

aphasia An acquired loss of ability to produce or understand language.

applied behavior analysis (ABA) A style of treatment that uses a series of trials to shape a desired behavior. Skills are broken down to their simplest components and taught through a system of reinforcement; prompts are given as needed when the child is learning a skill. As a skill is mastered the prompts are faded until the child can perform the task independently.

ataxia A lack of coordination of voluntary and involuntary muscles associated with problems in the cerebellum, leading to jerky, uncoordinated movements.

athetosis Involuntary, writhing movements that may be most noticeable in the face, neck, tongue, and hands, although it can affect any muscle group. Athetosis may occur in association with certain diseases, such as cerebral palsy or Rett disorder, or may be caused by certain medications.

atypical autism A general term for conditions that are close to but do not quite fit the set of conditions for autism. It is also referred to as pervasive developmental disorder–not otherwise specified.

aversives Behavioral methods employing punishment rather than positive reinforcement, often using physical pain.

axon Nerve fiber.

basal ganglia A series of specialized nerve cell structures located deep within the brain and responsible for movements.

behavior checklist Objective list that allows an observer to check for the existence of certain behaviors by observing the individual being evaluated.

behavior modification A technique of changing a person's behavior by carefully observing events before and after the behavior in question. The environment is manipulated to reinforce the desired responses, bringing about the desired change in behavior.

bradykinesia The slowing of motor movements due to dysfunction of the basal ganglia and related structures.

brain stem Part of the primitive part of the brain composed of midbrain, pons, and medulla that lies between the cerebrum and the spinal cord. The brain stem contains the reticular activating system and other key centers.

central nervous system A term that refers to the brain and the spinal cord.

cerebral cortex The outer region of the brain's cerebral hemispheres, comprised of gray matter and divided into four distinct sections: the frontal, temporal, occipital, and parietal lobes. The cerebral cortex is responsible for integrating higher mental functioning and conscious thought, sensations, and general movements.

chromosome One of the "packages" of genes and other DNA in the nucleus of a cell. Humans have 23 chromosome pairs, 46 in all. Each parent contributes one chromosome to each pair, so children get half of their chromosomes from their mothers and half from their fathers.

cognition The process of recognizing, interpreting, judging, reasoning, and knowing. Perception is considered a part of cognition by some psychologists, but not by others.

cognitive The process of knowing in the broadest sense, including perception, memory, and judgment.

cognitive deficit A perceptual, memory, or conceptual problem that interferes with learning.

cognitive retraining Developing or relearning the processes involved in thinking.

communication skills Consciously linking the meaning and the purpose of what a person says to what a person does.

coping skills The ability to deal with problems and difficulties by attempting to overcome them or accept them.

dendrite The shorter branches of the cell body of a neuron that makes contact with other neurons at synapses, ferrying nerve impulses from the neurons into the cell body.

discrimination   The ability to discern fine differences among stimuli, whether visual, auditory, tactile, or so on.

DNA   The substance contained within chromosomes whose base sequence encodes an individual's genetic information.

dopamine   A chemical messenger (neurotransmitter) in the brain that controls movement and balance, and that is essential to the proper functioning of the central nervous system.

echolalia   The repetition or parroting of words or phrases.

electroencephalogram (EEG)   A test that uses electrodes placed on the scalp to record electrical brain activity. It is often used to diagnose seizure disorders or to look for abnormal brain wave patterns.

emotional lability   Exhibiting rapid and drastic changes in emotions (such as laughing, crying, anger) without apparent reason.

fine motor skills   The use of small muscle groups for controlled movements, particularly in object manipulation.

frustration tolerance   The ability to deal with frustrating events in daily life without becoming angry or aggressive.

gait apraxia   The loss of the ability to consciously execute the movements required to coordinate walking, resulting in unsteadiness, toe walking, a jerky gait, and balance problems.

gene   Piece of DNA that contains the information for making a specific protein.

genome   All the DNA contained in an organism or a cell; includes both the DNA and chromosomes within the nucleus and the DNA outside the nucleus.

gross motor   Movement that involves balance, coordination, and large muscle activity.

homeobox genes   Genes found in almost all animals that control how and where parts of the body develop. Active very early in life, these genes tell other genes when to act and when to stop.

hot spots   Areas on chromosomes where mutations, activity, or recombination occurs with unusually high frequency.

hyperlexia   The ability to read at an early age. To be hyperlexic, a child does not need to understand what he or she is reading.

hypotonia   Low muscle tone.

identical twins   Twins formed from the splitting of the same fertilized egg, so they share 100 percent of their genetic material.

individualized educational program (IEP)   A written education plan for a school-aged child with disabilities, developed by a team of professionals and the child's parents. The IEP is based on a multidisciplinary evaluation of the child, describes how the child is presently doing, what the child's learning needs are, and what services the child will need. It is reviewed and updated yearly.

macrocephaly   A condition in which the head circumference is above the 97th percentile.

nucleus   The central cell structure that houses chromosomes.

perseveration   Compulsively repeating movement or speech, or sticking to one idea or task.

prefrontal area   The brain location for processes of foresight, abstract thinking, and judgment.

proprioceptive   Capable of receiving stimuli originating in muscles, tendons, and other internal tissues.

serotonin   A neurotransmitter that is found especially in the brain, blood, and stomach lining of mammals. People with autism tend to have abnormally high levels of serotonin.

stereotypies   Inappropriate, persistent, involuntary repetition of body postures, actions, or speech patterns that may be rhythmic, coordinated, and without purpose. Stereotypies are associated with a variety of brain and behavior disorders, such as Rett disorder, Tourette syndrome, obsessive-compulsive disorder, and autism.

synapse   The tiny space separating one neuron from another.

tactile   The ability to receive and interpret stimuli through contact with the skin.

SUGGESTED READING

ADHD AND AUTISM

Kennedy, Diane, and Rebecca Banks. *The ADHD Autism Connection: A Step Toward More Accurate Diagnoses and Effective Treatments.* New York: Waterbrook Press, 2002.

ADULTS WITH AUTISM

Barnard, Judith et al. *Ignored or Ineligible: the Reality for Adults with Autistic Spectrum Disorders.* London: National Autistic Society, 2001.

Barnhill, Gena. *Right Address ... Wrong Planet: Children with Asperger Syndrome Becoming Adults.* Shawnee Mission, Kans.: Autism Asperger Publishing Company, 2002.

Bicknell, A. *Independent Living for Adults with Autism and Asperger Syndrome: A Guide for Families of People with Autistic Spectrum Disorders.* London: National Autistic Society, 1999.

Hane, Ruth Elaine Joyner et al. *Ask and Tell: Self-Advocacy and Disclosure for People on the Autism Spectrum.* Shawnee Mission, Kans.: Autism Asperger Publishing Company, 2004.

Harrington, Kathie. *For Parents and Professionals: Autism in Adolescents and Adults.* East Moline, Ill.: LinguiSystems, Inc., 1998.

Holmes, David. *Autism in Adulthood.* New York: Routledge, 1996.

———. *Autism Through the Lifespan: The Eden Model.* Bethesda, Md.: Woodbine House, 1998.

Howlin, Patricia. *Autism: Preparing for Adulthood.* New York: Routledge, 1996.

Johnson, Malcolm. *Managing with Asperger Syndrome: A Practical Guide for White Collar Professionals.* London: Jessica Kingsley Publishers, 2004.

Lawson, Wendy. *Build Your Own Life: A Self-Help Guide for Individuals with Asperger Syndrome.* London: Jessica Kingsley Publishers, 2003.

Matson, Johnny L., ed. *Autism in Children and Adults: Etiology, Assessment, and Intervention.* Pacific Grove, Calif.: Brooks/Cole, 1994.

Meyers, K., and B. Briesman, eds. *Children Grow Up: Autism in Adolescents and Adults.* Lawrenceville, N.J.: COSAC Press, 1986.

Morgan, Hugh. *Adults with Autism: A Guide to Theory and Practice.* New York: Cambridge University Press, 1996.

Slater-Walker, Gisela, and Christopher Slater-Walker. *An Asperger Marriage.* London: Jessica Kingsley Publishers, 2002.

Stanford, Ashley. *Asperger Syndrome and Long-Term Relationships.* London: Jessica Kingsley Publishers, 2003.

Tremelloni, Laura. *Arctic Spring: Potential for Growth in Adults with Psychosis and Autism.* London: Karnac Books, 2005.

ADVOCACY

Budde, J., ed. *Advocacy and Autism.* Lawrence: University of Kansas Press, 1977.

Hane, Ruth Elaine Joyner et al. *Ask and Tell: Self-Advocacy and Disclosure for People on the Autism Spectrum.* Shawnee Mission, Kans.: Autism Asperger Publishing Company, 2004.

ART TALENT AND ART THERAPY

Davalos, Sandra R. *Making Sense of Art: Sensory-Based Art Activities for Children with Autism, Asperger Syndrome, and Pervasive Developmental Disorders.* Shawnee Mission, Kans.: Autism Asperger Publishing Company, 1999.

Evans, Kathy, and Janek Dubowski. *Art Therapy with Children on the Autistic Spectrum: Beyond Words.* London: Jessica Kingsley Publishers, 2001.

Kellman, Julia. *Autism, Art, and Children: The Stories We Draw.* Westport, Conn.: Bergin & Garvey, 2001.

Lerman, Jonathan. *Jonathan Lerman: The Drawings of a Boy with Autism.* New York: George Braziller, 2002.

Selfe, Lorna. *Nadia: A Case of Extraordinary Drawing Ability in an Autistic Child.* London: Academic Press, 1977.

———. *Normal and Anomalous Representational Drawing Ability in Children.* London: Academic Press, 1983.

ASPERGER'S SYNDROME

Addison, Anne. *One Small Starfish*. Arlington, Tex.: Future Horizons, 2002.

Attwood, Anthony. *Asperger's Syndrome: A Guide for Parents and Professionals*. London: Jessica Kingsley Publishers, 1998.

Bashe, Patricia Romanowski et al. *The OASIS Guide to Asperger Syndrome: Completely Revised and Updated: Advice, Support, Insight, and Inspiration*. New York: Crown, 2005.

Birch, Jen. *Congratulations! It's Asperger Syndrome*. London: Jessica Kingsley Publishers, 2003.

Blakemore-Brown, Lisa. *Reweaving the Autistic Tapestry— Autism, Asperger's Syndrome and ADHD*. London: Jessica Kingsley Publishers, 2001.

Bogdashina, Olga. *Communication Issues in Autism and Asperger Syndrome: Do We Speak the Same Language?* London: Jessica Kingsley Publishers, 2004.

Bolick, Theresa. *Asperger Syndrome and Adolescence: Helping Preteens and Teens Get Ready for the Real World*. Gloucester, Mass.: Fair Winds Press, 2004.

———. *Asperger Syndrome and Young Children: Building Skills for the Real World; For People Who Know and Care for Three-to-Seven-Year-Olds*. Gloucester, Mass.: Fair Winds Press, 2004.

Boyd, Brenda. *Parenting a Child with Asperger Syndrome: 200 Tips and Strategies*. London: Jessica Kingsley Publishers, 2003.

Brock, C. *Able Autistic Pupils Transferring to Mainstream Secondary School*. Nottingham: The University of Nottingham, 1991.

Cohen, Jeffrey. *The Asperger Parent: How to Raise a Child with Asperger Syndrome and Maintain Your Sense of Humor*. Shawnee Mission, Kans.: Autism Asperger Publishing Company, 2002.

Coucouvanis, Judith. *Super Skills: A Social Skills Group Program for Children with Asperger Syndrome, High-Functioning Autism and Related Challenges*. Shawnee Mission, Kans.: Autism Asperger Publishing Company, 2005.

Delfos, Martine. *A Strange World-Autism, Asperger's Syndrome and PDD-NOS: A Guide For Parents, Partners, Professional Carers, and People with ASDS*. London: Jessica Kingsley Publishers, 2005.

Deudney, C. *Asperger Syndrome in Your Classroom*. London: The National Autistic Society, 2001.

Deudney, C., and A. Shah. *Mental Health and Asperger Syndrome*. London: The National Autistic Society, 2001.

Elliott, Lisa B. *Embarrassed Often … Ashamed Never*. Shawnee Mission, Kans.: Autism Asperger Publishing Company, 2002.

Faherty, Catherine. *What Does It Mean to Me*. Arlington, Tex.: Future Horizons, 2000.

Fling, Echo R. *Eating an Artichoke: A Mother's Perspective on Asperger Syndrome*. London: Jessica Kingsley Publishers, 2000.

Freeman, Sabrina K., and Lorelei Dake. *Teach Me Language: A Language Manual for Children with Autism, Asperger's Syndrome and Related Developmental Disorders*. Langley, BC, Canada: SKF Books, 1996.

———. *The Companion Exercise Forms for Teach Me Language*. Langley, BC, Canada: SKF Books, 1997.

Frith, Uta, ed. *Autism and Asperger's Syndrome*. Cambridge: Cambridge University Press, 1994.

Gagnon, Elisa. *Power Cards: Using Special Interests to Motivate Children and Youth with Asperger Syndrome and Autism*. Shawnee Mission, Kans.: Autism Asperger Publishing Co., 2001.

Garrison, William. *Small Bargains: Children in Crisis and the Meaning of Parental Love*. New York: Simon & Schuster, 1993.

Ghaziuddin, Mohammad. *Mental Health Aspects of Autism and Asperger Syndrome*. London: Jessica Kingsley Publishers, 2005.

Gillberg, Christopher. *A Guide to Asperger Syndrome*. Cambridge: Cambridge University Press, 2002.

Gutstein, Steven. *Autism/Asperger's: Solving the Relationship Puzzle*. Arlington, Tex.: Future Horizons, 2001.

Gutstein, Steven, and Rachelle K. Sheely. *Relationship Development Intervention with Children, Adolescents and Adults: Social and Emotional Development Activities for Asperger Syndrome, Autism, PDD and NLD*. London: Jessica Kingsley Publishers, 2002.

Hadcroft, Will. *The Feeling's Unmutual: Growing up with Asperger Syndrome (Undiagnosed)*. London: Jessica Kingsley Publishers, 2004.

Hall, Kenneth. *Asperger Syndrome, the Universe and Everything*. London: Jessica Kingsley Publishers, 2000.

Harpur, John, Maria Lawlor, and Michael Fitzgerald. *Succeeding in College with Asperger Syndrome*. London: Jessica Kingsley Publishers, 2004.

Hartnett, Martha Kennedy. *Choosing Home: Deciding to Homeschool with Asperger's Syndrome*. London: Jessica Kingsley Publishers, 2004.

Hays, Marilyn, and Veronica Zysk, eds. *Working Together for a Brighter Future: A Unique Approach for Educating High-Functioning Students with Autism*. Arlington, Tex.: Future Horizons, 1996.

Hesmondhalgh, Matthew, and Christine Breakey. *Access and Inclusion for Children with Autistic Spectrum Disorders: Let Me In*. London: Jessica Kingsley Publishers, 2001.

Hewetson, Ann. *The Stolen Child: Aspects of Autism and Asperger Syndrome*. Westport, Conn.: Bergin & Garvey, 2002.

Howlin, Patricia. *Children with Autism and Asperger Syndrome: A Guide for Practitioners and Carers.* New York: John Wiley & Sons, 1998.

Jackson, Jacqui. *Multicoloured Mayhem: Parenting the Many Shades of Adolescence, Autism, Asperger Syndrome and AD/HD.* London: Jessica Kingsley Publishers, 2004.

Jackson, Luke, and Tony Attwood. *Freaks, Geeks and Asperger Syndrome: A User Guide to Adolescence.* London: Jessica Kingsley Publishers, 2002.

Jacobsen, Paula. *Asperger Syndrome and Psychotherapy: Understanding Asperger Perspectives.* London: Jessica Kingsley Publishers, 2003.

Jensen, Audra. *When Babies Read: A Practical Guide to Helping Young Children with Hyperlexia, Asperger Syndrome and High-functioning Autism.* London: Jessica Kingsley Publishers, 2005.

Johnson, Malcolm. *Managing With Asperger Syndrome: A Practical Guide for White Collar Professionals.* London: Jessica Kingsley Publishers, 2004.

Jones, G. *Educational Provision for Children with Autism and Asperger Syndrome: Meeting Their Needs.* London: David Fulton, 2001.

Klin, Ami, Fred R. Volkmar, and Sara S. Sparrow, eds. *Asperger Syndrome.* New York: Guilford Press, 2000.

LaSalle, Barbara. *Finding Ben: A Mother's Journey Through the Maze of Asperger's.* New York: McGraw-Hill, 2003.

Lawson, Wendy. *Build Your Own Life: A Self-Help Guide for Individuals with Asperger Syndrome.* London: Jessica Kingsley Publishers, 2003.

Ledgin, Norm. *Asperger's and Self-Esteem: Insight and Hope through Famous Role Models.* Arlington, Tex.: Future Horizons, 2002.

Leventhal-Belfer, Laurie, and Cassandra Coe. *Asperger Syndrome in Young Children: A Developmental Approach for Parents and Professionals.* London: Jessica Kingsley Publishers, 2004.

Lovecky, Deirdre V. *Different Minds: Gifted Children with AD/HD, Asperger Syndrome, and Other Learning Deficits.* London: Jessica Kingsley Publishers, 2004.

Martinovitch, Judith. *Creative Expressive Activities and Asperger's Syndrome: Social and Emotional Skills and Positive Life Goals for Adolescents and Young Adults.* London: Jessica Kingsley Publishers, 2005.

McAfee, Jeanette. *Navigating the Social World: A Curriculum for Individuals with Asperger's Syndrome, High Functioning Autism and Related Disorders.* Arlington, Tex.: Future Horizons, 2001.

McCabe, Patrick, Estelle McCabe, and Jared McCabe. *Living and Loving with Asperger Syndrome: Family Viewpoints.* London: Jessica Kingsley Publishers, 2003.

Mertz, Gretchen. *Help for the Child with Asperger's Syndrome: A Parent's Guide to Negotiating the Social Service Maze.* London: Jessica Kingsley Publishers, 2004.

Molloy, Harvey, and Latika Vasil. *Asperger Syndrome, Adolescence, and Identity: Looking Beyond the Label.* London: Jessica Kingsley Publishers, 2004.

Moore, Susan Thompson. *Asperger Syndrome and the Elementary School Experience: Practical Solutions for Academic and Social Difficulties.* Shawnee Mission, Kans.: Autism Asperger Publishing Co., 2002.

Moyes, Rebecca A. *Incorporating Social Goals in the Classrooms: A Guide for Teachers and Parents with High Functioning Autism and Asperger Syndrome.* London: Jessica Kingsley Publishers, 2001.

Myles, Brenda Smith. *Children and Youth with Asperger Syndrome: Strategies for Success in Inclusive Settings.* Thousand Oaks, Calif.: Corwin Press, 2005.

Myles, Brenda Smith, and Diane Adreon. *Asperger Syndrome and Adolescence: Practical Solutions for School Success.* Shawnee Mission, Kans.: Autism Asperger Publishing Co., 2001.

Myles, Brenda Smith et al. *Asperger Syndrome and Sensory Issues: Practical Solutions for Making Sense of the World.* Shawnee Mission, Kans.: Autism Asperger Publishing Company, 2000.

Myles, Brenda Smith, and Richard L. Simpson. *Asperger Syndrome: A Guide for Educators and Parents.* Austin, Tex.: Pro-Ed, 2003.

Myles, Brenda Smith, and Jack Southwick. *Asperger Syndrome and Difficult Moments: Practical Solutions for Tantrums, Rage, and Meltdowns.* Shawnee Mission, Kans.: Autism Asperger Publishing Co., 1999.

Newport, Jerry. *Your Life Is Not a Label: A Guide to Living Fully with Autism and Asperger's Syndrome.* Arlington, Tex.: Future Horizons, 2001.

Newport, Jerry, and Mary Newport. *Autism-Asperger's and Sexuality: Puberty and Beyond.* Arlington, Tex.: Future Horizons, 2002.

Osborne, Lawrence. *American Normal.* New York: Copernicus Books, 2002.

Ozonoff, Sally, Geraldine Dawson, and James McPartland. *A Parent's Guide to Asperger Syndrome and High-Functioning Autism: How to Meet the Challenges and Help Your Child Thrive.* New York: Guilford Press, 2002.

Powers, Michael D., and Janet Poland. *Asperger Syndrome and Your Child: A Parent's Guide.* New York: Harper, 2002.

Prior, Margot, ed. *Learning and Behavior Problems in Asperger Syndrome.* New York: Guilford Press, 2003.

Pyles, Lise. *Hitchhiking Through Asperger Syndrome.* London: Jessica Kingsley Publishers, 2001.

———. *Homeschooling the Child with Asperger Syndrome: Real Help for Parents Anywhere and on Any Budget.* London: Jessica Kingsley Publishers, 2004.

Rhode, Maria, and Trudy Klauber. *The Many Faces of Asperger's Syndrome.* London: Karnac Books, 2004.

Rodman, Karen. *Asperger Syndrome and Adults … Is Anyone Listening? Essays and Poems and Partners, Parents and Family Members of Adults with Asperger's Syndrome.* London: Jessica Kingsley Publishers, 2003.

Romanowski, Patricia Bashe, and Barbara L. Kirby. *The OASIS Guide to Asperger Syndrome: Advice, Support, Insights, and Inspiration, Completely Revised and Updated.* New York: Crown Publishing, 2005.

Sainsbury, Clare. *The Martian in the Playground: Understanding the Schoolchild with Asperger's Syndrome.* Bristol: Lucky Duck Publishing Ltd., 2000.

Sanders, Robert S., Jr. *On My Own Terms: My Journey with Asperger's.* London: Armstrong Valley Publishing, 2004.

Schopler, Eric, Gary Mesibov, and Linda J. Kunce, eds. *Asperger Syndrome or High-Functioning Autism.* New York: Plenum Publishing, 1998.

Schreibman, Laura. *The Science and Fiction of Autism.* Cambridge, Mass.: Harvard University Press, 2005.

Sicile-Kira, Chantal. *Autism Spectrum Disorders: The Complete Guide to Understanding Autism, Asperger's Syndrome, Pervasive Developmental Disorder, and Other ASD.* New York: Perigee Books, 2003.

Sohn, Alan, and Cathy Grayson. *Parenting Your Asperger Child: Individualized Solutions for Teaching Your Child Practical Skills.* New York: Penguin, 2005.

Stanford, Ashley. *Asperger Syndrome and Long-Term Relationships.* London: Jessica Kingsley Publishers, 2003.

Stanton, Mike. *Learning to Live with High Functioning Autism: A Parent's Guide for Professionals.* London: Jessica Kingsley Publishers, 2000.

Stewart, Kathryn. *Helping a Child with Nonverbal Learning Disorder or Asperger's Syndrome: A Parent's Guide.* Oakland, Calif.: New Harbinger Publications, 2002.

Stillman, William. *The Everything Parent's Guide to Children with Asperger's Syndrome: Help, Hope, and Guidance.* Cincinnati, Ohio: Adams Media Corporation, 2005.

Stoddart, Kevin P. *Children, Youth and Adults with Asperger Syndrome: Integrating Multiple Perspectives.* London: Jessica Kingsley Publishers, 2005.

Stuart-Hamilton, Ian. *An Asperger Dictionary of Everyday Expressions.* London: Jessica Kingsley Publishers, 2004.

Szatmari, Peter. *A Mind Apart: Understanding Children with Autism and Asperger Syndrome.* New York: Guilford Press, 2004.

Thomas, George et al. *Asperger Syndrome—Practical Strategies for the Classroom: A Teacher's Guide.* Shawnee Mission, Kans.: Autism Asperger Publishing Co., 2002.

Webb, James T. et al. *Misdiagnosis and Dual Diagnosis of Gifted Children and Adults: ADHD, Bipolar, OCD, Asperger's, Depression, and Other Disorders.* Phoenix, Ariz.: Great Potential Press, 2005.

Welton, Jude. *Can I Tell You about Asperger Syndrome: A Guide for Friends and Family.* London: Jessica Kingsley Publishers, 2003.

Willey, Liane Holliday, ed. *Asperger Syndrome in Adolescence: Living with the Ups, the Downs and Things in Between.* London: Jessica Kingsley Publishers, 2003.

———. *Asperger Syndrome in the Family: Redefining Normal.* London: Jessica Kingsley Publishers, 2001.

———. *Pretending to Be Normal: Living with Asperger's Syndrome.* London: Jessica Kingsley Publishers, 1999.

Williams, Chris, and Barry Wright. *How to Live with Autism and Asperger Syndrome: Practical Strategies for Parents and Professionals.* London: Jessica Kingsley Publishers, 2004.

Winter, Matt. *Asperger Syndrome: What Teachers Need to Know.* London: Jessica Kingsley Publishers, 2003.

Wrobel, Mary. *Taking Care of Myself: A Personal Curriculum for Young People with Autism/Asperger's.* Arlington, Tex.: Future Horizons, 2003.

ASSISTANCE DOGS

Gross, Patty Dobbs. *The Golden Bridge: A Guide to Assistance Dogs for Children Challenged by Autism or Other Developmental Disabilities.* West Lafayette, Ind.: Purdue University Press, 2005.

AUTISM SPECTRUM DISORDER/ PDD

Ariel, Cindy. *Voices from the Spectrum: Parents, Grandparents, Siblings, People with Autism, and Professionals Share Their Wisdom.* London: Jessica Kingsley Publishers, 2006.

Bruey, Carolyn Thorwarth. *Demystifying Autism Spectrum Disorders: A Guide to Diagnosis for the Parents and Professionals.* Bethesda, Md.: Woodbine House, 2004.

Fleisher, Marc. *Survival Strategies for People on the Autism Spectrum.* London: Jessica Kingsley Publishers, 2005.

Fovel, J. Tyler. *The ABA Program Companion: Organizing Quality Programs for Children With Autism and PDD.* New York: DRL Books, 2002.

Gutstein, Steven, and Rachelle K. Sheely. *Relationship Development Intervention with Children, Adolescents and Adults: Social and Emotional Development Activities for Asperger Syndrome, Autism, PDD and NLD.* London: Jessica Kingsley Publishers, 2002.

Heflin, L. Juane, and Donna Alaimo. *Autism Spectrum Disorders: Effective Instructional Practices.* Englewood Cliffs, N.J.: Prentice Hall, 2006.

Hewitt, Sally. *Specialist Support Approaches to Autism Spectrum Disorder Students in Mainstream Settings.* London: Jessica Kingsley Publishers, 2004.

Prelock, Patricia. *Autism Spectrum Disorders: A Communication-Based Handbook.* Austin, Tex.: Pro-Ed, 2006.

Quinn, Barbara, and Anthony Malone. *Pervasive Developmental Disorder: An Altered Perspective.* London: Jessica Kingsley Publishers, 2000.

Sicile-Kira, Chantal. *Autism Spectrum Disorders: The Complete Guide to Understanding Autism, Asperger's Syndrome, Pervasive Developmental Disorder, and Other ASD.* New York: Perigee Books, 2003.

———. *Adolescents on the Autism Spectrum: A Parent's Guide to the Cognitive, Social, Physical, and Transition Needs of Teenagers with Autism Spectrum Disorders.* New York: Perigee, 2006.

Smith, Melinda J. *Teaching Playskills to Children with Autistic Spectrum Disorder.* New York: DRL Books, 2001.

Sussman, Fern. *More Than Words: Helping Parents Promote Communication and Social Skills in Children with Autism Spectrum Disorder.* Toronto: Hanen Centre, 1999.

Volkmar, Fred. *Handbook of Autism and Pervasive Developmental Disorders.* New York: John Wiley & Sons, 2005.

Yapko, Diane. *Understanding Autism Spectrum Disorders: Frequently Asked Questions.* London: Jessica Kingsley Publishers, 2003.

Zager, Dianne E. Berkell. *Autism Spectrum Disorders: Identification, Education, and Treatment.* Hillsdale, N.J.: Lawrence Erlbaum Associates, 2004.

Zysk, Veronica, and Ellen Notbohm. *1001 Great Ideas for Teaching or Raising Children with ASD.* Arlington, Tex.: Future Horizons, 2004.

AUTISTIC SAVANTS

Hermelin, Beate. *Bright Splinters of the Mind: A Personal Story of Research with an Autistic Savant.* London: Jessica Kingsley Publishers, 2001.

Treffert, Darold A. *Extraordinary People: Understanding Savant Syndrome.* New York: Harper and Row, 1989.

BEHAVIOR AND BEHAVIOR ANALYSIS

Austin, John, and James E. Carr, eds. *Handbook of Applied Behavior Analysis.* Reno, Nev.: Context Press, 2000.

Bellack, Allan S., Michael Hersen, and Alan E. Kazdin. *International Handbook of Behavior Modification and Therapy.* New York: Plenum Publishing, 1990.

Bérard, Guy. *Hearing Equals Behavior.* New Canaan, Conn.: Keats Publishing, 1993.

Clements, John, and Ewa Zarkowska. *Behavioral Concerns and Autistic Spectrum Disorders: Explorations and Strategies for Change.* London: Jessica Kingsley Publishers, 2000.

Dalrymple, Nancy J. *Helpful Responses to Some of the Behaviors of Individuals with Autism.* Bloomington: Indiana Resource Center for Autism, 1992.

———. *Helping People with Autism Manage Their Behavior.* Bloomington: Indiana Resource Center for Autism, 1993.

Davis, Bill, and Wendy Goldband Schunick. *Dangerous Encounters: Avoiding Perilous Situations with Autism.* London: Jessica Kingsley Publishers, 2002.

Dickinson, Paul, and Liz Hannah. *It Can Get Better: Dealing with Common Behavior Problems in Your Young Autistic Child.* London: National Autistic Society, 1998.

Fouse, Beth, and Maria Wheeler. *A Treasure Chest of Behavioral Strategies for Individuals with Autism.* Arlington, Tex.: Future Horizons, 1997.

Fovel, J. Tyler. *The ABA Program Companion: Organizing Quality Programs for Children with Autism and PDD.* New York: DRL Books, 2002.

Foxx, Richard M. *Decreasing Behaviors of Persons with Severe Retardation and Autism.* Champaign, Ill.: Research Press, 1982.

Ghezzi, Patrick M., W. Larry Williams, and James E. Carr. *Autism: Behavior-Analytic Perspectives.* Reno, Nev.: Context Press, 1999.

Grandin, Temple, and Catherine Johnson. *Animals in Translation: Using the Mysteries of Autism to Decode Animal Behavior.* New York: Harvest Books, 2006.

Harris, Sandra L., and Mary Jane Weiss. *Right from the Start: Behavioral Intervention for Young Children with Autism.* Bethesda, Md.: Woodbine House, 1998.

Howlin, Patricia, ed. *Behavioral Approaches to the Treatment of Children.* Cambridge: Cambridge University Press, 1998.

Keenan, Mickey. *Applied Behaviour Analysis and Autism: Building a Future Together.* London: Jessica Kingsley Publishers, 2005.

Leaf, Ron, and John McEachin, eds. *A Work in Progress: Behavioral Management Strategies and a Curriculum for Intensive Behavioral Treatment of Autism.* New York: Different Roads to Learning, 1999.

Legge, Brenda. *Can't Eat, Won't Eat: Dietary Difficulties and Autistic Spectrum Disorders.* London: Jessica Kingsley Publishers, 2001.

Lovaas, O. Ivar. *Behavioral Problems of Autism: Experimental Analysis of Autism.* New York: Irvington Publications, 1986.

———. *The Autistic Child: Language Development through Behavior Modification.* New York: Irvington Publishers, Inc., 1977.

Maurice, Catherine, Gina Green, and Richard Foxx, eds. *Making a Difference: Behavioral Intervention for Autism.* Austin, Tex.: Pro Ed, 2001.

Maurice, Catherine, Gina Green, and Stephen Luce, eds. *Behavioral Intervention for Young Children with Autism: A Manual for Parents and Professionals.* Austin, Tex.: Pro-Ed, 1996.

Miller, Arnold, and Eileen Eller-Miller. *From Ritual to Repertoire: A Cognitive Developmental Systems Approach with Behavior Disordered Children.* New York: John Wiley & Sons, 1989.

Myles, Brenda Smith, and Jack Southwick. *Asperger Syndrome and Difficult Moments: Practical Solutions for Tantrums, Rage, and Meltdowns.* Shawnee Mission, Kans.: Autism Asperger Publishing Co., 1999.

Prior, Margot, ed. *Learning and Behavior Problems in Asperger Syndrome.* New York: Guilford Press, 2003.

Richman, Shira. *Raising a Child with Autism: A Guide to Applied Behavior Analysis for Parents.* London: Jessica Kingsley Publishers, 2000.

Whitaker, Philip. *Challenging Behaviour and Autism: Making Sense—Making Progress.* London: National Autistic Society, 2001.

THE BRAIN

Baron-Cohen, Simon. *Mindblindness: An Essay on Autism and Theory of Mind.* Cambridge, Mass.: MIT Press, 1995.

Baron-Cohen, Simon, Helen Tager-Flusberg, and Donald Cohen. *Understanding Other Minds: Perspectives from Developmental Cognitive Neuroscience.* New York: Oxford University Press, 2000.

Bauman, Margaret L., and Thomas L. Kemper. *The Neurobiology of Autism.* Baltimore, Md.: Johns Hopkins University Press, 2005.

Broman, Sarah H., and Jordan Grafman, eds. *Atypical Cognitive Deficits in Developmental Disorders: Implications for Brain Function.* Hillsdale, N.J.: Lawrence Erlbaum Associates, 1994.

Coleman, Mary. *The Neurology of Autism.* London: Oxford University Press, 2005.

DeFelice, Karen L. *Enzymes for Autism and Other Neurological Conditions.* London: Jessica Kingsley Publishers, 2002.

Gilberg, Christopher. *The Biology of the Autistic Syndromes,* 3rd ed. Cambridge: Cambridge University Press, 2000.

Moldin, Steven. *Neurobiology of Autism in the Post-genomic Era.* London: CRC Press, 2005.

CHILDHOOD DISINTEGRATIVE DISORDER (CDD)

Catalano, Robert A. *When Autism Strikes: Families Cope with Childhood Disintegrative Disorder.* New York: Plenum Publishing, 1998.

CIVIL RIGHTS AND AUTISM

National Autistic Society. *Autism: Rights in Reality: How People with Autism Spectrum Disorders and Their Families Are Still Missing out on Their Rights.* London: National Autistic Society, 2003.

COLLEGE AND AUTISM

Harpur, John, Maria Lawlor, and Michael Fitzgerald. *Succeeding in College with Asperger Syndrome.* London: Jessica Kingsley Publishers, 2004.

Prince-Hughes, Dawn. *Aquamarine Blue 5: Personal Stories of College Students with Autism.* Athens, Ohio: Swallow Press, 2002.

COMMUNICATION

Berger, Carol Lee. *Facilitated Communication and Technology Guide.* Eugene, Ore.: New Breakthroughs, 1994.

———. *Facilitated Communication Guide.* Eugene, Ore.: New Breakthroughs, 1992.

———. *Facilitated Communication Guide and Materials.* Eugene, Ore.: New Breakthroughs, 1992.

———. *Facilitated Communication Guide, Volume 2.* Eugene, Ore.: New Breakthroughs, 1993.

Beukelman, David R., and Pat Mirenda. *Augmentative and Alternative Communication,* 2nd ed. Baltimore, Md.: Paul H. Brookes, 1998.

Biklen, Douglas. *Communication Unbound: How Facilitated Communication Is Challenging Traditional Views of Autism and Ability/Disability.* New York: Teachers College Press, 1993.

Biklen, Douglas, and Don Cardinal, eds. *Contested Words, Contested Science: Unraveling the Facilitated Communication Controversy.* New York: Teachers College Press, 1997.

Bondy, Andy, and Lori Frost. *A Picture's Worth: PECS and Other Visual Communication Strategies in Autism.* Bethesda, Md.: Woodbine House, 2001.

Brandl, Cherlene. *Facilitated Communication: Case Studies—See Us Smart!* Ann Arbor, Mich.: Robbie Dean Press, 1999.

Butler, Katherine G., ed. *Severe Communication Disorders: Intervention Strategies.* Gaithersburg, Md.: Aspen Publishers, 1993.

Cafiero, Joanne. *Meaningful Exchanges for People with Autism: An Introduction to Augmentative and Alternative Communication.* Bethesda, Md.: Woodbine House, 2005.

Churchill, Don W. *Language of Autistic Children.* Washington: V. H. Winston & Sons, 1978.

Crossley, Rosemary. *Facilitated Communication Training.* New York: Teachers College Press, 1994.

————. *Speechless: Facilitating Communication for People without Voices*. New York: E. P. Dutton, 1997.

Donnellan, Anne M., and Martha R. Leary. *Movement Differences and Diversity in Autism/Mental Retardation: Appreciating and Accommodating People with Communication Challenges*. Madison, Wisc.: DRI Press, 1995.

Eastham, David. *Understand*. Ottawa: Oliver Pate, 1985.

Eastham, Margaret, and Anne Grice, eds. *Silent Words: The Story of David Eastham*. Ottawa: Oliver Pate, 1992.

Fay, Warren H., and Adriana Luce Scholer. *Emerging Language in Autistic Children*. Baltimore, Md.: University Park Press, 1980.

Freeman, Sabrina K., and Lorelei Dake. *Teach Me Language: A Language Manual for Children with Autism, Asperger's Syndrome and Related Developmental Disorders*. Langley, BC, Canada: SKF Books, 1996.

————. *The Companion Exercise Forms for Teach Me Language*. Langley, BC, Canada: SKF Books, 1997.

Hewett, David, and Melanie Nind, eds. *Access to Communication: Developing the Basics of Communication with People with Severe Learning Difficulties Using Intensive Interaction*. London: David Fulton, 1994.

————. *Interaction in Action: Reflections on the Use of Intensive Interaction*. London: David Fulton, 1998.

Hinerman, Paige Shaughnessy. *Teaching Autistic Children to Communicate*. Rockville, Md.: Aspen Systems Corp., 1983.

Lovaas, Ivar. *The Autistic Child: Language Development through Behavior Modification*. New York: Irvington Publishers, Inc., 1977.

MacDonald, James D. *Communicating Partners: 30 Years of Building Responsive Relationships with Late-Talking Children including Autism, Asperger's Syndrome (ASD), Down Syndrome, and Typical Development*. London: Jessica Kingsley Publishers, 2004.

Martin, Russell. *Out of Silence: An Autistic Boy's Journey into Language and Communication*. New York: Penguin Books, 1995.

McClannahan, Lynn E. *Teaching Conversation to Children with Autism: Scripts and Script Fading*. Bethesda, Md.: Woodbine House, 2005.

Ogletree, Billy T. *How to Use Augmentative and Alternative Communication (Pro Ed Series on Autism Spectrum Disorders)*. Austin, Tex.: Pro Ed, 2005.

Potter, Carol, and Chris Whittaker. *Enabling Communication in Children with Autism*. London: Jessica Kingsley Publishers, 2001.

Prelock, Patricia. *Autism Spectrum Disorders: A Communication-Based Handbook*. Austin, Tex.: Pro-Ed, 2006.

Rapin, Isabelle, and Lorna Wing. *Preschool Children with Inadequate Communication: Developmental Language Disorder, Autism, Mental Deficiency*. Cambridge: Cambridge University Press, 1996.

Richard, Jesse et al. *First Hand: Personal Accounts of Breakthroughs in Facilitated Communicating*. Madison, Wisc.: DRA Press, 1993.

Rocha, Adriana, and Kristi Jorde. *A Child of Eternity: An Extraordinary Young Girl's Message from the World Beyond*. New York: Ballantine Books, 1995.

St. John, Patricia. *The Secret Language of Dolphins*. New York: Summit Books, 1991.

Sonders, Susan Aud. *Giggle Time—Establishing the Social Connection: A Program to Develop the Communication Skills of Children with Autism, AS, and PDD*. London: Jessica Kingsley Publishers, 2002.

Sussman, Fern. *More Than Words: Helping Parents Promote Communication and Social Skills in Children with Autism Spectrum Disorder*. Toronto: Hanen Centre, 1999.

Twachtman-Cullen, Diane. *A Passion to Believe: Autism and the Facilitated Communication Phenomenon*. Boulder, Colo.: Westview Press, 1998.

CREATIVITY AND AUTISM

Fitzgerald, Michael. *Autism and Creativity: Is There a Link Between Autism in Men and Exceptional Ability*. New York: Brunner-Routledge, 2004.

DIAGNOSIS

Bruey, Carolyn Thorwarth. *Demystifying Autism Spectrum Disorders: A Guide to Diagnosis for the Parents and Professionals*. Bethesda, Md.: Woodbine House, 2004.

Exkorn, Karen Siff. *The Autism Sourcebook: Everything You Need to Know about Diagnosis, Treatment, Coping, and Healing*. New York: Regan Books, 2005.

Gillberg, Christopher, ed. *Diagnosis and Treatment of Autism*. New York: Plenum, 1989.

Glasberg, Beth. *Functional Behavior Assessment for People with Autism: Making Sense of Seemingly Senseless Behavior*. Bethesda, Md.: Woodbine House, 2005.

Hochman, Jacques, and Pierre Ferrari. *Imitation, identification chez l'enfant autiste*. Paris: Bayard editions, 1992.

Klin, Ami, and Fred Volkmar. *Asperger's Syndrome: Guidelines for Assessment and Diagnosis*. Pittsburgh, Pa.: Learning Disabilities Association of America, 1996.

Krug, David A., Joel R. Arick, and Patricia J. Almond. *Autism Screening Instrument for Educational Planning*. Los Angeles: Western Psychological Services, 1993.

Ledgin, Norm. *Diagnosing Jefferson*. Arlington, Tex.: Future Horizons, 2000.

Matson, Johnny L., ed. *Autism in Children and Adults: Etiology, Assessment, and Intervention*. Pacific Grove, Calif.: Brooks/Cole, 1994.

Rapoport, Judith, and Deborah R. Ismond. *DSM-IV Training Guide for Diagnosis of Childhood Disorders*, 4th ed. New York: Brunner-Routledge, 1996.

Schopler, Eric, and Gary B. Mesibov. *Diagnosis and Assessment in Autism.* New York: Plenum Press, 1988.

Stone, Wendy. *Does My Child Have Autism?* New York: Jossey Bass Wiley, 2006.

Trevarthen, Colwyn, Kenneth J. Aitken, and Despina Padoudi. *Children with Autism: Diagnosis and Intervention to Meet Their Needs.* London: Jessica Kingsley Publishers, 1998.

Waltz, Mitzi. *Autistic Spectrum Disorders: Understanding the Diagnosis and Getting Help.* Sebastopol, Calif.: O'Reilly Media, 2002.

DIET, ALLERGY, AND AUTISM

Callahan, Mary. *Fighting for Tony.* New York: Simon & Schuster, 1987.

Fenster, Carol. *Gluten-Free 101: Easy, Basic Dishes Without Wheat.* Centennial Colo.: Savory Palate, 2003.

Hagman, Bette. *The Gluten-Free Gourmet Bakes Bread: More than 200 Wheat-Free Recipes.* New York: Owl Books, 2000.

———. *The Gluten-Free Gourmet Cooks Comfort Foods: Creating Old Favorites with the New Flours.* New York: Henry Holt, 2004.

———. *The Gluten-Free Gourmet Cooks Fast and Healthy: Wheat-Free and Gluten-Free with Less Fuss and Less Fat.* New York: Owl Books, 2000.

———. *The Gluten-free Gourmet Makes Dessert: More Than 200 Wheat-free Recipes for Cakes, Cookies, Pies and Other Sweets.* New York: Owl Books, 2003.

———. *More from the Gluten-Free Gourmet.* New York: Owl Books, 2000.

Jackson, Luke, and Marilyn Le Breton. *A User Guide to the GF/CF Diet for Autism, Asperger Syndrome and AD/HD.* London: Jessica Kingsley Publishers, 2001.

Kendall, Roger V. *Building Wellness With Dmg: How a Breakthrough Nutrient Gives Cancer, Autism and Cardiovascular Patients a Second Chance at Health.* New York: Bookworld Services, 2003.

Korn, Danna. *Wheat-Free, Worry-Free: The Art of Happy, Healthy Gluten-Free Living.* Carlsbad, Calif.: Hay House, 2002.

Le Breton, Marilyn, and Rosemary Kessick. *The AiA Gluten and Dairy Free Cookbook.* London: Jessica Kingsley Publishers, 2002.

———. *Diet Intervention and Autism: Implementing the Gluten Free and Casein Free Diet for Autistic Children and Adults: A Practical Guide for Parents.* London: Jessica Kingsley Publishers, 2001.

Legge, Brenda. *Can't Eat, Won't Eat: Dietary Difficulties and Autistic Spectrum Disorders.* London: Jessica Kingsley Publishers, 2001.

Lowell, Jax Peters. *Against the Grain: The Slightly Eccentric Guide to Living Well Without Gluten or Wheat (The Gluten-Free Bible).* New York: Henry Holt, 1996.

Nambudripad, Devi S. *Say Good-Bye to Allergy-Related Autism.* New York: Delta Publishers, 1999.

Ryberg, Roben. *The Gluten-Free Kitchen: Over 135 Delicious Recipes for People with Gluten Intolerance or Wheat Allergy.* New York: Three Rivers Press, 2000.

Sanderson, Sherry. *Incredible Edible Gluten-Free Food for Kids: 150 Family-Tested Recipes.* Bethesda, Md.: Woodbine House, 2003.

Sarros, Connie. *Wheat-Free, Gluten-Free Dessert Cookbook.* New York: McGraw-Hill, 2003.

Savill, Antoinette. *Gluten, Wheat, and Dairy Free Cookbook.* New York: Thorsons Pub., 2000.

Shattock, Paul, Dawn Savery, and Paul Whiteley. *Autism as a Metabolic Disorder.* Sunderland, UK: Autism Research Unit, 1997.

Shaw, William et al. *Biological Treatments for Autism and PDD.* Manhattan, Kans.: Sunflower Press, 1997.

Washburn, Donna, and Heather Butt. *The Best Gluten-Free Family Cookbook.* Tonawanda, N.Y.: Robert Rose, 2003.

EDUCATION

Adams, Janice. *Autism-P.D.D.: Creative Ideas during the School Years.* Ontario, Canada: Adams Publications, 1995.

Barnard, Judith et al. *Autism in Schools: Crisis or Challenge.* London: National Autistic Society, 2002.

Barnard, Judith et al. *Inclusion and Autism: Is It Working?* London: National Autistic Society, 2000.

Beaney, Joy, and Penny Kershaw. *Inclusion in the Primary Classroom: Support Materials for Children with Autistic Spectrum Disorders.* London: National Autistic Society, 2003.

Bondy, Andrew S. *The Pyramid Approach to Education.* Cherry Hill, N.J.: Pyramid Educational Consultants, 1996.

Bowley, Agatha H. *The Young Handicapped Child: Educational Guidance for the Young Cerebral Palsied, Deaf, Blind, and Autistic Child.* London: E & S Livingstone, 1969.

Brereton, Avril, and Bruce J. Tonge. *Pre-schoolers with Autism: An Education and Skills Training Programme for Parents, Manual for Clinicians.* London: Jessica Kingsley Publishers, 2005.

Brock, C. *Able Autistic Pupils Transferring to Mainstream Secondary School.* Nottingham: The University of Nottingham, 1991.

Burkowsky, Mitchell R., ed. *Parents and Teachers Guide to the Care of Autistic Children.* Syracuse, N.Y.: Systems Educators, Inc., 1970.

California Department of Education. *Best Practices for Designing and Delivering Effective Programs for Individuals with Autistic Spectrum Disorders.* Los Angeles: California Department of Education, 1997.

Carrier, Denise M. *Chase of a Lifetime: A Journey through Therapeutic and Academic Strategies for Children on the Autism Spectrum.* Lincoln, Nebr.: iUniverse, 2003.

Collins, Michael, Judith Gould, and Richard Mills. *Common Ground*. London: National Autistic Society, 1996.

Dalrymple, Nancy J., and Barbara Porco. *Functional School Activities I*. Bloomington, Ind.: Indiana Resource Center for Autism, 1989.

Davis, Kimberly. *Adapted Physical Education for Students with Autism*. Springfield, Ill.: Charles C. Thomas, 1990.

Deudney, C. *Asperger Syndrome in Your Classroom*. London: The National Autistic Society, 2001.

Domina, Bryant. *Principles of Success for the Classroom Teacher of the Autistic Impaired*. Grandville, Mich.: Individual Educational Systems, 1998.

———. *A Practical Guide to Effective Programming for the Autistic Impaired: A Book for Educators and Parents*. Grandville, Mich.: Individual Educational Systems, 1994.

Dowty, Terri, and Kitt Cowlishaw, eds. *Home Educating Our Autistic Spectrum Children: Paths Are Made by Walking*. London: Jessica Kingsley Publishers, 2002.

Duran, Elva. *Teaching the Moderately and Severely Handicapped Student and Autistic Adolescent (with Particular Attention to Bilingual Children)*. Springfield, Ill.: Charles C. Thomas, 1988.

Duran, Elva, and Lou Brown. *Vocational Training and Employment of the Moderately and Severely Handicapped and Autistic Adolescent with Particular Emphasis to Bilingual Special Ed*. Springfield, Ill.: Charles C. Thomas, 1992.

Duran, Elva, and Diane Cordero De Noriega. *Teaching Students with Moderate/Severe Disabilities, Including Autism: Strategies for Second Language Learners in Inclusive Settings*. Springfield, Ill.: Charles C. Thomas, 1996.

Ernsperger, Lori. *Keys to Success for Teaching Students with Autism*. Arlington, Tex.: Future Horizons, 2003.

Fouse, Beth. *Creating a Win-Win IEP for Students with Autism! A How-To Manual for Parents and Educators*. Arlington, Tex.: Future Horizons, 1999.

Fullerton, Ann et al. *Higher Functioning Adolescents and Young Adults with Autism: a Teacher's Guide*. Austin, Tex.: Pro Ed, 1996.

Gray, Carol. *What's Next? Preparing the Student with Autism or Other Developmental Disabilities for Success in the Community*. Arlington, Tex.: Future Horizons, 1992.

Hannah, Liz. *Teaching Young Children with Autistic Spectrum Disorders to Learn: A Practical Guide for Parents and Staff in Mainstream Schools and Nurseries*. London: The National Autistic Society, 2001.

Hays, Marilyn, and Veronica Zysk, eds. *Working Together for a Brighter Future: A Unique Approach for Educating High-Functioning Students with Autism*. Arlington, Tex.: Future Horizons, 1996.

Heflin, L. Juane, and Donna Alaimo. *Autism Spectrum Disorders: Effective Instructional Practices*. Englewood Cliffs, N.J.: Prentice Hall, 2006.

Hewitt, Sally. *Specialist Support Approaches to Autism Spectrum Disorder Students in Mainstream Settings*. London: Jessica Kingsley Publishers, 2004.

Howlin, Patricia, Simon Baron-Cohen, and Julia Hadwin. *Teaching Children with Autism to Mind-Read: A Practical Guide for Teachers and Parents*. New York: John Wiley & Sons, 1998.

Jones, Glenys. *Educational Provision for Children with Autism and Asperger Syndrome: Meeting Their Needs*. London: David Fulton Publishers, 2002.

Jordan, Rita. *Autism with Severe Learning Difficulties*. London: Souvenir Press Ltd., 2002.

Jordan, Rita, and Stuart Powell. *Understanding and Teaching Children with Autism*. New York: Wiley, 1995.

Kitahara, Kiyo. *Daily Life Physical Education for Autistic Children: A Record of the Homogeneous Guidance Given at Musashino Higashi Gakuen School*. Boston, Mass.: Nimrod Press, 1984.

Kluth, Paula. *You're Going to Love This Kid: Teaching Students with Autism in the Inclusive Classroom*. Baltimore, Md.: Paul H. Brookes, 2003.

Knoblock, Peter, ed. *Teaching and Mainstreaming Autistic Children*. Denver, Colo.: Love Publishing Company, 1982.

Koegel, Robert L., Arnold Rincover, and Andrew L. Egel. *Educating and Understanding Autistic Children*. San Diego: College-Hill Press, 1982.

Larkey, Sue. *Making It a Success: Practical Strategies and Worksheets for Teaching Students with Autism Spectrum Disorder*. London: Jessica Kingsley Publishers, 2005.

Lord, Catherine, and James McGee, eds. *Educating Children With Autism*. Washington, D.C.: National Academy Press, 2001.

Lovaas, O. Ivar. *Teaching Individuals with Developmental Delays: Basic Intervention Techniques*. Austin, Tex.: Pro Ed, 2002.

Magnusen, Christy L. *Teaching Children with Autism and Related Spectrum Disorders: An Art and a Science*. London: Jessica Kingsley Publishers, 2005.

McConnell, Kathleen, and Gail Ryser. *Practical Ideas That Really Work for Students with Autism Spectrum Disorders*. Austin, Tex.: Pro Ed, 2000.

McCracken, M. *A Circle of Children: A Teacher's Dedication and Love*. Philadelphia: Lippincott, 1973.

Meyer, Naomi. *The Journey with Joshua: Educating My Autistic Child*. Lakewood, N.J.: Bristol, Rhein & Englander, 1994.

Moore, Susan Thompson. *Asperger Syndrome and the Elementary School Experience: Practical Solutions for Academic & Social Difficulties*. Shawnee Mission, Kans.: Autism Asperger Publishing Co., 2002.

Moyes, Rebecca A. *Addressing the Challenging Behavior of Children with High-Functioning Autism/Asperger Syn-*

drome in the Classroom: A Guide for Teachers and Parents. London: Jessica Kingsley Publishers, 2002.

———. *Incorporating Social Goals in the Classrooms: A Guide for Teachers and Parents with High Functioning Autism and Asperger Syndrome.* London: Jessica Kingsley Publishers, 2001.

———. *I Need Help with School!* Arlington, Tex.: Future Horizons, 2003.

Powell, Stuart, ed. *Helping Children with Autism to Learn.* London: David Fulton Publishers, 2000.

Prior, Margot, ed. *Learning and Behavior Problems in Asperger Syndrome.* New York: Guilford Press, 2003.

Quill, Kathleen Ann. *Teaching Children with Autism: Strategies to Enhance Communication and Socialization.* New York: Delmar, 1995.

Scheuermann, Brenda, and Jo Webber. *Autism: Teaching Does Make a Difference.* Florence, Ky.: Wadsworth Publishing, 2001.

Scott, Jack, Claudia Clark, and Michael P. Brady. *Students with Autism: Characteristics and Instructional Programming for Special Educators.* Florence, Ky.: Singular Publishing Group, 1997.

Sewell, Karen. *Breakthroughs: How to Reach Students with Autism.* Verona, Wisc.: The Attainment Company, 1998.

Siegel, Bryna. *Helping Children with Autism Learn: A Guide to Treatment Approaches for Parents and Professionals.* New York: Oxford University Press, 2003.

Wagner, Sheila. *Inclusive Programming for Elementary Students With Autism.* Arlington, Tex.: Future Horizons, 1999.

———. *Inclusive Programming for Middle School Students With Autism.* Arlington, Tex.: Future Horizons, 2001.

Winter, Matt. *Asperger Syndrome: What Teachers Need to Know.* London: Jessica Kingsley Publishers, 2003.

Zysk, Veronica, and Ellen Notbohm. *1001 Great Ideas for Teaching or Raising Children with ASD.* Arlington, Tex.: Future Horizons, 2004.

EMPLOYMENT ISSUES

Duran, Elva, and Lou Brown. *Vocational Training and Employment of the Moderately and Severely Handicapped and Autistic Adolescent with Particular Emphasis to Bilingual Special Ed.* Springfield, Ill.: Charles C. Thomas, 1992.

Fast, Yvona. *Employment for Individuals with Asperger Syndrome or Non-Verbal Learning Disability: Stories and Strategies.* London: Jessica Kingsley Publishers, 2004.

Grandin, Temple, and Kate Duffy. *Developing Talents: Careers for Individuals with Asperger Syndrome and High-Functioning Autism.* Shawnee Mission, Kans.: Autism Asperger Publishing, 2004.

Gray, Carol. *What's Next? Preparing the Student with Autism or Other Developmental Disabilities for Success in the Community.* Arlington, Tex.: Future Horizons, 1992.

Hane, Ruth Elaine Joyner et al. *Ask and Tell: Self-Advocacy and Disclosure for People on the Autism Spectrum.* Shawnee Mission, Kans.: Autism Asperger Publishing Company, 2004.

Harris, Sandra L., and Jan S. Handleman, eds. *Preschool Education Programs for Children with Autism.* Austin, Tex.: Pro Ed, 2000.

Hawkins, Gail. *How To Find Work That Works for People with Asperger Syndrome: The Ultimate Guide for Getting People With Asperger Syndrome into the Workplace (and Keeping Them There!).* London: Jessica Kingsley Publishers, 2004.

Johnson, Malcolm. *Managing with Asperger Syndrome: A Practical Guide for White Collar Professionals.* London: Jessica Kingsley Publishers, 2004.

Meyer, Roger. *Asperger Syndrome Employment Workbook: An Employment Workbook for Adults with Asperger Syndrome.* London: Jessica Kingsley Publishers, 2001.

Mithaug, Dennis E. *How to Teach Prevocational Skills to Severely Handicapped Persons.* Austin, Tex.: Pro Ed, 1981.

Smith, Marcia Datlow, Ronald G. Belcher, and Patricia D. Juhrs. *A Guide to Successful Employment for Individuals with Autism.* Baltimore, Md.: Paul H. Brookes, 1995.

FERAL CHILDREN

Craig, Eleanor. *One, Two, Three . . . The Story of Matt, A Feral Child.* New York: McGraw-Hill, 1991.

Gaspard-Itard, Jean-Marc. *The Wild Boy of Aveyron.* Appleton, Wisc.: Appleton-Century-Crofts, Meridith Publishing Co., 1962.

Lane, Harlan L., and Richard Pillard. *The Wild Boy of Burundi: A Study of an Outcast Child.* New York: Random House, 1978.

GENERAL

Alvarez, Anne, and Susan Reid, eds. *Autism And Personality; Findings from the Tavistock Autism Workshop.* New York: Routledge, 1999.

Autism Society of America. *Autism Society of America 1993 Handbook.* Silver Spring, Md.: Autism Society of America, 1993.

Autism Society of North Carolina. *Autism Primer: Twenty Questions and Answers, 3rd edition.* Raleigh, N.C.: Autism Society of North Carolina, 1998.

Balsamo, Thomas, and Sharon Rosenbloom. *Souls: Beneath and Beyond Autism.* New York: McGraw-Hill, 2003.

Baron-Cohen, Simon, and Patrick Bolton. *Autism: The Facts.* Oxford: Oxford University Press, 1993.

Baron-Cohen, Simon, Helen Tager-Flusberg, and Donald J. Cohen. *Understanding Other Minds; Perspectives from Autism.* New York: Oxford University Press, 1993.

Bérard, Guy. *Hearing Equals Behavior.* New Canaan, Conn.: Keats Publishing, 1993.

Berkell, Dianne E. *Autism: Identification, Education and Treatment.* Hillsdale, N.J.: Lawrence Erlbaum Associates, 1992.

Bettelheim, Bruno. *The Empty Fortress: Infantile Autism and the Birth of the Self.* New York: The Free Press, 1967.

Beyer, Jannik, and Lone Gammeltoft. *Autism and Play.* London: Jessica Kingsley Publishers, 1999.

Bosch, Gerhard. *Der fruhkindliche Autismus.* Berlin: Springer, 1962.

———. *Infantile Autism: A Clinical and Phenomenological-Anthropological Approach Taking Language as the Guide.* New York: Springer-Verlag, 1970.

Boucher, Jill. *Autism.* London: Sage Publications, 2005.

Brauner, Alfred. *L'enfant dereel.* Toulouse: Privat, 1986.

Buttner, Claudia. *Autistische Sprachstorungen.* Hurth: Gabel, 1995.

Chassman, Marilyn. *One-on-One: Working with Low-Functioning Children with Autism and Other Developmental Disabilities.* Verona, Wisc.: IEP Resources, 1999.

Clo, E. *Autismo Infantile.* Troina, Italy: Oasi Editrice, 1996.

Cohen, Donald J., and Anne M. Donnellan, ed. *Handbook of Autism and Pervasive Developmental Disorders.* New York: John Wiley & Sons, 2005.

Cohen, Judith H. *Succeeding with Autism: Hear My Voice.* London: Jessica Kingsley Publishers, 2005.

Cohen, Shirley. *Targeting Autism: What We Know, Don't Know, and Can Do to Help Young Children with Autism and Related Disorders.* Berkeley: University of California Press, 2002.

Coleman, Mary, ed. *The Autistic Syndromes.* New York: American Elsevier Publishing Co., 1976.

Delfos, Martine. *A Strange World—Autism, Asperger's Syndrome and PDD-NOS: A Guide for Parents, Partners, Professional Carers, and People with ASDS.* London: Jessica Kingsley Publishers, 2005.

Doman, Glen. *What to Do about Your Brain-injured Child: Or Your Brain-damaged, Mentally Retarded, Mentally Deficient, Cerebral-palsied, Epileptic, Autistic, Athetoid, Hyperactive, Attention Deficit Disordered, Developmentally Delayed, Down's Child.* Garden City Park, N.Y.: Square One Publishers, 2005.

Durig, Alexander. *How to Understand Autism: The Easy Way.* London: Jessica Kingsley Publishers, 2002.

Fordham, Michael. *The Self and Autism.* London: William Heineman Medical Books Ltd., 1976.

Frith, Uta. *Autism: Explaining the Enigma.* Oxford: Basil Blackwell, 2003.

Gabriels, Robin L., and Dina E. Hill, eds. *Autism: From Research to Individualized Practice.* London: Jessica Kingsley Publishers, 2002.

Ghaziuddin, Mohammad. *Mental Health Aspects of Autism and Asperger Syndrome.* London: Jessica Kingsley Publishers, 2005.

Gillingham, Gail. *Autism, Handle with Care.* Palo Alto: Tacit Publishing, 2001.

———. *Autism: A New Understanding!* Palo Alto: Tacit Publishing, Inc., 2000.

Grubar, J. C. *Autismo e integrazione.* Rome, Italy: Phoenix, 1996.

Gupta, Vidya Bhushan, ed. *Autistic Spectrum Disorders in Children.* Florence, Ky.: Marcel Dekker, 2004.

Happe, Francesca G. E. *Autism: An Introduction to Psychological Theory.* Cavendish, Australia: UCL Press, 1994.

Herbaudiere, Denise. *Cati, ou, Les sentiers de la vie: une enfant autiste a l'age adulte.* Paris: P. Belfond, 1991.

Hesmondhalgh, Matthew, and Christine Breakey. *Access and Inclusion for Children with Autistic Spectrum Disorders: Let Me In.* London: Jessica Kingsley Publishers, 2001.

Hill, David A., and Martha R. Leary. *Movement Disturbance: A Clue to Hidden Competencies in Persons Diagnosed with Autism and Other Developmental Disabilities.* Madison, Wisc.: DRI Press, 1993.

Hobson, R. Peter. *Autism and the Development of the Mind.* Hillsdale, N.J.: Lawrence Erlbaum Associates Ltd., 1993.

Hodgdon, Linda. *Solving Behavior Problems in Autism (Visual Strategies Series).* Troy, Mich.: Quirk Roberts Publishing, 1999.

Johnson, Mary Donnet, and Sherry Henshaw Corden. *Beyond Words: The Successful Inclusion of a Child with Autism.* Knoxville, Tenn.: Merry Pace Press, 2004.

Jordan, Rita. *Autistic Spectrum Disorders: An Introductory Handbook for Practitioners.* London: David Fulton Publishers, 1999.

Jordan, Rita, and Glenys Jones. *Meeting Needs of Children with Autistic Spectrum Disorders.* London: David Fulton Publishers, 1999.

Kaplan, Lawrence. *Diagnosis Autism: Now What?* Draper, Utah: Etham Books, 2005.

Kehrer, Hans E. *Autismus: diagnostische, therapeutische und soziale Aspekte.* Heidelberg, Germany: Asanger, 1995.

———. *Praktische Verhaltenstherapie bei geistig Behinderten. Ein Leitfaden fur Betreuer.* Dortmund, Germany: Modernes Lernen, 1997.

Lempp, Reinhart. *Vom Verlust der Fahigkeit, sich selbst zu betrachten: eine entwicklungspsychologische Erklarung der Schizophrenie und des Autismus.* Bern: H. Huber, 1992.

Lenchitz, Ken. *Autism and Post-Traumatic Stress Disorder. Ending Autistic Fixation.* Springfield, Ill.: Charles C. Thomas Pub., 2001.

Mesibov, Gary B., Lynn W. Adams, and Laura G. Klinger. *Autism: Understanding the Disorder.* New York: Plenum Publishing Corp., 1997.

Morgan, Sam B. *The Unreachable Child: An Introduction to Early Childhood Autism.* Memphis: Memphis State University Press, 1981.

Morton-Cooper, Alison. *Health Care and the Autism Spectrum: A Guide for Health Professionals, Parents and Carers.* London: Jessica Kingsley Publishers, 2004.

Murray-Slutsky, Carolyn, and Betty Paris. *Exploring the Spectrum of Autism and Pervasive Developmental Disorders: Intervention Strategies.* Morganville N.J.: Therapy Skill Builders, 2000.

Naseef, R. A. *Special Children, Challenged Parents: The Struggles and Rewards of Raising a Child with a Disability.* Baltimore, Md.: Paul H. Brookes, 2001.

National Autistic Society. *Beyond Rain Man: Experiences of and Attitudes Towards Autism.* London: National Autistic Society, 1996.

Ozonoff, Sally, Sally J. Rogers, and Robert L. Hendren. *Autism Spectrum Disorders: A Research Review for Practitioners.* Washington, D.C.: American Psychiatric Press, 2003.

Peacock, G., A. Forrest, and R. Mills. *Autism: The Invisible Children.* London: National Autistic Society, 1996.

Perron, Roger, and Denys Ribas. *Autismes de l'enfance.* Paris: Presses universitaires de France, 1994.

Quinn, Campion. *100 Questions & Answers about Autism.* London: Jones & Bartlett Publications, 2005.

Rastelli, Linda, and Lito Tajeda-Flores. *Understanding Autism for Dummies.* New York: John Wiley & Sons, 2003.

Ratey, John J., and Catherine Johnson. *Shadow Syndromes.* New York: Random House, 1998.

Ritvo, Edward R. *Understanding the Nature of Autism and Asperger's Disorder: Forty Years along the Research Trail.* London: Jessica Kingsley Publishers, 2005.

Russell, James. *Autism as an Executive Disorder.* New York: Oxford University Press, 1998.

Ryaskin, O. T. *Focus on Autism Research.* Hauppauge, N.Y.: Nova Science Publishers, 2005.

———. *Trends in Autism Research.* Hauppauge, N.Y.: Nova Science Publishers, 2005.

Schopler, Eric, and Gary B. Mesibov, eds. *High-functioning Individuals with Autism.* New York: Plenum Press, 1992.

Seach, Diana. *Interactive Play for Children with Autism.* London: Routledge, 2006.

Sigman, Marian, and Lisa Capps. *Children with Autism: A Developmental Perspective.* Cambridge, Mass.: Harvard University Press, 1997.

Stillman, William. *Demystifying the Autistic Experience: A Humanistic Introduction for Parents, Caregivers, and Educators.* London: Jessica Kingsley Publishers, 2002.

Volkmar, Fred R. et al., eds. *Handbook of Autism and Pervasive Developmental Disorders, Volume One, Diagnosis, Development, Neurobiology, and Behavior.* New York: John Wiley & Sons, 2005.

Volkmar, Fred R. et al., eds. *Handbook of Autism and Pervasive Developmental Disorders, Volume Two, Assessment, Interventions, and Policy.* New York: John Wiley & Sons, 2005.

Volkmar, Fred R., and Lisa A. Wiesner. *Healthcare for Children on the Autism Spectrum: A Guide to Medical, Nutritional, and Behavioral Issues.* Bethesda, Md.: Woodbine House, 2004.

Waterhouse, Stella. *A Positive Approach to Autism.* London: Jessica Kingsley Publishers, 1999.

Wetherby, Amy M., and Barry M. Prizant, eds. *Autism Spectrum Disorders: A Transactional Developmental Perspective.* Baltimore, Md.: Paul H. Brookes, 2000.

Williams, Donna. *Autism: an Inside-Out Approach: An Innovative Look at the "Mechanics" of "Autism" and Its Developmental Cousins.* London: Jessica Kingsley Publishers, 1996.

Wolfberg, Pamela J. *Play and Imagination in Children with Autism.* New York: Teachers College Press, 1999.

Zelan, Karen. *Between Their World and Ours: Breakthroughs with Autistic Children.* New York: St. Martin's Press, 2003.

Zysk, Veronica. *The Best of Autism Digest: Outstanding Selections from over Four Years of Issues.* Arlington, Tex.: Future Horizons, 2005.

Zysk, Veronica, and Ellen Notbohm. *1001 Great Ideas for Teaching or Raising Children with ASD.* Arlington, Tex.: Future Horizons, 2004.

GROUP HOMES

Holmes, David. *Establishing Group Homes for Adults with Autism.* Princeton, N.J.: Eden Press, 1985.

HISTORY OF AUTISM

Houston, Rab A., and Uta Frith. *Autism in History: The Case of Hugh Blair of Borgue C. 1708–1765.* Malden, Mass.: Blackwell Pub., 2000.

Gaspard-Itard, Jean-Marc. *The Wild Boy of Aveyron.* Appleton, Wisc.: Appleton-Century-Crofts, Meridith Publishing Co., 1962.

HOMEOPATHY/NATURAL MEDICINE

Lansky, Amy L. *Impossible Cure: The Promise of Homeopathy.* Portola Valley, Calif.: R.L. Ranch Press, 2003.

Marohn, Stephanie. *The Natural Medicine Guide to Autism.* Charlottesville, Va.: Hampton Roads Publishing Company, 2002.

Seifert, Cheryl D. *Holistic Interpretation of Autism: A Theoretical Framework.* Lanham, Md.: University Press of America, 1990.

Woodward, Bob, and Marga Hogenboom. *Autism: A Holistic Approach.* Edinburgh, Scotland: Floris Books, 2001.

HOMESCHOOLING

Hartnett, Martha Kennedy. *Choosing Home: Deciding to Homeschool with Asperger's Syndrome.* London: Jessica Kingsley Publishers, 2004.

Pyles, Lisa. *Homeschooling the Child with Asperger Syndrome: Real Help for Parents Anywhere and on Any Budget.* London: Jessica Kingsley Publishers, 2004.

MENTAL RETARDATION AND AUTISM

Kraijer, Dirk W. *Autism and Autistic-like Conditions in Mental Retardation.* Netherlands: Swets & Zeitlinger, 1997.

MUSIC AND AUTISM

Cameron, Lindsley. *The Music of Light: The Extraordinary Story of Hikari and Kenzaburo Oe.* New York: Simon & Schuster, 1998.

Serafina Poch Blasco. *Musicoterapia para niños autistas: historia de la musicoterapia española.* Madrid: Poch Blasco, 1973.

NONVERBAL LEARNING DISORDERS

Gutstein, Steven, and Rachelle K. Sheely. *Relationship Development Intervention with Children, Adolescents and Adults: Social and Emotional Development Activities for Asperger Syndrome, Autism, PDD and NLD.* London: Jessica Kingsley Publishers, 2002.

Stewart, Kathryn. *Helping a Child with Nonverbal Learning Disorder or Asperger's Syndrome: A Parent's Guide.* Oakland, Calif.: New Harbinger Publications, 2002.

OCCUPATIONAL THERAPY AND AUTISM

Miller-Kuhaneck, Heather, ed. *Autism: A Comprehensive Occupational Therapy Approach.* Bethesda, Md.: American Occupational Therapy Association, 2004.

PARENTING

Aarons, Maureen, and Tessa Gittens. *The Handbook of Autism: A Guide for Parents and Professionals.* New York: Routledge, 1999.

Abrams, Philip, and Leslie Henriques. *The Autistic Spectrum Parents' Daily Helper: A Workbook for You and Your Child.* Berkeley, Calif.: Ulysses Press, 2004.

Adams, Janice. *Autism-P.D.D.: Introducing Strategies for Parents and Professionals.* Chicago: Adams Press, 1995.

Autism Society of America. *How They Grow: A Handbook for Parents of Young Children with Autism.* Silver Spring, Md.: Autism Society of America, 1990.

Boushey, Ann. *Parent to Parent: Information and Inspiration for Parents Dealing with Autism and Asperger's Syndrome.* London: Jessica Kingsley Publishers, 2004.

Boyd, Brenda. *Parenting a Child with Asperger Syndrome: 200 Tips and Strategies.* London: Jessica Kingsley Publishers, 2003.

Brill, Marlene Targ. *Keys to Parenting the Child with Autism.* Hauppauge, N.Y.: Barron's, 2001.

Burkowsky, Mitchell R., ed. *Parents and Teachers Guide to the Care of Autistic Children.* Syracuse, N.Y.: Systems Educators, Inc., 1970.

Catalano, Robert A. *When Autism Strikes: Families Cope with Childhood Disintegrative Disorder.* New York: Plenum Publishing, 1998.

Cohen, Jeffrey. *The Asperger Parent: How to Raise a Child with Asperger Syndrome and Maintain Your Sense of Humor.* Shawnee Mission, Kans.: Autism Asperger Publishing Company, 2002.

Dillon, Kathleen M. *Living with Autism: The Parents' Stories.* Boone, N.C.: Parkway, 1995.

Downey, Martha Kate. *If You've Ever Wanted to Crawl in the Closet with an OREO: Tips for Parenting a Child with Special Needs.* San Francisco: Books by MK, 2004.

Everard, Peggie. *Involuntary Strangers: Autism: The Problems Faced by Parents.* London: John Clare Books, 1980.

Garrison, William. *Small Bargains: Children in Crisis and the Meaning of Parental Love.* New York: Simon & Schuster, 1993.

Gray, David E. *Autism and the Family: Problems, Prospects, and Coping with the Disorder.* Springfield, Ill.: Charles C. Thomas, 1998.

Hamilton, Lynn. *Facing Autism: Giving Parents Reason for Hope and Guidance for Help.* New York: Waterbrook Press, 2000.

Hannah, Liz. *Teaching Young Children with Autistic Spectrum Disorders to Learn: A Practical Guide for Parents and Staff in Mainstream Schools and Nurseries.* London: The National Autistic Society, 2001.

Harland, Kelly. *A Will of His Own: Reflections on Parenting a Child with Autism.* Bethesda, Md.: Woodbine House, 2002.

Harrington, Kathie. *For Parents and Professionals: Autism in Adolescents & Adults.* East Moline, Ill.: LinguiSystems, Inc., 1998.

Hart, Charles A. *A Parent's Guide to Autism: Answers to the Most Common Questions.* New York: Pocket Book Publishers, 1993.

———. *Without Reason: A Family Copes with Two Generations of Autism.* New York: Harper & Row, 1989.

Holland, Olga. *The Dragons of Autism: Autism as a Source of Wisdom.* London: Jessica Kingsley Publishers, 2002.

Ives, Martine, and Nell Munro. *Caring for a Child with Autism: A Practical Guide for Parents.* London: Jessica Kingsley Publishers, 2002.

Janzen, Janice E. *Autism: Facts and Strategies for Parents.* Morganville, N.J.: Therapy Skill Builders, 1999.

Johnson, Catherine. *A Parent's Guide to Autism: Essential Help for Understanding Your Child's Condition and Finding Treatment That Makes a Difference.* New York: Owl Books, 2006.

Keenan, Mickey, Ken P. Kerr, and Karola Dillenburger, eds. *Parents' Education as Autism Therapists: Applied Behavior Analysis in Context.* London: Jessica Kingsley Publishers, 1999.

Kozloff, Martin A. *Reaching the Autistic Child: A Parent Training Program.* Cambridge, Mass.: Brookline Books, 1998.

Lane, Dara. *Small Miracles Day by Day: A Guide for Parents of Individuals with Low Functioning Autism.* Internet: Virtualbookworm.com, 2003.

Lavin, J. L. *Special Kids Need Special Parents: A Resource for Parents of Children with Special Needs.* New York: Berkley Books, 2001.

Matthews, Joan Lord, and James Williams. *The Self-Help Guide for Special Kids and Their Parents.* London: Jessica Kingsley Publishers, 2000.

Maurice, Catherine, Gina Green, and Stephen Luce, eds. *Behavioral Intervention for Young Children with Autism: A Manual for Parents and Professionals.* Austin, Tex.: Pro-Ed, 1996.

McCabe, Patrick, Estelle McCabe, and Jared McCabe. *Living and Loving with Asperger Syndrome: Family Viewpoints.* London: Jessica Kingsley Publishers, 2003.

Mertz, Gretchen. *Help for the Child with Asperger's Syndrome: A Parent's Guide to Negotiating the Social Service Maze.* London: Jessica Kingsley Publishers, 2004.

Mialaret, Gerald. *Dancing with Dragons: An Entire Family's Insights into a Disability.* Arlington, Tex.: Future Horizons, 1996.

Moor, Julia. *Playing, Laughing and Learning with Children on the Autism Spectrum: A Practical Resource of Play Ideas for Parents and Carers.* London: Jessica Kingsley Publishers, 2002.

National Autistic Society. *The Autistic Spectrum: A Parent's Guide.* London: National Autistic Society, 2001.

Ozonoff, Sally, Geraldine Dawson, and James McPartland. *A Parent's Guide to Asperger Syndrome and High-Functioning Autism: How to Meet the Challenges and Help Your Child Thrive.* New York: Guildford Press, 2002.

Powers, Michael D., ed. *Children with Autism: A Parent's Guide.* Bethesda, Md.: Woodbine House, 2000.

Randall, Peter, and Jonathan Parker. *Supporting the Families of Children with Autism.* New York: John Wiley, 1999.

Richman, Shira. *Raising a Child with Autism: A Guide to Applied Behavior Analysis for Parents.* London: Jessica Kingsley Publishers, 2000.

Satkiewicz-Grayhardt, Viki, Barbara Peerenboom, and Roxanne Campbell. *Crossing Bridges: A Parent's Perspective on Coping after a Child Is Diagnosed with Autism/PDD.* Poughkeepsie, N.Y.: Potential Unlimited Publishing, 1996.

Schopler, Eric. *Parent Survival Manual: A Guide to Crisis Resolution in Autism and Related Developmental Disorders.* New York: Plenum Press, 1995.

Schopler, Eric, and Gary B. Mesibov, eds. *The Effects of Autism on the Family.* New York: Plenum Press, 1984.

Small, Mindy, and Lisa Kontente. *Everyday Solutions: A Practical Guide for Families of Children with Autism Spectrum Disorder.* Shawnee Mission, Kans.: Autism Asperger Publishing Company, 2003.

Sohn, Allan, and Cathy Grayson. *Parenting Your Asperger Child: Individualized Solutions for Teaching Your Child Practical Skills.* New York: Perigee, 2005.

Steere, Cathy. *Too Wise To Be Mistaken, Too Good To Be Unkind: Christian Parents Contend with Autism.* Sand Springs, Okla.: Grace and Truth Books, 2000.

Tilton, Adelle Jameson. *The Everything Parent's Guide to Children with Autism: Know What to Expect, Find the Help You Need, and Get Through the Day.* Cincinnati: Adams Media Corporation, 2004.

Williams, Chris, and Barry Wright. *How to Live with Autism and Asperger Syndrome: Practical Strategies for Parents and Professionals.* London: Jessica Kingsley Publishers, 2004.

Wing, Lorna. *The Autistic Spectrum: A Guide for Parents and Professionals.* London: Constable and Robinson, 2003.

Wiseman, Nancy. *Could It Be Autism? A Parent's Guide to the First Signs and Next Steps.* New York: Broadway, 2006.

Zysk, Veronica, and Ellen Notbohm. *1001 Great Ideas for Teaching or Raising Children with ASD.* Arlington, Tex.: Future Horizons, 2004.

PDD-NOS

Delfos, Martine. *A Strange World—Autism, Asperger's Syndrome and PDD-NOS: A Guide for Parents, Partners, Professional Carers, and People with ASDS.* London: Jessica Kingsley Publishers, 2005.

Kephart, Beth. *A Slant of Sun: One Child's Courage.* New York: W.W. Norton, 1998.

PERSONAL ACCOUNTS OF AUTISM

Adams, Christina. *A Real Boy: A True Story of Autism, Early Intervention, and Recovery.* New York: Berkley Trade, 2005.

Andron, Linda. *Our Journey through High Functioning Autism and Asperger Syndrome: A Roadmap.* London: Jessica Kingsley Publishers, 2001.

Arendt, Lusia. *Living and Working with Autism.* London: National Autistic Society, 1992.

Axline, Virginia Mae. *Dibs in Search of Self.* New York: Ballantine, 1964.

Ayres, A. et al. *Love, Jean: Inspiration for Families Living with Dysfunction of Sensory Integration.* Santa Rosa, Calif.: Crestport Press, 2004.

Barron, Judy, and Sean Barron. *There's a Boy in Here.* New York: Avon Books, 2002.

Betts, Carolyn. *A Special Kind of Normal.* New York: Scribner, 1983.

Bettelheim, Bruno. *A Home for the Heart.* New York: Knopf, 1974.

Billington, Tom. *Separating, Losing and Excluding Children: Narratives of Difference.* London: Falmer Press, 2000.

Blackman, Lucy. *Lucy's Story: Autism and Other Adventures.* London: Jessica Kingsley Publishers, 2001.

Brantlinger, Ellen, Susan M. Klein, and Samuel L. Guskin. *Fighting for Darla: Challenges for Family Care and Professional Responsibility: The Case Study of a Pregnant Adolescent with Autism.* New York: Teachers College Press, 1994.

Brunett, Rhonda. *From Autism to All-Star.* Carol Stream, Ill.: Specialty Publishing Company, 2004.

Buten, Howard. *Through the Glass Wall: Journeys into the Closed-Off Worlds of the Autistic.* New York: Bantam, 2005.

Callahan, Mary. *Fighting for Tony.* New York: Simon & Schuster, 1987.

Cameron, Lindsley. *The Music of Light: The Extraordinary Story of Hikari and Kenzaburo Oe.* New York: Simon & Schuster, 1998.

Carrier, Denise M. *Chase of a Lifetime: A Journey through Therapeutic and Academic Strategies for Children on the Autism Spectrum.* Internet: iUniverse, 2003.

Christopher, William, and Barbara Christopher. *Mixed Blessings.* Nashville: Abingdon Press, 1989.

Collins, Paul. *Not Even Wrong: Adventures in Autism.* London: Bloomsbury USA, 2004.

Copeland, James. *For the Love of Ann.* London: Arrow Books, 1973.

Cutler, Eustacia. *Thorn in My Pocket: Temple Grandin's Mother Tells the Family Story.* Arlington, Tex.: Future Horizons, 2004.

Davis, Bill, and Wendy Goldband Schunick. *Breaking Autism's Barriers: A Father's Story.* London: Jessica Kingsley Publishers, 2001.

Deckmar, Maud. *My Son Fred: Living with Autism.* London: Jessica Kingsley Publishers, 2004.

Dillon, Kathleen M. *Living with Autism: The Parents' Stories.* Boone, N.C.: Parkway, 1995.

Downey, Martha Kate. *If You've Ever Wanted to Crawl in the Closet with an OREO: Tips for Parenting a Child with Special Needs.* San Francisco: Books by MK, 2004.

Eastham, David. *Understand.* Ottawa: Oliver Pate, 1985.

Eastham, Margaret, and Anne Grice, eds. *Silent Words: The Story of David Eastham.* Ottawa: Oliver Pate, 1992.

Edelson, Stephen M., and Bernard Rimland, eds. *Treating Autism: Parent Stories of Hope and Success.* San Diego: Autism Research Institute, 2003.

Edgar, Joanna. *Love, Hope and Autism.* London: National Autistic Society, 1999.

Elliott, Lisa B. *Embarrassed Often … Ashamed Never.* Shawnee Mission, Kans.: Autism Asperger Publishing Company, 2002.

Everard, Peggie. *Involuntary Strangers: Autism: The Problems Faced by Parents.* London: John Clare Books, 1980.

Faherty, Catherine. *What Does It Mean to Me.* Arlington, Tex.: Future Horizons, 2000.

Fling, Echo R. *Eating an Artichoke: A Mother's Perspective on Asperger Syndrome.* London: Jessica Kingsley Publishers, 2000.

Frankland, Mark. *Freddie the Weaver: The Boy Who Fought to Join the World.* London: Sinclair-Stevenson, 1995.

Gerlach, Elizabeth King. *Just This Side of Normal: Glimpses of a Life with Autism.* Eugene, Ore.: Four Leaf Press, 1999.

Gerland, Gunilla. *A Real Person: Life on the Outside.* London: Souvenir Press, 1997.

Giddan, Normal, and Jane J. Giddan. *Autistic Adults at Bittersweet Farm.* Binghamton, N.Y.: Haworth Press, 1990.

Giesbrecht, Penny Rosell. *Where Is God When a Child Suffers?* Internet: Hannibal Books, 1988.

Gilpin, R. Wayne, ed. *Laughing and Loving with Autism: A Collection of "Real Life" Warm & Humorous Stories.* Arlington, Tex.: Future Horizons, 1993.

———. *More Laughing and Loving with Autism.* Arlington, Tex.: Future Horizons, 1994.

Grandin, Temple. *Thinking in Pictures: And Other Reports from My Life with Autism.* New York: Doubleday, 1996.

Grandin, Temple, and Margaret Scariano. *Emergence: Labeled Autistic.* New York: Warner Books, 1996.

Green, Phyllis J. D., and Patricia M. Apple. *Spinning Straw: The Jeff Apple Story.* Ontario: Diverse City Press, 1999.

Greenfield, Josh. *A Client Called Noah: A Family Journey Continued.* New York: Harcourt Brace Jovanovich, 1986.

———. *A Place for Noah.* New York: Harcourt, 1989.

Hadcroft, Will. *The Feeling's Unmutual: Growing up with Asperger Syndrome (Undiagnosed).* London: Jessica Kingsley Publishers, 2004.

Harland, Kelly. *A Will of His Own: Reflections on Parenting a Child with Autism.* Bethesda, Md.: Woodbine House, 2002.

Hart, Charles A. *Without Reason: A Family Copes with Two Generations of Autism.* New York: Harper & Row, 1989.

Hermelin, Beate. *Bright Splinters of the Mind: A Personal Story of Research with an Autistic Savant.* London: Jessica Kingsley Publishers, 2001.

Hewetson, Ann. *Laughter And Tears: A Family's Journey to Understanding the Autism Spectrum.* London: Jessica Kingsley Publishers, 2005.

Hickman, L. *Living in My Skin: The Insider's View of Life with a Special Needs Child.* San Antonio, Tex.: Communication Skill Builders, 2000.

Holland, Olga. *The Dragons of Autism: Autism as a Source of Wisdom.* London: Jessica Kingsley Publishers, 2002.

Hughes, Robert. *Running with Walker: A Memoir.* London: Jessica Kingsley Publishers, 2003.

Hundley, Joan Martin. *The Small Outsider: The Story of an Autistic Child.* Sydney, Australia: Angus and Robertson, 1971.

Jackson, Luke. *Freaks, Geeks and Asperger Syndrome: A User Guide to Adolescence.* London: Jessica Kingsley Publishers, 2002.

Johnson, Carol Sue, and Julia Crowder. *Autism: From Tragedy to Triumph.* Boston: Branden Books, 1994.

Johnson, Rene. *Winter's Flower.* Bloomington, Ill.: Rain-Tree, 1992.

Junker, Karin Stensland. *The Child in the Glass Ball.* New York: Abingdon Press, 1964.

Karasik, Paul, and Judy Karasik. *The Ride Together: A Brother and Sister's Memoir of Autism in the Family.* New York: Washington Square, 2003.

Kaufman, Barry Neil. *Happiness is a Choice.* New York: Ballantine, 1994.

———. *A Miracle to Believe In.* Garden City, N.Y.: Doubleday, 1981.

———. *Son-Rise.* New York: Warner, 1997.

Kaufman, Barry N., and Raun Kaufman. *Son-Rise: The Miracle Continues.* Novato, Calif.: H.J. Kramer, 1995.

Kephart, Beth. *A Slant of Sun: One Child's Courage.* New York: W.W. Norton, 1998.

Lambert, Phyllis Haywood. *Turning Every Stone: Autism with Love—A Mother's Journal.* Whispering Pines, N.C.: Scots Plaid Press, 1990.

LaSalle, Barbara. *Finding Ben: A Mother's Journey through the Maze of Asperger's.* New York: McGraw-Hill, 2003.

Lawson, Wendy. *Life Behind Glass: A Personal Account of Autism Spectrum Disorder.* New South Wales, Australia: Southern Cross University Press, 1998.

———. *Understanding and Working with the Spectrum of Autism: An Insider's View.* London: Jessica Kingsley Publishers, 2001.

Ledgin, Norm. *Diagnosing Jefferson.* Arlington, Tex.: Future Horizons, 2000.

Lindelien, Keli. *Gift from My Son: Autism Redefined.* Charlottesville Va.: Hampton Roads Publishing, 2004.

Lovell, Ann. *In A Summer Garment: The Experience of an Autistic Child.* London: Lion Publishing, 1983.

Martin, Earle P., Jr. *Dear Charlie—A Grandfather's Love Letter to His Grandson with Autism.* Arlington, Tex.: Future Horizons, 2000.

Matthews, Joan Lord, and James Williams. *The Self-Help Guide for Special Kids and their Parents.* London: Jessica Kingsley Publishers, 2000.

Maurice, Catherine. *Let Me Hear Your Voice: A Family's Triumph over Autism.* New York: Ballantine, 1994.

McDermott, J. *Babyface: A Story of Heart and Bones.* Bethesda, Md.: Woodbine House, 2000.

McDonnell, Jane Taylor, and Paul McDonnell. *News from the Border: A Mother's Memoir of Her Autistic Son.* New York: Ticknor & Fields, 1997.

McKean, Thomas A. *Light on the Horizon: A Deeper View from Inside the Autism Puzzle.* Arlington, Tex.: Future Horizons, 1996.

———. *Soon Will Come The Light: A View from Inside the Autism Puzzle.* Arlington, Tex.: Future Horizons, 1994.

McPherson, Sandra. *The Spaces Between Birds: Mother/Daughter Poems, 1967–1995.* Middletown, Conn.: Wesleyan University Press, 1996.

Meyer, Donald J., ed. *Uncommon Fathers: Reflections on Raising a Child with a Disability.* Bethesda, Md.: Woodbine House, 1995.

Meyer, Naomi. *The Journey with Joshua: Educating My Autistic Child.* Lakewood, N.J.: Bristol, Rhein & Englander, 1994.

Mialaret, Gerald. *Dancing with Dragons: An Entire Family's Insights into a Disability.* Arlington, Tex.: Future Horizons, 1996.

Miedzianik, David. *My Autobiography.* Raleigh: Autism Society of North Carolina, 1993.

Miller, Jean Kearns. *Women from Another Planet: Our Lives in the Universe of Autism.* Portland, Ore.: 1stBooks Library, 2003.

Mukhopadhyay, Tito R. *Beyond the Silence: My Life, The World, and Autism.* London: National Autistic Society, 2000.

————. *The Mind Tree: A Miraculous Child Breaks the Silence of Autism.* London: Arcade Books, 2003.

Naseef, Robert A. *Special Children, Challenged Parents: The Struggles and Rewards of Raising a Child with a Disability.* Secaucus, N.J.: Birch Lane Press, 1997.

Newport, Jerry, and Mary Newport. *Mozart and the Whale: An Asperger's Love Story.* Washington, D.C.: Touchstone, 2006.

O'Neil, Jasmine Lee. *Through the Eyes of Aliens: A Book about Autistic People.* London: Jessica Kingsley Publishers, 1998.

Oe, Kenzaburo. *A Healing Family.* Japan: Kodansha International, 2001.

Overton, Jennifer. *Snapshots of Autism: A Family Album.* London: Jessica Kingsley Publishers, 2003.

Paradiz, Valerie. *Elijah's Cup: A Family's Journey into the Community and Culture of High-Functioning Autism and Asperger's Syndrome.* New York: Free Press, 2002.

Park, Clara Claiborne. *Exiting Nirvana: A Daughter's Life with Autism.* Boston: Back Bay Books, 2002.

————. *The Siege: The First Eight Years of an Autistic Child with an Epilogue, 15 Years Later.* Boston, Mass.: Little, Brown, 1990.

Pinney, Rachel, Mimi Schlachter, and Anthea Courtenay. *Bobby: Breakthrough of a Special Child.* New York: St. Martin's/Marek, 1983.

Post, Connie. *Seasons of Love, Seasons of Loss.* 1992.

Prince-Hughes, Dawn. *Songs of the Gorilla Nation: My Journey through Autism.* New York: Three Rivers Press, 2005.

Prince-Hughes, Dawn, ed. *Aquamarine Blue 5: Personal Stories of College Students with Autism.* Athens, Ohio: Swallow Press, 2002.

Rankin, Kate. *Growing up Severely Autistic: They Call Me Gabriel.* London: Jessica Kingsley Publishers, 2000.

Reed, Dan. *Paid for the Privilege: Hearing the Voices of Autism.* Madison, Wisc.: DRI Press, 1996.

Richard, Jesse et al. *First Hand: Personal Accounts of Breakthroughs in Facilitated Communicating.* Madison, Wisc.: DRA Press, 1993.

Rocha, Adriana, and Kristi Jorde. *A Child of Eternity: An Extraordinary Young Girl's Message from the World Beyond.* New York: Ballantine Books, 1995.

Sanders, Robert S., Jr. *On My Own Terms: My Journey with Asperger's.* London: Armstrong Valley Publishing, 2004.

————. *Overcoming Asperger's: Personal Experience & Insight.* London: Armstrong Valley Publishing, 2002.

Schneider, Edgar. *Living the Good Life with Autism.* London: Jessica Kingsley Publishers, 2002.

Schulze, Craig B. *When Snow Turns to Rain: One Family's Struggle to Solve the Riddle of Autism.* Rockville, Md.: Woodbine House, 1993.

Sellin, Birger. *I Don't Want to Be Inside Me Anymore.* New York: HarperCollins, 1996.

————. *In Dark Hours I Find My Way: Messages from an Autistic Mind.* London: Victor Gollancz, 1995.

Shaw, Jean. *I'm Not Naughty—I'm Autistic: Jodi's Journey.* London: Jessica Kingsley Publishers, 2002.

Shore, Stephen. *Beyond the Wall: Personal Experiences with Autism.* Shawnee Mission, Kans.: Autism Asperger Publishing Co., 2002.

Simpson, Wallis A. *My Andrew: Day-to-Day Living with an ASD Child.* Internet: iUniverse, 2004.

Skye, Liane Gentry. *Turn Around, Bright Eyes—Snapshots from a Voyage out of Autism's Silence.* Otsego, Mich.: PageFree Publishing, 2002.

Sperry, Virginia Walker, and Sally Provence. *Fragile Success: Nine Autistic Children, Childhood to Adulthood.* North Haven, Conn.: Archon Books, 1995.

Sroussi, Karyn. *Unraveling the Mystery of Autism & PDD: A Mother's Story of Research and Recovery.* New York: Simon & Schuster, 2000.

Stacey, Patricia. *The Boy Who Loved Windows: Opening the Heart and Mind of a Child Threatened with Autism.* Philadelphia: DaCapo Press, 2003.

Stehli, Annabel. *The Sound of a Miracle, A Child's Triumph over Autism.* New York: Doubleday, 1997.

Stehli, Annabel, ed. *Sound of Falling Snow: Children's Stories of Recovery from Autism & Related Disorders.* Santa Rosa, Calif.: Beaufort Books, 2004.

Tantam, Digby. *A Mind of One's Own.* London: National Autism Society, 1999.

Vuletic, Ljiljana, Michel Ferrari, and Teodor Mihail. *Transfer Boy: Perspectives on Asperger Syndrome.* London: Jessica Kingsley Publishers, 2005.

Waites, Junee, and Helen Swinbourne. *Smiling at Shadows: A Mother's Journey Raising an Autistic Child.* Berkeley Calif.: Ulysses Press, 2002.

Wheatley, Thelma. *My Sad Is All Gone: A Family's Triumph over Violent Autism.* Lancaster, Ohio: Lucky Press, 2004.

Whelan, Kevin. *Izzy Baia.* San Diego: Marino Books, 1998.

Willey, L. H. *Pretending to Be Normal: Living with Asperger's Syndrome,* 1st ed. London: Jessica Kingsley Publishers, 1999.

Willey, Liane Holliday, ed. *Asperger Syndrome in Adolescence: Living with the Ups, the Downs and Things in Between.* London: Jessica Kingsley Publishers, 2003.

————. *Asperger Syndrome in the Family: Redefining Normal.* London: Jessica Kingsley Publishers, 2001.

————. *Pretending to Be Normal: Living with Asperger's Syndrome.* London: Jessica Kingsley Publishers, 1999.

Williams, Donna. *Everyday Heaven: Journeys Beyond the Stereotypes of Autism.* London: Jessica Kingsley Publishers, 2004.

————. *Like Color to the Blind: Soul Searching and Soul Finding.* New York: Times Books, 1996.

————. *Nobody Nowhere: The Extraordinary Autobiography of an Autistic.* New York: Random House, 1992.

———. *Not Just Anything.* Arlington, Tex.: Future Horizons, 1995.

———. *Somebody Somewhere: Breaking Free from the World of Autism.* London: Jessica Kingsley Publishers, 1995.

PRESCHOOL

Harris, Sandra, L., and Jan S. Handleman, eds. *Preschool Education Programs for Children with Autism.* Austin, Tex.: Pro Ed, 2000.

Janert, Sibylle. *The Autistic Child in Preschool: A Practical Handbook for Nursery Workers and Early Years Teachers.* London: Jessica Kingsley Publishers, 1997.

Rapin, Isabelle, and Lorna Wing. *Preschool Children with Inadequate Communication: Developmental Language Disorder, Autism, Mental Deficiency.* Cambridge: Cambridge University Press, 1996.

Schopler, Eric, Mary Elizabeth Van Bourgondien, and Marie M. Bristol. *Preschool Issues in Autism.* New York: Plenum Press, 1993.

RELATIONSHIPS

Aston, Maxine. *Aspergers in Love: Couple Relationships and Family Affairs.* London: Jessica Kingsley Publishers, 2003.

———. *The Other Half of Asperger Syndrome: A Guide to an Intimate Relationship with a Partner Who Has Asperger Syndrome.* London: Autism Asperger Publishing Company, 2002.

Gutstein, Steven E., and Rachelle K. Sheely. *Relationship Development Intervention with Children, Adolescents and Adults.* London: Jessica Kingsley Publishers, 2002.

RETT DISORDER AND AUTISM

Haas, Richard H., Isabelle Rapin, and Hugo W. Moser. *Rett Syndrome and Autism.* St. Louis: Year Book Medical Pub., 1988.

RUBELLA AND AUTISM

Chess, Stella, Sam J. Korn, and Paulina B. Fernandez. *Psychiatric Disorders of Children with Congenital Rubella.* New York: Brunner/Mazel, 1971.

SCHIZOPHRENIA AND AUTISM

Matson, Johnny L. *Chronic Schizophrenia and Adult Autism: Issues in Diagnosis, Assessment, and Psychological Treatment.* New York: Springer, 1989.

SELF-INJURIOUS BEHAVIOR

Favell, Judith E., and James W. Greene. *How to Treat Self-Injurious Behavior.* Austin, Tex.: Pro Ed, 1980.

SENSORY INTEGRATION PROBLEMS

Anderson, Johanna. *Sensory Motor Issues in Autism.* Odessa, Fla.: Psychological Corp., 1999.

Ayres, Jean. *Sensory Integration and the Child.* Los Angeles, Calif.: Western Psychological Services, 1979.

Ayres, A. et al. *Love, Jean: Inspiration for Families Living with Dysfunction of Sensory Integration.* Santa Rosa, Calif.: Crestport Press, 2004.

Bogdashina, Olga. *Sensory Perceptual Issues in Autism: Different Sensory Experiences, Different Perceptual Worlds.* London: Jessica Kingsley Publishers, 2003.

Delacato, Carl H. *The Ultimate Stranger: the Autistic Child.* Garden City, N.Y.: Doubleday, 1974.

Fisher, Anne G., Elizabeth A. Murray, and Anita C. Bundy. *Sensory Integration: Theory and Practice.* Philadelphia: F. A. Davis, 1991.

Huebner, Ruth A. *Autism: A Sensorimotor Approach to Management.* Gaithersburg, Md.: Aspen Publishers, 2000.

Myles, Brenda Smith et al. *Asperger Syndrome and Sensory Issues: Practical Solutions for Making Sense of the World.* Shawnee Mission, Kans.: Autism Asperger Publishing Company, 2000.

Trott, Maryann Colby, Susan Winndock, and Marci Laurel. *SenseAbilities: Understanding Sensory Integration.* Morganville, N.J.: Therapy Skill Builders, 1993.

Williams, Donna. *Autism and Sensing: The Unlost Instinct.* London: Jessica Kingsley Publishers, 1998.

Yack, Ellen, Shirley Sutton, and Paula Aquilla. *Building Bridges through Sensory Integration: Occupational Therapy for Children with Autism and Pervasive Developmental Disorder.* Toronto: Sensory Resources, 2003.

SEXUAL ISSUES AND AUTISM

Dalrymple, Nancy J., Susan Gray, and Lisa Ruble. *Sex Education: Issues for the Person with Autism.* Bloomington, Ind.: Indiana Resource Center for Autism, 1991.

Lawson, Wendy. *Sex, Sexuality and the Autism Spectrum.* London: Jessica Kingsley Publishers, 2005.

Newport, Jerry, and Mary Newport. *Autism—Asperger's and Sexuality: Puberty and Beyond.* Arlington, Tex.: Future Horizons, 2002.

Slater-Walker, Gisela, and Christopher Slater-Walker. *An Asperger Marriage.* London: Jessica Kingsley Publishers, 2002.

Stanford, Ashley. *Asperger Syndrome and Long-Term Relationships.* London: Jessica Kingsley Publishers, 2003.

SIBLINGS

Bishop, Beverly. *My Friend with Autism: A Coloring Book for Peers and Siblings.* Arlington, Tex.: Future Horizons, 2003.

Harris, Sandra. *Siblings of Children with Autism: A Guide for Families.* Bethesda, Md.: Woodbine House, 2003.

Hart, Charles A. *Without Reason: A Family Copes With Two Generations of Autism.* New York: Harper & Row, 1989.

Jacobs, Barbara. *Loving Mr. Spock: Understanding an Aloof Lover. Could It Be Asperger's Syndrome?* Arlington, Tex.: Future Horizons, 2004.

Karasik, Paul, and Judy Karasik. *The Ride Together: A Brother and Sister's Memoir of Autism in the Family.* New York: Washington Square, 2003.

McHugh, M. *Special Siblings: Growing up with Someone with a Disability.* Baltimore, Md.: Paul H. Brookes, 2002.

Meyer, Donald. *Views From Our Shoes: Growing up with a Brother or Sister with Special Needs.* Bethesda, Md.: Woodbine House, 1997.

Rosenberg, Marsha Sarah. *Coping When a Brother or Sister Is Autistic.* New York: Rosen Publishing Group, 2000.

Siegel, Bryna, and Stuart C. Silverstein. *What about Me? Growing up with a Developmentally Disabled Sibling.* New York: Perseus Publishing, 2001.

SLEEP PROBLEMS AND AUTISM

Durand, V. Mark. *Sleep Better! A Guide to Improving Sleep for Children with Special Needs.* Baltimore, Md.: Paul H. Brookes, 1998.

SOCIAL SKILLS AND AUTISM

Coucouvanis, Judith. *Super Skills: A Social Skills Group Program for Children with Asperger Syndrome, High-Functioning Autism and Related Challenges.* Shawnee Mission, Kans.: Autism Asperger Publishing Company, 2005.

Gutstein, Steven, and Rachelle K. Sheely. *Relationship Development Intervention with Children, Adolescents and Adults: Social and Emotional Development Activities for Asperger Syndrome, Autism, PDD and NLD.* London: Jessica Kingsley Publishers, 2002.

Martinovitch, Judith. *Creative Expressive Activities And Asperger's Syndrome: Social And Emotional Skills And Positive Life Goals for Adolescents And Young Adults.* London: Jessica Kingsley Publishers, 2005.

McAfee, Jeanette. *Navigating the Social World: A Curriculum for Individuals with Asperger's Syndrome, High Functioning Autism and Related Disorders.* Arlington, Tex.: Future Horizons, 2001.

Moore, Susan Thompson. *Asperger Syndrome and the Elementary School Experience: Practical Solutions for Academic & Social Difficulties.* Shawnee Mission, Kans.: Autism Asperger Publishing Co., 2002.

Moyes, Rebecca A. *Incorporating Social Goals in the Classrooms: A Guide for Teachers and Parents with High Functioning Autism and Asperger Syndrome.* London: Jessica Kingsley Publishers, 2001.

Quill, Kathleen Ann. *Do-Watch-Listen-Say: Social and Communication Intervention for Children With Autism.* Baltimore, Md.: Paul H. Brookes Publishers, 2000.

Sicile-Kira, Chantal. *Adolescents on the Autism Spectrum: A Parent's Guide to the Cognitive, Social, Physical, and Transition Needs of Teenagers with Autism Spectrum Disorders.* New York: Perigee, 2006.

Simpson, Richard, Brenda Smith Myles, and Gary M. Sasso. *Social Skills for Students with Autism.* Arlington, Va.: Council for Exceptional Children, 1997.

Slater-Walker, Gisela, and Christopher Slater-Walker. *An Asperger Marriage.* London: Jessica Kingsley Publishers, 2002.

Sonders, Susan Aud. *Giggle Time—Establishing the Social Connection: A Program to Develop the Communication Skills of Children with Autism, AS, and PDD.* London: Jessica Kingsley Publishers, 2002.

Sussman, Fern. *More Than Words: Helping Parents Promote Communication and Social Skills in Children with Autism Spectrum Disorder.* Toronto: Hanen Centre, 1999.

Weiss, Mary Jane, and Sandra L. Harris. *Reaching Out, Joining In: Teaching Social Skills to Young Children with Autism.* Bethesda, Md.: Woodbine House, 2001.

Winner, Michelle Garcia. *Inside Out: What Makes the Person with Social-cognitive Deficits Tick.* London: Jessica Kingsley Publishers, 2002.

———. *Thinking about You, Thinking about Me: Philosophy and Strategies for Facilitating the Development of Perspective Taking for Students with Social Cognitive Deficits.* London: Jessica Kingsley Publishers, 2003.

Wolfberg, Pamela J., and Adriana L. Schuler. *Peer Play and the Autism Spectrum: The Art of Guiding Children's Socialization and Imagination.* Shawnee Mission, Kans.: Autism Asperger Publishing Company, 2003.

TEACCH METHOD

Mesibov, Gary B., Victoria Shea, and Eric Schopler. *The TEACCH Approach to Autism Spectrum Disorders.* New York: Plenum, 2004.

Mesibov, Gary, and Marie Howley. *Accessing the Curriculum for Pupils with Autistic Spectrum Disorders: Using the*

TEACCH Programme to Help Inclusion. London: David Fulton Publishers, 2003.

Peeters, Theo. *Autism: From Theoretical Understanding to Educational Intervention.* Lewisville, Tex.: J. A. Majors Company, 1997.

Rollett, Brigitte, and Ursula Kastner-Koller. *Praxisbuch Autismus: Ein Leitfaden fuer Eltern, Erzieher, Lehrer und Therapeuten.* Stuttgart, Germany: Fischer, 1994.

TEENS AND AUTISM

Bolick, Theresa. *Asperger Syndrome and Adolescence: Helping Preteens & Teens Get Ready for the Real World.* Gloucester, Mass.: Fair Winds Press, 2004.

Brantlinger, Ellen, Susan M. Klein, and Samuel L. Guskin. *Fighting for Darla: Challenges for Family Care and Professional Responsibility: The Case Study of a Pregnant Adolescent with Autism.* New York: Teachers College Press, 1994.

Fullerton, Ann et al. *Higher Functioning Adolescents and Young Adults with Autism: A Teacher's Guide.* Austin, Tex.: Pro Ed, 1996.

Gray, Carol. *What's Next? Preparing the Student with Autism or Other Developmental Disabilities for Success in the Community.* Arlington, Tex.: Future Horizons, 1992.

Gutstein, Steven, and Rachelle K. Sheely. *Relationship Development Intervention with Children, Adolescents and Adults: Social and Emotional Development Activities for Asperger Syndrome, Autism, PDD and NLD.* London: Jessica Kingsley Publishers, 2002.

Harrington, Kathie. *For Parents and Professionals: Autism in Adolescents and Adults.* East Moline, Ill.: LinguiSystems, Inc., 1998.

Jackson, Jacqui. *Multicoloured Mayhem: Parenting the Many Shades of Adolescence, Autism, Asperger Syndrome and AD/HD.* London: Jessica Kingsley Publishers, 2004.

Jackson, Luke, and Tony Attwood. *Freaks, Geeks and Asperger Syndrome: A User Guide to Adolescence.* London: Jessica Kingsley Publishers, 2002.

Martinovitch, Judith. *Creative Expressive Activities and Asperger's Syndrome: Social and Emotional Skills and Positive Life Goals for Adolescents and Young Adults.* London: Jessica Kingsley Publishers, 2005.

Meyers, K., and B. Briesman, eds. *Children Grow Up: Autism in Adolescents and Adults.* Lawrenceville, N.J.: COSAC Press, 1986.

Molloy, Harvey, and Latika Vasil. *Asperger Syndrome, Adolescence, and Identity: Looking Beyond the Label.* London: Jessica Kingsley Publishers, 2004.

Myles, Brenda Smith. *Children and Youth with Asperger Syndrome: Strategies for Success in Inclusive Settings.* Thousand Oaks, Calif.: Corwin Press, 2005.

Myles, Brenda Smith, and Diane Adreon. *Asperger Syndrome and Adolescence: Practical Solutions for School Success.*

Shawnee Mission, Kans.: Autism Asperger Publishing Company, 2001.

Newport, Jerry, and Mary Newport. *Autism—Asperger's and Sexuality: Puberty and Beyond.* Arlington, Tex.: Future Horizons, 2002.

Palmer, Ann. *Realizing the College Dream with Autism or Asperger Syndrome: A Parent's Guide to Student Success.* London: Jessica Kingsley Publishers, 2005.

Porco, Barbara. *Growing Towards Independence by Learning Functional Skills and Behaviors.* Bloomington, Ind.: Indiana Resource Center for Autism, 1989.

Prince-Hughes, Dawn. *Aquamarine Blue 5: Personal Stories of College Students with Autism.* Athens, Ohio: Swallow Press, 2002.

Schopler, Eric, and Gary B. Mesibov. *Autism in Adolescents and Adults.* New York: Plenum Press, 1983.

———. *The Autistic Child through Adolescence.* New York: Plenum Press, 1982.

Sicile-Kira, Chantal. *Adolescents on the Autism Spectrum: A Parent's Guide to the Cognitive, Social, Physical, and Transition Needs of Teenagers with Autism Spectrum Disorders.* New York: Perigee, 2006.

Willey, Liane Holliday, ed. *Asperger Syndrome in Adolescence: Living with the Ups, the Downs and Things in Between.* London: Jessica Kingsley Publishers, 2003.

TOILET TRAINING

Wheeler, Maria. *Toilet Training for Individuals with Autism and Related Disorders: A Comprehensive Guide for Parents and Teachers.* London: Jessica Kingsley Publishers, 1999.

TREATMENT METHODS

Aarons, Maureen, and Tessa Gittens. *Autism: A Social Skills Approach for Children and Adolescents.* London: Winslow, 1998.

Alecson, Deborah Golden. *Alternative Treatments for Children Within.* New York: NTC Publishing Group, 1999.

Alvarez, Anne. *Live Company: Psychoanalytic Psychotherapy with Autistic, Borderline, Deprived, and Abused Children.* London: Tavistock/Routledge, 1992.

Alvin, Juliette, and Auriel Warwick. *Music Therapy for the Autistic Child.* New York: Oxford University Press, 1991.

Anderson, Margaret. *Tales from the Table: Five Accounts of Love as Interventions with Children on the Autistic Spectrum.* London: Jessica Kingsley Publishers, 2006.

Austin, John, and James E. Carr, eds. *Handbook of Applied Behavior Analysis.* Reno, Nev.: Context Press, 2000.

Axline, Virginia Mae. *Play Therapy: The Inner Dynamics of Childhood.* London: Churchill Livingston, 1989.

Bachrach, Ann et al. *Developmental Therapy for Young Children with Autistic Characteristics.* State College, Pa.: University Park Press, 1978.

Baker, Jed. *The Autism Social Skills Picture Book.* Arlington, Tex.: Future Horizons, 2003.

———. *Social Skills Training for Children and Adolescents with Asperger Syndrome and Social-Communications Problems.* Shawnee Mission, Kans.: Autism Asperger Publishing Company, 2003.

Baker, Linda J., and Lawrence A. Welkowitz. *Asperger's Syndrome: Intervening in Schools, Clinics, and Communities.* Hillsdale, N.J.: Lawrence Erlbaum Associates, 2004.

Baker, Sidney. *Autism: Effective Biomedical Treatments (Have We Done Everything We Can for This Child? Individuality in an Epidemic).* San Diego: Autism Research Institute, 2005.

Baker, Sidney M., and Jon Pangborn. *Defeat Autism Now! Clinical Options Manual for Physicians*, 1999.

Barthelemy, C., L. Hameury, and G. Lelord. *L'autisme de l'enfant. La Therapie d'echange et de developpement.* Paris: E.S.F., 1995.

Bellack, Allan S., Michael Hersen, and Alan E. Kazdin. *International Handbook of Behavior Modification and Therapy.* New York: Plenum Publishing, 1990.

Berger, Dorita. *Music Therapy, Sensory Integration, and the Autistic Child.* London: Jessica Kingsley Publishers, 2002.

Broer, Ted. *Maximum Solutions for ADD, Learning Disabilities and Autism: Natural Treatments of ADD, ADHD, and Autism.* Lake Mary, Fla.: Creation House, 2002.

Buron, Kari Dunn, and Mitzi Curtis. *Incredible 5-Point Scale: Assisting Students with Autism Spectrum Disorders in Understanding Social Interactions and Controlling Their Emotional Responses.* Shawnee Mission, Kans.: Autism Asperger Publishing Company, 2004.

Butler, Katherine G., ed. *Severe Communication Disorders: Intervention Strategies.* Gaithersburg, Md.: Aspen Publishers, 1993.

Carlton, Stella. *The Other Side of Autism: A Positive Approach.* Worcester, Mass.: The Self Publishing Association Ltd., 1993.

Carrier, Denise M. *Chase of a Lifetime: A Journey through Therapeutic and Academic Strategies for Children on the Autism Spectrum.* Lincoln, Neb.: iUniverse, 2003.

Christopher, William, and Barbara Christopher. *Mixed Blessings.* Nashville, Tenn.: Abingdon Press, 1989.

Cipolloni, David C. *An Extraordinary Silence: The Emergence of a Deeply Disturbed Child.* Westport, Conn.: Bergin & Garvey, 1993.

Coffey, Hubert S., and Louise L. Wiener. *Group Treatment of Autistic Children.* Englewood Cliffs, N.J.: Prentice Hall, 1967.

Cohen, Shirley. *Targeting Autism: What We Know, Don't Know, and Can Do to Help Young Children with Autism and Related Disorders.* Berkeley: University of California Press, 2002.

Corbier, Jean-Ronel. *Optimal Treatment for Children with Autism and Other Neuropsychiatric Conditions.* Lincoln, Neb.: iUniverse, 2005.

Coyne, Phyllis, Colleen Nyberg, and Mary Lou Vandenburg. *Developing Leisure Time Skills for Persons with Autism: A Practical Approach for Home, School and Community.* Arlington, Tex.: Future Horizons, 1999.

Dalrymple, Nancy J. *Helpful Responses to Some of the Behaviors of Individuals with Autism.* Bloomington: Indiana Resource Center for Autism, 1992.

———. *Helping People with Autism Manage Their Behavior.* Bloomington: Indiana Resource Center for Autism, 1993.

Delmolino, Lara, and Sandra L. Harris. *Incentives for Change: Motivating People with Autism Spectrum Disorders to Learn and Gain Independence.* Bethesda, Md.: Woodbine House, 2004.

DePalma, Valerie, and Marci Wheeler. *Learning Self-Care Skills.* Bloomington: Indiana Resource Center for Autism, 1991.

Dolnick, Edward. *Madness on the Couch: Blaming the Victim in the Heyday of Psychoanalysis.* New York: Simon & Schuster, 1998.

Edelson, Stephen B. *Conquering Autism: Reclaiming Your Child through Natural Therapies.* New York: Kensington, 2003.

Edelson, Stephen M., and Bernard Rimland, eds. *Treating Autism: Parent Stories of Hope and Success.* San Diego: Autism Research Institute, 2003.

Edwards, Judith, ed. *Being Alive: Building on the Work of Anne Alvarez.* New York: Brunner-Routledge, 2001.

Elliott, Lisa B. *Embarrassed Often ... Ashamed Never.* Shawnee Mission, Kans.: Autism Asperger Publishing Company, 2002.

Ellis, Kathryn, ed. *Autism: Professional Perspectives and Practice.* London: Chapman & Hall, 1990.

Exkorn, Karen Siff. *The Autism Sourcebook: Everything You Need to Know about Diagnosis, Treatment, Coping, and Healing.* New York: Regan Books, 2005.

Fouse, Beth, and Maria Wheeler. *A Treasure Chest of Behavioral Strategies for Individuals with Autism.* Arlington, Tex.: Future Horizons, 1997.

Foxx, Richard M. *Decreasing Behaviors of Persons with Severe Retardation and Autism.* Champaign, Ill.: Research Press, 1982.

Gagnon, Elisa. *Power Cards: Using Special Interests to Motivate Children and Youth with Asperger Syndrome and Autism.* Shawnee Mission, Kans.: Autism Asperger Publishing Company, 2001.

Gerdtz, John, and Joel Bergman. *Autism: A Practical Guide for Those Who Help Others.* New York: Continuum Pub Group, 1990.

Gerlach, Elizabeth K. *Autism Treatment Guide.* Arlington, Tex.: Future Horizons, 2003.

Giddan, Jane J., and Norman S. Giddan. *European Farm Communities for Autism.* Toledo: Medical College of Ohio Press, 1993.

Giles, T. R. *Handbook of Effective Psychotherapy.* New York: Plenum, 1993.

Gillberg, Christopher, ed. *Diagnosis and Treatment of Autism.* New York: Plenum, 1989.

Greenspan, Stanley I., Serena Weider, and Robin Simons. *The Child with Special Needs: Encouraging Intellectual and Emotional Growth.* Boston: Addison-Wesley, 1998.

Groden, Gerald, and M. Grace Baron, eds. *Autism: Strategies for Change: A Comprehensive Approach to the Education and Treatment of Children with Autism and Related Disorders.* New York: Amereon Press, 1991.

Guralnick, Michael J., ed. *The Effectiveness of Early Intervention.* Baltimore, Md.: Paul H. Brookes, 1996.

Gutstein, Steven E., and Rachelle K. Sheely. *Relationship Development Intervention with Children, Adolescents and Adults.* London: Jessica Kingsley Publishers, 2002.

Hedges, Lawrence E. *Working the Organizing Experience: Transforming Psychotic, Schizoid, and Autistic States.* Northvale, N.J.: Jason Aronson, 1994.

Howlin, Patricia. *Children with Autism and Asperger Syndrome: A Guide for Practitioners and Carers.* New York: John Wiley & Sons, 1998.

Howlin, Patricia et al. *Treatment of Autistic Children.* New York: John Wiley & Sons, 1987.

Howlin, Patricia, Simon Baron-Cohen, and Julia Hadwin. *Teaching Children with Autism to Mind-Read: A Practical Guide for Teachers and Parents.* New York: John Wiley & Sons, 1998.

Huebner, Ruth A. *Autism: A Sensorimotor Approach to Management.* Gaithersburg, Md.: Aspen Publishers, 2000.

Janert, Sibylle. *Reaching the Young Autistic Child: Reclaiming Non-Autistic Potential through Communicative Strategies and Games.* London: Free Association Books, 2000.

Johnson, Catherine. *A Parent's Guide to Autism: Essential Help for Understanding your Child's Condition and Finding Treatment That Makes a Difference.* New York: Owl Books, 2006.

Koegel, Lynn Kern, and Claire LaZebnik. *Overcoming Autism.* New York: Viking Press, 2004.

Koegel, Robert L., and Lynn Kern Koegel, eds. *Teaching Children with Autism: Strategies For Initiating Positive Interactions and Improving Learning Opportunities.* Baltimore, Md.: Paul H. Brookes, 1995.

Lehman, Jill Fain, Rebecca Klaw, and Gavin Peebles. *From Goals to Data and Back Again: Adding Backbone to Developmental Intervention for Children With Autism.* London: Jessica Kingsley Publishers, 2003.

Lockshin, Stephanie B., Jennifer M. Gillis, and Raymond G. Romanczyk. *Helping Your Child with Autism Spectrum Disorder: A Step-By-Step Workbook for Families.* Oakland, Calif.: New Harbinger Publications, 2005.

Luiselli, James K., and Michael J. Cameron, eds. *Antecedent Control: Innovative Approaches to Behavioral Support.* Baltimore, Md.: Paul H. Brookes, 1998.

Matson, Johnny L., ed. *Autism in Children and Adults: Etiology, Assessment, and Intervention.* Pacific Grove, Calif.: Brooks/Cole, 1994.

McCandless, J. *Children with Starving Brains: A Medical Treatment Guide for Autism Spectrum Disorder.* North Bergen, N.J.: Bramble, 2003.

McClannahan, Lynn E., and Patricia J. Krantz. *Activity Schedules for Children with Autism: Teaching Independent Behavior.* Bethesda, Md.: Woodbine House, 1999.

Mesibov, Gary B., Victoria Shea, and Eric Schopler. *The TEACCH Approach to Autism Spectrum Disorders.* New York: Plenum, 2004.

Mesibov, Gary, and Marie Howley. *Accessing the Curriculum for Pupils with Autistic Spectrum Disorders: Using the TEACCH Programme to Help Inclusion.* London: David Fulton, 2003.

Miller, Arnold and Eileen Eller-Miller. *From Ritual to Repertoire: A Cognitive Developmental Systems Approach with Behavior Disordered Children.* New York: John Wiley & Sons, 1989.

Nambudripad, Dr. Devi S. *Say Good-Bye to Allergy Related Autism.* New York: Delta Publishers, 1999.

Savner, Jennifer, and Brenda Smith Myles. *Making Visual Supports Work in the Home and Community: Strategies for Individuals with Autism and Asperger Syndrome.* Shawnee Mission, Kans.: Autism Asperger Publishing Company, 2000.

Schopler, Eric et al., eds. *The Research Basis for Autism Intervention.* New York: Plenum, 2001.

Siegel, Bryna. *Helping Children With Autism Learn: A Guide to Treatment Approaches for Parents and Professionals.* London: Oxford University Press, 2003.

———. *The World of the Autistic Child: Understanding and Treating Autistic Spectrum Disorders.* New York: Oxford University Press, 1996.

Simons, Jeanne, and Sabine Oishi. *The Hidden Child: The Linwood Method for Reaching the Autistic Child.* Kensington, Md.: Woodbine House, 1987.

Simpson, Richard L. *Autism Spectrum Disorders: Intervention and Treatment for Children and Youth.* Thousand Oaks, Calif.: Corwin Press, 2004.

Tsai, Luke. *Taking the Mystery out of Medications in Autism/ Asperger's Syndromes.* Arlington, Tex.: Future Horizons, 2001.

VACCINES AND AUTISM

Converse, Judy. *When Your Doctor Is Wrong: Hepatitis B Vaccine and Autism.* Philadelphia: Xlibris Corporation, 2002.

Kirby, David. *Evidence of Harm: Mercury in Vaccines and the Autism Epidemic: A Medical Controversy.* New York: St. Martin's Griffin, 2006.

Miller, Neil Z. *Vaccines, Autism and Childhood Disorders: Crucial Data That Could Save Your Child's Life.* Santa Fe, N. Mex.: New Atlantean Press, 2003.

YOUNG CHILDREN AND AUTISM

Brereton, Avril, and Bruce J. Tonge. *Pre-schoolers with Autism: An Education And Skills Training Programme for Parents, Manual For Clinicians.* London: Jessica Kingsley Publishers, 2005.

Cumine, Val, Julia Leach, and Gill Stevenson. *Autism in the Early Years: A Practical Guide.* London: David Fulton Publishers, 2000.

Deudney, Christine, and Lynda Tucker. *Autistic Spectrum Disorders in Young Children: A Guide for Early Years Practitioners.* London: National Autistic Society, 2003.

Harris, Sandra L., and Jan S. Handleman, eds. *Preschool Education Programs for Children with Autism.* Austin, Tex.: Pro Ed, 1993.

Harris, Sandra L., and Mary Jane Weiss. *Right from the Start: Behavioral Intervention for Young Children with Autism.* Bethesda, Md.: Woodbine House, 1998.

Janert, Sibylle. *The Autistic Child in Preschool: A Practical Handbook for Nursery Workers and Early Years Teachers.* London: Jessica Kingsley Publishers, 1997.

———. *Reaching the Young Autistic Child: Reclaiming Non-Autistic Potential through Communicative Strategies and Games.* London: Free Association Books, 2000.

Jensen, Audra. *When Babies Read: A Practical Guide to Helping Young Children with Hyperlexia, Asperger Syndrome and High-functioning Autism.* London: Jessica Kingsley Publishers, 2005.

Johnson, Mary Donnet and Sherry Henshaw Corden. *Beyond Words: The Successful Inclusion of a Child with Autism.* Knoxville, Tenn.: Merry Pace Press, 2004.

Kathiresan, M. Davi. *The ABC's of Autism.* Lansing, Mich.: Autism Society of Michigan, 2000.

Leventhal-Belfer, Laurie, and Cassandra Coe. *Asperger Syndrome in Young Children: A Developmental Approach for Parents and Professionals.* London: Jessica Kingsley Publishers, 2004.

Maurice, Catherine, Gina Green, and Stephen Luce, eds. *Behavioral Intervention for Young Children with Autism: A Manual for Parents and Professionals.* Austin, Tex.: Pro Ed, 1996.

Newman, Sarah. *Small Steps Forward: Using Games and Activities to Help Your Pre-School Child with Special Needs.* London: Jessica Kingsley Publishers, 1999.

Sainsbury, Clare. *The Martian in the Playground: Understanding the Schoolchild with Asperger's Syndrome.* Bristol: Lucky Duck Publishing Ltd., 2000.

Wall, Kate. *Autism and Early Years Practice: A Guide for Early Years Professionals, Teachers and Parents.* London: Paul Chapman Educational Publishing, 2004.

INDEX

Page numbers in **boldface** indicate major treatment of a topic.

A

AAP. *See* American Academy of Pediatrics
ABA. *See* applied behavior analysis
ABC (autism behavior checklist) 11, **18–19,** 20
ability test **1,** 101–102
    nonverbal 113
abuse (shaken baby syndrome) 143–144
Achenbach, Thomas M. 1
Achenbach Childhood Behavior Checklist (CBCL) **1**
activities of daily living **1,** 58
ADA (Americans with Disabilities Act) **4**
    and ability tests 1
adaptive living skills **1–2,** 6–7
adaptive skill areas 112–113
ADD. *See* attention deficit disorder
ADHD. *See* attention deficit hyperactivity disorder
ADI-R (Autism Diagnostic Interview-Revised) 11, **19,** 24, 33, 138
adolescents 25–26, 37
ADOS (autism diagnostic observation scale) 11, **19–20,** 24, 33–34, 138
adults
    with autism **2**
    with autism spectrum disorders 27
Advisory Committee on Immunization Practices 96
advocacy groups 166–167
age of onset viii
aggression

in Asperger's syndrome 11
in autism spectrum disorders iv–v, 22
in autistic disorder 109
valproate for 281
AIT. *See* auditory integration training
akathisia **2**
Alabama 16, 184, 192–193
Alabama Autism Surveillance Program (AASP) 16
Alaska 193–194
allergy to cow's milk **2–3**
aloofness **3**
alprazolam 41, 45–46, 112
American Academy of Family Physicians (AAFP)
    on research with children 277
    on safety of vaccines 160
American Academy of Neurology, on autism screening v
American Academy of Pediatrics (AAP)
    on auditory integration training 39
    on autism screening v
    on facilitated communication 60, 80
    on patterning 121–122
    on safety of vaccines 31, 96, 160
American Association of People with Disabilities 173
American Association of University Affiliated Programs for Persons with Developmental Disabilities 171
American Association on Mental Retardation 171
American Bar Association 174

American Board of Psychiatry and Neurology (ABPN) 117
American Hyperlexia Association 178–179
    American Musical Therapy Association 179–180
American Psychiatric Association (APA)
    DSM-IV-TR of viii, **64–65**
    on facilitated communication 60, 80
American Sign Language (ASL) **3–4,** 22, 57
American Sign Language Teachers Association 170
American Speech-Language-Hearing Association (ASHA) 170–171
Americans with Disabilities Act (ADA) **4**
    and ability tests 1
amitriptyline 5, 112
Anafranil. *See* clomipramine
Angelman, Harry 4
Angelman syndrome (AS) **4–5**
    diagnosis of 5
    genetics of 88, 90
    outlook in 5
    symptoms of 5
    treatment of 5
Angelman Syndrome Foundation 167
Animals in Translation (Grandin) 91
animal therapy **5,** 42, 67–68
antianxiety medications 111–112
antibiotics, oral, and autistic disorder 31
anticonvulsants. *See* antiepileptic medication
antidepressants **5,** 111–112
    for Asperger's syndrome 11

309

autistic disorder *(continued)*
  relationship development
    intervention for 38, 39
  screening instruments for v,
    33–34, **137–140**
  sensory problems in 40
  social skills training for 39
  social symptoms in 32, 34,
    103, 145–146
  speech-language therapy for
    39
  supplemental therapy for 42
  symptoms of 31–33
  TEACCH program for 38–39,
    67, 138, **153,** 182
  treatment of 35–42
  vaccinations and 30–31
  vision therapy for 42
*Autistic Disturbances of Affective
  Contact* (Kanner) 103
autistic savant **42–43,** 53–54, 57,
  115, 136
    Clemons, Alonzo **53–54**
    DeBlois, Tony **62–63**
    Lemke, Leslie **107–108**
    Peek, Kim **122–123**
    Pillault, Christophe **125**
    Wawro, Richard **162**
autoimmune system disorder **43**
aversive(s), definition of 284
aversive techniques **43–44,** 59
axon, definition of 284
Ayres, A. Jean 141, 181

B
Bailey, Anthony 139
Bandura, Albert 45
Barton, Marianne 138
basal ganglia 48
basic skills **45**
baths, Epsom salts **74–75,** 124
behavioral symptoms
  of autism spectrum disorders
    iv–v
  of autistic disorder 32, 34
behavioral therapy **45**
  for autistic disorder 37–38
  groups and resources on
    181–182
  for obsessive-compulsive
    disorder 118–119
  for oppositional defiant
    disorder 120

behavior analysis v
behavior analysis, applied (ABA)
  6–7, 25, 37, 38, 45
  adaptive living skills in 1–2,
    6–7
  definition of 284
  discrete trial training in v, 6,
    37, 38, 45, **65–67,** 153
  effectiveness of v–vi, 7, 25, 38
  goals and purpose of 7
  intensity of approach vi, 6, 66
  pivotal response training in
    116, 125
  positive behavior support in
    125–126
behavior checklists. *See also specific
tests*
  Achenbach Childhood
    Behavior Checklist (CBCL)
    1
  autism behavior checklist
    (ABC) 11, **18–19,** 20
  Checklist for Autism in
    Toddlers (CHAT) 23, 33,
    49–50, 137, 138
  Child Behavior Checklist **50**
  Connors Parent/Teacher Rating
    Scales–Revised **58**
  definition of 284
  Modified Checklist for Autism
    in Toddlers (M-CHAT) 23,
    33, **115,** 137, 138–139
behavior modification **45,** 284
benzodiazepines **45–46**
  for autistic disorder 41
  side effects of 46
Bérard, Guy 12, **46**
Bérard Auditory Integration
  Training 12, **46**
beta-blockers, for Asperger's
  syndrome 11
Bettelheim, Bruno **46–47**
Binet, Alfred 101
Bleuler, Eugen 93, 104
blood pressure medications 6, 111
body language 22, **47**
Boston Higashi school **47,** 61–62
Boston University 53, 55, 151, 275
boys v. girls 87
  in Asperger's syndrome 10, 87
  in autistic disorder 29, 87
  in childhood disintegrative
    disorder 51

in fragile X syndrome 84–85
in low-functioning autistic
  disorder 108
in oppositional defiant disorder
  120
in Rett disorder 131–132
bradykinesia, definition of 284
brain **47–48**
  and autism **48**
  inflammation of 99–100
brain stem 48, 284
brain tissue studies 28
Brick Township, New Jersey 55
Broca's aphasia 117
Buckley Amendment 80
bupropion 5, 41, 112
Burton, Richard 28

C
calcium 161
calendar calculating 43, 136
California 184–185, 197–199
camps, online resources on 183
Candida albicans 164
carbamazepine 6, 26, 140
  for Asperger's syndrome 11
  for autistic disorder 111
  side effects of 111
Carmen B. Pingree School for
  Children with Autism 18
CARS (childhood autism rating
  scale) 11, 24, 34, **50–51,** 137, 138
case history 49
casein 2–3, 26, 41, 65
casein-free diet **91** 282–283
CAST (Childhood Asperger
  Syndrome Test) 23, 33, **50,** 137,
  140
Catapres. *See* clonidine
CBCL (Achenbach Childhood
  Behavior Checklist) **1**
CDD. *See* childhood disintegrative
  disorder
celebrity family members, autistic
  28–29
Center for the Study of Autism
  49, 167–168, 168, 180
Centers for Disease Control and
  Prevention (CDC) 52
  on safety of vaccines 159–160
centers of excellence 52
central nervous system, definition
  of 284

symptoms of 84–85
treatment of 85–86
free and appropriate public
    education **86,** 99
Freud, Sigmund 93–94
friends **86**
frontal lobe 48
frustration tolerance, definition
    of 285
Full Circle Program 67
full inclusion **86**
functional magnetic resonance
    imaging (fMRI) **86**
furniture arrangement 135

G

gabapentin 6, 112
gait apraxia, definition of 285
galactosemia 89, 144
gamma-aminobutyric acid (GABA)
    pathway 90
Gardner, Howard 102
gender differences **87**
    in Asperger's syndrome 10,
        87
    in autistic disorder 29, 87
    in childhood disintegrative
        disorder 51
    in fragile X syndrome 84–85
    in low-functioning autistic
        disorder 108
    in oppositional defiant disorder
        120
    in Rett disorder 131–132
gene(s), definition of 285
genes and autism 27–28, **87–90,**
    279
genetic marker **90–91**
genetic-related groups and
    resources 178–179
genome 88, 285
Geodon. *See* ziprasidone
Georgia 187, 206–208
Gifted Hands, Inc. 54
Gilliam Autism Rating Scale **91**
girls v. boys 87
    in Asperger's syndrome 10, 87
    in autistic disorder 29, 87
    in childhood disintegrative
        disorder 51
    in fragile X syndrome 84–85
    in low-functioning autistic
        disorder 108

in oppositional defiant disorder
    120
in Rett disorder 131–132
gluten-free casein-free diet 26, **91**
    clinical trial on 282–283
gluten-free diet 26, 41, 63, 65, **91**
Goddard, Henry H. 101
Gould, Stephen J. 28
government funds, for adults with
    autism spectrum disorders 27
Grandin, Temple **91**
Granite Bay 55
Gray, Carol 147
Greenspan, Stanley 39, 82, 115,
    182
gross motor, definition of 285
group living, supervised 2, 27, 108
growth dysregulation hypothesis
    48
guanfacine, for Tourette syndrome
    155
guardianship **91**

H

Hagberg, Bengt 132
Haldol. *See* haloperidol
haloperidol **92,** 116
    for Asperger's syndrome 11
    for autism spectrum disorders
        26
    side effects of 92
    for Tourette syndrome 155
hand flapping iv, **92**
    in Angelman syndrome 5
    in autistic disorder 29
    in fragile X syndrome 84
handicap **92**
Hanks, Merton 28
Hawaii 187, 208–209
head size **92**
Head Start 70
health insurance and autism
    100–101
hearing loss 24
Heller's disease **92.** *See also*
    childhood disintegrative disorder
hemispheres of brain 47–48, 49
Henke, Tom 28
hereditary factors 27–28, 87–90
Higashi Institute for Professional
    Development 47
Higashi School (Boston) **47,**
    61–62

higher cognitive functions **93**
higher-order thinking **93**
high-functioning autistic disorder
    93, 109, 114
high school 25–26, 37
hippocampus, in auditory
    processing disorder 14
history of autism **93–94**
Hoffman, Dustin **94,** 122, 136
holding therapy **94**
homeobox (HOX) genes 88–89,
    285
horseback riding, therapeutic 5
hot spots, definition of 285
Howe, Samuel Gridley 148
HOXA1 gene 89
Human Dolphin Institute 67
hyperactivity **94**
    in Angelman syndrome 4–5
    antipsychotics for 6
    in Asperger's syndrome 11
    medications for 26
Hyperactivity Index 58
hyperlexia **94–95**
    advocacy/support group on
        178–179
    definition of 285
    diagnosis of 95
    symptoms of 95
    treatment and outlook in 95
hypothalamus 48
hypotonia, definition of 285

I

Idaho 187, 209–211
IDEA. *See* Individuals with
    Disabilities Education Act
identical twins, definition of 285
idiot savants 42–43, 136. *See also*
    autistic savant
IEE (independent education
    evaluation) **97**
IEP. *See* Individualized Education
    Program
IFSP (Individualized Family Service
    Program) 25, 37, **98**
IHP (Individualized Habilitation
    Program) **98**
Illinois 17, 187–188, 211–213
imipramine **96**
    for Asperger's syndrome 11
    side effects of 96
immediate echolalia 70